THE COMPLETE

Leaky Gut

Health & Diet Guide

Improve Everything from
Autoimmune Conditions to Eczema
by Healing Your Gut

INCLUDES **150** RECIPES

Dr. Makoto Trotter, BSc (Hons), ND
with **Doug Cook,** RD, MHSc

Robert
ROSE

For complete cataloguing information, see page 352.

Disclaimer

This book is a general guide only and should never be a substitute for the skill, knowledge and experience of
a qualified medical professional dealing with the facts, circumstances and symptoms of a particular case.

The nutritional, medical and health information presented in this book is based on the research, training
and professional experience of the authors, and is true and complete to the best of their knowledge. However,
this book is intended only as an informative guide for those wishing to know more about health, nutrition
and medicine; it is not intended to replace or countermand the advice given by the reader's personal
physician. Because each person and situation is unique, the authors and the publisher urge the reader to
check with a qualified health-care professional before using any procedure where there is a question as to
its appropriateness. A physician should be consulted before beginning any exercise program. The authors
and the publisher are not responsible for any adverse effects or consequences resulting from the use of
the information in this book. It is the responsibility of the reader to consult a physician or other qualified
health-care professional regarding his or her personal care.

This book contains references to products that may not be available everywhere. The intent of
the information provided is to be helpful; however, there is no guarantee of results associated with the
information provided. Use of brand names is for educational purposes only and does not imply endorsement.

The recipes in this book have been carefully tested by our kitchen and our tasters. To the best of our
knowledge, they are safe and nutritious for ordinary use and users. For those people with food or other
allergies, or who have special food requirements or health issues, please read the suggested contents of each
recipe carefully and determine whether or not they may create a problem for you. All recipes are used at the
risk of the consumer. We cannot be responsible for any hazards, loss or damage that may occur as a result of
any recipe use. For those with special needs, allergies, requirements or health problems, in the event of any
doubt, please contact your medical adviser prior to the use of any recipe.

Design and Production: Martina Hwang/PageWave Graphics Inc.
Editors: Bob Hilderley, Senior Editor, Health; Sue Sumeraj, Recipes
Medical editor: Joanna Odrowaz
Copy editor: Kelly Jones
Proofreader: Gillian Watts
Indexer: Gillian Watts
Nutrient analysis: Magda Fahmy
Illustrations: Kveta/threeinabox.com

Cover image: © istockphoto.com/belchonock

The publisher gratefully acknowledges the financial support of our publishing program by the Government
of Canada through the Canada Book Fund.

Published by Robert Rose Inc.
120 Eglinton Avenue East, Suite 800, Toronto, Ontario, Canada M4P 1E2
Tel: (416) 322-6552 Fax: (416) 322-6936
www.robertrose.ca

Printed and bound in USA

1 2 3 4 5 6 7 8 9 CKV 23 22 21 20 19 18 17 16 15

To my wife and daughter, who have been
beyond supportive of me in writing this book,
and for their radiant love and spirits.
And to my parents, who first showed me
that eating healthy food actually
does keep you healthy.

— *Makoto Trotter*

To my friends and family, who supported
me during the challenging times in my life,
enabling me to get to a place where I have
the skills to work on a project like this.
And to my mother and grandmother,
who introduced me to cooking.

— *Doug Cook*

Contents

Introduction

If you are reading this, you or someone you care about is likely ill and looking for help. By this time, you want straight answers — no small talk, just the facts. You may have become frustrated with your medical care. No one seems to know the true cause of your illness. Do you feel stuck in a treatment plan that appears to be going nowhere? Is there a piece of this puzzle that seems to be missing?

That missing piece may be leaky gut syndrome, also known as hyperpermeable gut. Leaky gut syndrome (LGS) is the common denominator to a diverse array of health conditions, ranging from irritable bowel syndrome to eczema, from thyroid disease to diabetes. In some cases, LGS instigates a disease condition in your body; in other cases, LGS perpetuates an existing disease condition; and in still other cases, LGS prevents the resolution of a disease. In all cases, LGS involves inflammation of tissues in the small intestine, also known as the gut, which typically results in damage to the lining of the gut and elsewhere in the body.

Not everybody responds the same way to leaky gut syndrome. We are all biologically different. We each have a different constitutional makeup, different tolerances, different stresses and different tendencies for pathologies that occur in different organ systems. We have different propensities to heal. There is no single universal approach that works for everyone. However, the treatment strategies presented in this book are safe and supportive for the majority of patients with a hyperpermeable gut. The lifestyle modifications, nutritional and herbal remedies, and diet plan and recipes we recommend will help settle your inflammation and help heal the lining of your gut.

These treatments require your participation in the healing process. Keep the big picture in mind. Step back

> **Leaky Gut Syndrome Dysfunctions**
>
> Leaky gut syndrome may be:
> - The trigger that sets off your ill health.
> - The factor that is making your disease last longer.
> - What is keeping you from getting better.

and observe your health trajectory. Keep this in mind in case your symptoms vary throughout the day. Fluctuations are normal, and can discourage you. Quantify your health as objectively as possible. If you notice that the intensity of symptoms has improved in a notable and measurable way (say, on a scale of 1 to 5) or that the frequency of inflammatory flare-ups has started to decrease, you are on the right track. Be patient and allow yourself a realistic timeline based on the intensity and duration of your condition. As a general rule, the longer you have been in a disease state, the deeper it is rooted in its pathology and the longer it will take to resolve. If you are improving overall, this is, of course, a good sign.

Some people heal very quickly while others respond slowly. In certain cases, you may not notice any perceivable improvements until you have followed a supportive nutritional and herbal treatment plan for several months, and then, at a certain point, your body responds and healing begins. Essentially, what you are doing through this process is providing support and the proper fuel to your immune system and digestive tract to encourage it to rebalance on its own.

Please be persistent, patient and self-aware throughout this process. If you are struggling to get results and feel that maybe you are lacking information to determine what is wrong, or if your condition is not improving, be sure to consult your health-care provider, who may recommend further tests to explain your specific problems. For complicated or unresponsive situations, this could be very helpful, but be aware that LGS is a disease state in the midst of ongoing research. At one time, LGS was not recognized as a disease state or syndrome, but in recent years, knowledge of this condition has grown as a result of evidence-based scientific studies and anecdotal evidence. The information provided in this book is based on the most recent scientific research and the experience of skilled practitioners. Having a better understanding of this syndrome and learning how to treat it more effectively may be the pieces of the puzzle that improve your health.

Be patient and allow yourself a realistic timeline based on the intensity and duration of your condition. As a general rule, the longer you have been in a disease state, the deeper it is rooted in its pathology and the longer it will take to resolve.

Acknowledgments

To the University of Waterloo, thank you for providing me with the knowledge base and work experience to better understand the complexities and wonder of life on a molecular plane.

To the Canadian College of Naturopathic Medicine, thank you for allowing me to take a big breath, step back and re-examine what I thought I knew and look at it with fresh eyes.

To my patients, thank you for being my best teachers and inspirations; for being open to learning and integrating new ideas; for having the courage to take steps in uncharted territory; and for making superhuman efforts to take the reins of your health into your own hands.

To Bob Dees and Bob Hilderley, thank you for having faith in my abilities and for your mentorship in guiding me through the book-writing process and the business of books.

To the amazing Robert Rose group of editors, publicists, illustrators and designers, thank you for turning my manuscript into something tangible and polished. Your expertise is invaluable.

And most importantly, to my wife, daughter and family, thank you for providing love, support, guidance and patience through this process; you are my everything.

— Makoto Trotter

Quick Guide to Managing Leaky Gut Syndrome

1. Consult with your health-care provider to assess your condition and review all potential treatment options.

2. Find a health-care provider who can recommend the most appropriate tests to determine whether you have leaky gut syndrome and provide direction on how to treat it.

3. Eat a whole foods diet, eliminating all processed foods and artificial ingredients.

4. Eliminate all caffeine, hot spices, black pepper and alcohol.

5. Avoid foods from the cruciferous vegetable family (arugula, bok choy, Brussels sprouts, collard greens, kale, mustard greens, radish, rutabaga, Swiss chard, turnips, watercress) and the onion family (chives, garlic, leeks, onions, shallots), as well as tomato sauces

6. Stick primarily to cooked foods, avoiding all raw meat, fish, vegetables and fruit.

7. Drink only room-temperature or warm liquids.

8. Design your main three meals around cooked peeled vegetables and/or fruit, naturally raised meat or fish and gluten-free whole grains.

continued on next page

9 Choose cooked peeled fruit, cooked peeled vegetables and/or skinless nuts, or foods made from these ingredients, for your snacks.

10 Eat every 2 to 3 hours, and stick to small to moderate-sized main meals with snacks in between.

11 Set time aside to relax and enjoy your meals, and ensure that you chew your food thoroughly.

12 Consult with your health-care provider to determine which supplements are appropriate for you. In general, the most important supplements for leaky gut syndrome are L-glutamine, probiotics, fish oils, turmeric, 5-HTP and zinc.

13 Prioritize stress reduction, a regular exercise regimen and quality sleep.

PART 1

Understanding Leaky Gut Syndrome

Progressive Onset

Rhonda was 34 when she first visited our clinic. She was a physically active, pleasant patient but she was working long hours at a stressful job and was not getting enough sleep. Her digestive problems had begun about 10 years ago, at age 25, and included abdominal pain, diarrhea (no bleeding), cramping and vomiting lasting for 1 to 2 days in episodes every 1 to 3 months. At the time, she was diagnosed with irritable bowel syndrome (IBS), but a few years later, the diagnosis was changed to Crohn's disease when a perianal abscess and fistula were discovered. Rhonda worked 14 to 15 hours per day and was not able to find time to prepare meals at home. Her daily diet was dominated by processed food — low-quality cafeteria food for lunch, takeout for dinner, usually no breakfast, and multiple cups of coffee each day. Not surprisingly, she suffered upper respiratory tract infections and required antibiotics two or three times per year. Her typical bowel movement pattern between flare-ups was four to five times per day, with loose, urgent stools.

This year was especially stressful for Rhonda because of the breakup of a long-term relationship and a death in the family. This may have triggered more severe symptoms. A few weeks before visiting us, she had an acute flare-up that involved fever, vomiting, diarrhea and abdominal pain to the extent that she needed to be hospitalized. The attending gastroenterologist prescribed the medication Remicade to control Rhonda's overactive immune response. This settled her symptoms for a week or so.

During this time, Rhonda developed thick, itchy, scaly psoriasis patches on her elbows and knees. This was our clue that she had leaky gut syndrome. Her digestive distress symptoms, combined with her skin irritation symptoms, indicated the typical pattern of development of leaky gut syndrome: a primary set of symptoms presenting at the site of their onset (gut), and a secondary set of symptoms presenting elsewhere in the body (skin) as foreign particles started permeating the gut wall into the bloodstream.

Rhonda was ready to make a change to her lifestyle if there was any chance of being "cured." After testing for food sensitivities, eliminating offending foods and making a long-term plan to adopt the Healthy Gut Diet Plan, Rhonda's daily bowel movements normalized. She has suffered only one flare-up during the past 3 years, with much milder symptoms. Her psoriasis is still present, but it's diminishing in size and intensity. She has expanded her food choices, and we added nutraceuticals — such as fish oils, probiotics, multivitamins and L-glutamine — to her diet to support her gut lining. Unfortunately, not all cases of leaky gut syndrome resolve so effectively.

CHAPTER 1

Deciphering Leaky Gut Syndrome

Leaky gut syndrome involves a malfunction of the filter between the stomach and the small intestine. LGS is not a disease with a single known cause or cure. There is no silver bullet. Rather, it is a syndrome involving a host of possible causes or factors and a corresponding number of possible treatments.

Leaky gut syndrome disrupts the normal function of the gut, the common name given to the small intestine, which comprises the duodenum, jejunum and ileum, stretching from the stomach to the large intestine, or bowel. In a healthy person, the tight junctions between cells in the intestines maintain the integrity of the lining of the gut, called the mucosa. These tight junctions help the intestinal wall to form a barrier that is able to protect against foreign material and pathogens entering the bloodstream while also allowing for the absorption of water, electrolytes and nutrients.

The intestinal wall also serves as a filter, determining what is and what is not allowed into your bloodstream. The cells of the intestinal mucosa are designed to be selective, absorbing essential nutrients as needed. If your

Did You Know?
Disease vs. Syndrome A disease can be defined as a health condition with predictable symptoms that can be related to a specific organ or system, whereas a syndrome is a health condition with a variety of symptoms that can be related to several body systems. In a disease, the cause is discernible. In a syndrome, such as leaky gut syndrome, the cause is a mystery or a puzzle.

FAQ

Q How can I have a leaky gut if my digestion is good?

A This is a common misunderstanding and it is based on the name of the condition, leaky gut syndrome. The problem does originate in the digestive tract, but this does not mean that digestive problems are always experienced. The malfunctioning mechanism in the lining of the small intestine is not something that you feel; rather, it can lead to many inflammatory diseases that present elsewhere in the body. These inflammatory diseases can present as digestive problems, but not always.

Key Terms

The medical language used to describe leaky gut syndrome can be challenging at the outset. You may want to bookmark this glossary and refer to it from time to time when new terms are introduced.

Allergen: An allergen is a substance that triggers a hypersensitivity response in the body. In the context of this book, we are looking at food allergens of the "IgG class" (immunoglobulin G class) that trigger a reaction that presents as a delayed sensitivity (compared to the classic food allergy response of acute hives, swelling and/or anaphylaxis).

Antigen: An antigen is a substance that provokes a response by the immune system. An allergen is a type of antigen, but an antigen does not have to be an allergen. For example, bacteria and viruses may be antigens that trigger an immune response but not an allergic response.

Autoimmunity: Autoimmunity is the action of the immune system attacking its own tissues. An autoimmune disease is a condition that develops as the result of an autoimmunity response.

Blood/brain barrier: This is the highly selective junction between the blood and brain. Only certain substances with appropriate characteristics can cross from the circulatory system into the fluids surrounding the brain.

Hyperpermeability: Hyperpermeability is the dysfunctional state of increased penetration across a selective barrier, such as the gut wall in the context of leaky gut syndrome.

Immune system: The immune system is the body system that protects you against foreign bodies that may lead to infection or disease.

Inflammation: Inflammation is initiated by the immune system in response to a damaging stimulus, such as infection, physical irritation or trauma. In an attempt to rid itself of the damaging stimulus, the capillaries dilate and the affected area can become red, swollen, hot and painful.

Metabolism: Metabolism can be divided into two parts: catabolism breaks down organic matter to create energy, and anabolism uses that energy to construct cell components. These processes are required for physiological functioning, maintenance, growth, reproduction and adaptation.

Mucosa: Mucosa is the cellular lining of a body cavity (including lungs, nasal passage and mouth, plus urinary, reproductive and digestive tracts) and is made up of moist mucous membranes.

Pathogen: A pathogen is an agent that triggers a disease or infection. A pathogen is a type of antigen. Examples of pathogens are bacteria and viruses.

Peristalsis: Peristalsis is the rhythmic movement of the smooth muscles lining the digestive tract that helps to move food from one end to the other.

Tight junctions: Tight junctions are the spot welds between cells that help them to function as a barrier. This barrier forces foreign molecules to be absorbed into the cells rather than moving between them.

Villi: Villi are fingerlike inward projections of the intestinal wall that serve to increase the absorptive surface area of the digestive tract.

gut is in good health, nutrients are transported directly through the cells of the intestinal mucosa; if your gut is in poor health, nutrients trickle away — or "leak" — through the spaces between these cells and become waste.

Hyperpermeability

How effectively the tight junctions "spot-weld" the mucosal cells determines the permeability of the gut. If the cells become abnormally permeable, or leaky, the result can be LGS. As the name suggests, the gut "leaks" material into the bloodstream, which triggers inflammation that can appear in many systems besides the digestive, or gastrointestinal, system. Leaky gut is the origin of the problem but not always the site where symptoms appear.

Leaky gut is the origin of the problem but not always the site where symptoms appear.

Body Systems Affected by Hyperpermeability

Hyperpermeability can instigate or perpetuate many different conditions and diseases within the various body systems.

- **Cardiovascular diseases and conditions:** headache, heart disease, vasculitis, hypertension, pericarditis
- **Central nervous system conditions:** migraine, chronic fatigue syndrome, fibromyalgia, fatigue, anxiety, depression, schizophrenia, mood disorders, autism spectrum disorder, multiple sclerosis
- **Digestive conditions and diseases:** irritable bowel syndrome (IBS), inflammatory bowel disease (IBD), Crohn's disease, ulcerative colitis, constipation, diarrhea, celiac disease, acid reflux disease (GERD), food sensitivities
- **Endocrine (hormonal) conditions:** diabetes types 1 and 2, irregular menses, premenstrual syndrome, heavy menses, low libido, erectile dysfunction, suboptimal thyroid function, adrenal fatigue, polycystic ovarian syndrome
- **Immune system conditions:** autoimmune conditions, multiple food sensitivities, recurrent or chronic infections

- **Integumentary (skin) conditions:** eczema, psoriasis, severe acne, seborrhea, hives
- **Musculoskeletal system:** rheumatoid arthritis, joint pain, muscle pain
- **Respiratory system:** asthma, chronic congestion, cardiopulmonary disease (COPD)

Diseases Associated with Hyperpermeability

Recent studies have shown that more and more diseases appear to be associated with a hyperpermeable gut. Increased permeability has been connected to several gastrointestinal disorders and systemic illnesses:

- **Acute sepsis:** Patients with acute sepsis (infection of the blood or tissues that can cause disease) have abnormal gut permeability as well as an impaired ability to absorb nutrients from the intestinal lumen (the tunnel through which food passes).
- **Dysbiosis:** Bacterial overgrowth can cause dysbiosis (microbial imbalance) in the small intestine, which may trigger leaky gut syndrome.
- **Insulin resistance and metabolism:** One consequence of gut permeability is an increase in blood endotoxins (toxins secreted by bacteria). This has been observed in obese patients, who may have increased insulin resistance and altered metabolic states.
- **Liver cirrhosis:** Patients with advanced liver cirrhosis are at risk of peritonitis (infection of the abdomen) and systemic endotoxemia (bacterial toxins in the blood, leading to shock), which may be associated with

Childhood Diseases

Leaky gut syndrome has been implicated in the development of several systemic childhood diseases that may start as early as infancy. The disruption of tight junctions in a hyperpermeable gut has been connected to:

- Allergies
- Asthma
- Autism
- Inflammatory bowel disease
- Systemic inflammatory response syndrome (SIRS, or sepsis)
- Type 1 diabetes

increased gut permeability because of changes in the tight junctions in the intestinal wall.

- **Obesity:** Obesity is associated with increased gut permeability.

Other conditions connected to leaky gut syndrome include burn trauma, HIV and Parkinson's disease.

Inflammation

Leaky gut syndrome is also associated with certain inflammatory conditions that disrupt the intestinal barrier. Increased gut permeability contributes to these complications by dampening the ability of the immune system to fight off the infection. The tight junctions can

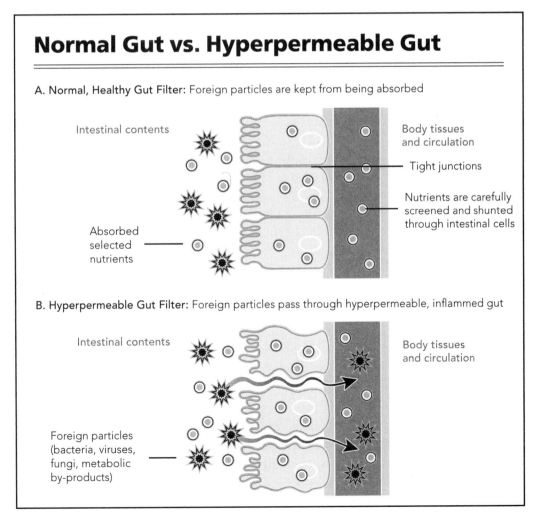

Normal Gut vs. Hyperpermeable Gut

A. Normal, Healthy Gut Filter: Foreign particles are kept from being absorbed

Intestinal contents

Body tissues and circulation

Tight junctions

Nutrients are carefully screened and shunted through intestinal cells

Absorbed selected nutrients

B. Hyperpermeable Gut Filter: Foreign particles pass through hyperpermeable, inflammed gut

Intestinal contents

Body tissues and circulation

Foreign particles (bacteria, viruses, fungi, metabolic by-products)

House Analogy for Inflammation

A good analogy for the outward presentation of inflammation is water damage to a house caused by a leaking internal pipe. Eczema (an inflammatory skin condition) is analogous to the bubbling, discolored paint on the damaged walls. If this is treated simply by sanding and repainting (the same as using prescription anti-inflammatory creams), the root cause of the problem is not addressed and the symptoms will recur. Waterlogged, weakened support beams can be viewed as arthritis, and the spreading rust on the leaky pipe as an inflamed bowel.

The way to approach this is to first determine that the cause of the problem is water damage (leaky gut syndrome) and then go to the source and fix the leaky pipe (heal the gut). The other symptoms will eventually improve as the moisture dries up (as the inflammation clears in the body).

As antibodies trap and eliminate foreign substances, even healthy tissues can become inflamed.

be affected by inflammation that pushes the cells apart. If some of the "spot welds," or adhesions, are displaced, the integrity of the gut filter is compromised and the intestinal wall becomes more porous. Particles that would normally be filtered out by the mucosal cells are absorbed into the bloodstream via the microscopic spaces between cells. These particles include food allergens, metabolic waste by-products and environmental pathogens (bacteria, viruses, fungi and parasites). These particles can disrupt the health of the body as they cross the barrier between the blood and the brain, known as the blood/brain barrier. Your immune system is stocked with antibodies designed to nullify these invaders. As antibodies trap and eliminate foreign substances, even healthy tissues can become inflamed.

Chronic Inflammation

Inflammation can cause havoc in many different systems. For example, inflammation in the digestive tract can trigger irritable bowel syndrome, inflammation of the skin can trigger eczema, and inflammation of the joint capsules can trigger arthritis. If the antibodies become overworked, the result is chronic inflammatory response. As your body continues to try to break down and dispose of these various intruders, it creates by-products that can cause or contribute to systemic, chronic inflammation. This can affect the way your body functions by depleting your energy and enabling recurrent infections.

Autoimmune Conditions

Chronic inflammation can also lead to autoimmune conditions, in which the immune system confuses its message and attacks itself. There is a genetic component to autoimmune disease, but there are also environmental, lifestyle and diet triggers that can activate these genes.

LGS shares many symptoms with these common autoimmune diseases. Leaky gut syndrome can also instigate and perpetuate these conditions:

- Ankylosing spondylitis
- Crohn's disease
- Glomerulonephritis
- Graves' disease
- Hashimoto's disease
- Multiple sclerosis
- Pernicious anemia
- Psoriasis
- Rheumatoid arthritis
- Scleroderma
- Sjögren's syndrome
- Systemic lupus erythematosus
- Type 1 diabetes
- Ulcerative colitis

There is a genetic component to autoimmune disease, but there are also environmental, lifestyle and diet triggers that can activate these genes.

River Analogy for Permeability

To better understand the effects of disrupted permeability, picture a large river (your intestines) flowing through a town (your body). The river is reinforced with walls (levees and spillways). A malfunction of the spillways (a leaky, or hyperpermeable, gut) causes the river to overflow, flooding the town. The malfunction of the spillways becomes increasingly difficult to manage because the flooding limits access to the water controls. Within the town, resources are spread thin as emergency vehicles (your compromised immune system) are overwhelmed and their abilities are restricted. Chaos ensues and communications are disrupted (your immune system signals are misinterpreted and you develop an autoimmune disease). In the same way, reestablishing a healthy gut should repair the floodgates that trigger and perpetuate disease and prevent you from healing.

Anatomy of the Gut

Location of Small and Large Intestine

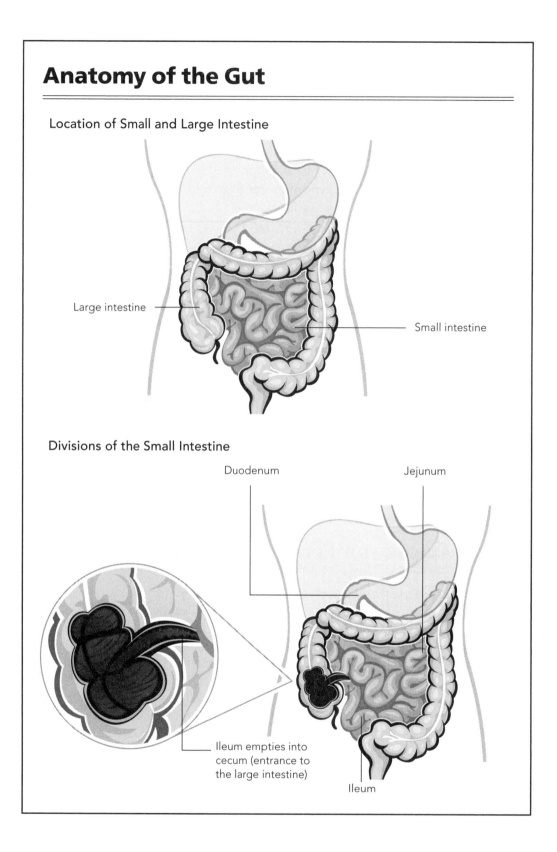

Large intestine

Small intestine

Divisions of the Small Intestine

Duodenum

Jejunum

Ileum empties into
cecum (entrance to
the large intestine)

Ileum

The Anatomy of the Digestive Tract

How we digest food has an impact on the development of a hyperpermeable gut. The digestive tract runs from the mouth to the anus, with several stops in between. Along the way, various parts can spring a leak.

Mouth to Gut

Digestion starts in the mouth with the mechanical breakdown of food by chewing and the chemical action of salivary enzymes. When you swallow, peristalsis (the rhythmic wavelike action of the smooth muscles that line the digestive tract) moves the bolus (chewed ball of food) through the esophagus to the stomach.

The stomach, followed by the gut, is the first line of defense against pathogens and allergens. Powerful gastric acids and enzymes in the stomach break down the food into smaller particles.

Small Intestine

From the stomach, the chyme (the mass of semi-digested food mixed with gastric juices) is transferred into the duodenum, the first section of the small intestine. In the duodenum, the gastric acid is neutralized and additional enzymes from the pancreas, as well as bile from the gallbladder, further break down fats, proteins and carbohydrates in the chyme.

The small intestine plays a major role in the absorption of nutrients from ingested food. An average adult's small intestine is about 20 feet long, which provides a long contact period for nutrient absorption. The shape of the lining of the small intestine increases its capacity to absorb food. The lining has small fingerlike villi that project into the intestinal lumen (the tunnel through which food passes). These villi have another layer of even smaller projections, called microvilli. The combined surface area of the villi and microvilli maximizes the ability of the small intestine to absorb nutrients.

Did You Know?

Digestive Choreography
The digestive system is constantly working to ensure that secreted enzymes break down food into manageable particles for us to properly absorb and assimilate. If one of these many carefully choreographed digestive functions is disrupted, it can initiate a process that triggers inflammation, which lays the groundwork for leaky gut syndrome.

Principal Parts of the Gastrointestinal Tract

The gastrointestinal system can be seen as a long pipe, or tract, that begins at the mouth and ends at the anus, with separate sections throughout that each have a particular function.

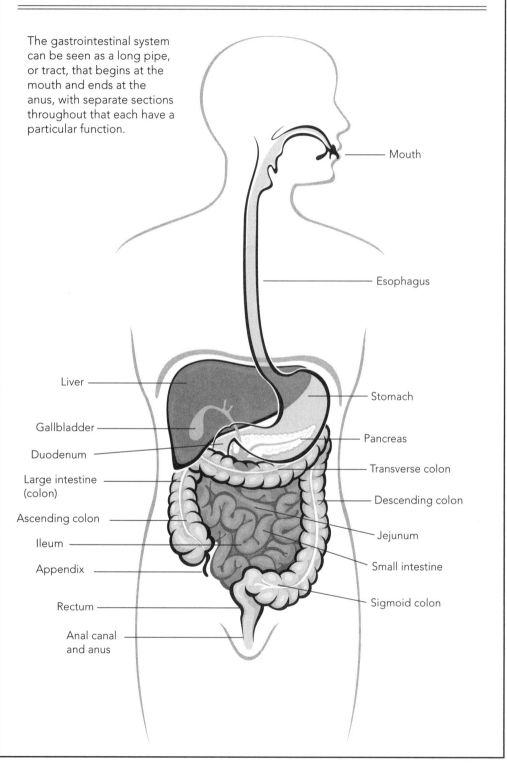

Mouth

Esophagus

Liver

Stomach

Gallbladder

Pancreas

Duodenum

Transverse colon

Large intestine (colon)

Descending colon

Ascending colon

Jejunum

Ileum

Small intestine

Appendix

Sigmoid colon

Rectum

Anal canal and anus

Peristalsis

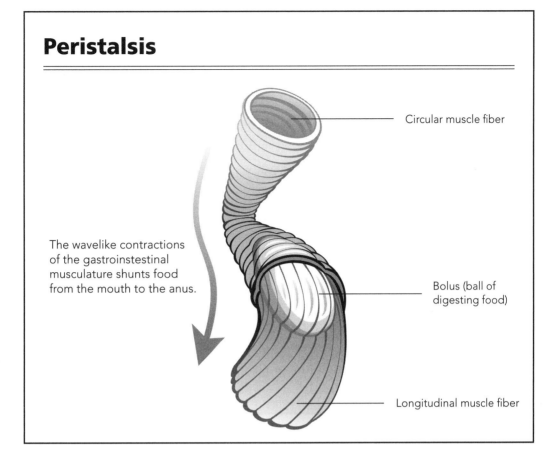

Circular muscle fiber

The wavelike contractions of the gastroinstestinal musculature shunts food from the mouth to the anus.

Bolus (ball of digesting food)

Longitudinal muscle fiber

Nutrient absorption takes place mainly in the jejunum, or the middle of the small intestine, and in the last section, the ileum. The jejunum is slightly shorter than the ileum, but together the two parts make up most of the small intestine. They are the primary sites of leaky gut. As well, IBS-C (irritable bowel syndrome with constipation) and active inflammatory bowel disease (IBD) occur in the small intestine.

Large Intestine

The large intestine, or colon, is about 4 to 5 feet long. The colon is involved mainly in reabsorbing water and eliminating waste materials to form the feces, which exit through the rectum via the anus. Compared to the small intestine, the large intestine is much less likely to develop gut hyperpermeability. However, the large intestine may be involved in certain cases of altered gut permeability, such as IBS-D (irritable bowel syndrome with chronic diarrhea) and inactive ulcerative colitis.

Did You Know?

LGS Paradoxes

Leaky gut syndrome can manifest as one of many health conditions and diseases. Some people with leaky gut syndrome may experience digestive symptoms, and others may not. For example, you can have eczema and perfect digestion, but the eczema may be the result of leaky gut syndrome. Leaky gut syndrome is not just a condition of the gut, although it is a condition that originates in the gut.

Bicycle Maintenance Analogy for LGS

Leaky gut syndrome seems to slowly weaken not only the gastrointestinal system but also other body systems. Think of this as riding a bicycle with tires that are starting to leak in many places. You have a few tire patches that you can use to seal up the holes. You know this is not the solution to fixing the leaks, but it can help you to keep riding. You also have to adjust how you ride the bike. To compensate for the air leaks, you may need to be more cautious and ride more slowly. You can keep going — just not as well. This less-than-optimal functioning is equivalent to a diseased state.

Dysfunctional State

Leaky gut syndrome would be easy to understand if it manifested only in the gastrointestinal system. However, LGS is not specific to the gut, which makes this condition so perplexing. It is far more pervasive and much more complex than inflammatory bowel disease or irritable bowel syndrome. LGS is an underlying dysfunctional state that can manifest itself in other body systems and can contribute to a variety of diseases. Leaky gut syndrome starts and maintains many disease processes. In the case of digestive disease, the ramifications of leaky gut syndrome are more intuitively understood — the discomfort is in the gut, after all. However, it may be more difficult to see the connection between leaky gut syndrome and those diseases of organs or systems that are neither close by nor closely associated with the intestines.

LGS is an underlying dysfunctional state that can manifest itself in other body systems and can contribute to a variety of diseases.

Imbalance

LGS not only appears capable of upsetting the digestive system but can also upset the balance of other body systems essential for good health. Our body systems and their organs communicate with each other in an effort to achieve an internal balance known as homeostasis.

For example, to maintain this homeostatic state, your brain (an organ) communicates with the nervous system and communicates beyond this system to organs in other systems.

Body systems are constantly checking in with each other and monitoring other systems to maintain a balanced internal environment, despite changes in the external environment. When you are ill, your normal healthy physiology is thrown off balance by a trigger. Triggers are environmental factors that may negatively affect your normal physiology or activate certain genetic predispositions. The study of how genes are activated by environmental stimuli is termed "epigenetics." When such an imbalance happens, homeostasis finds a way to compensate so that you can continue to function. The result is that you may still feel ill as homeostasis maintains the disease process and may even lead to new health problems.

When you are ill, your normal healthy physiology is thrown off balance by a trigger. Triggers are environmental factors that may negatively affect your normal physiology or activate certain genetic predispositions.

Recovery

In a healthy, balanced state, your body should recover fully from an acute illness. However, if you don't lead a healthy lifestyle and you don't eat a healthy diet, you may be thrown out of balance, even if you are symptom-free. Being free of disease does not mean being in a state of wellness, and a stressor of the right intensity could shock your body into a new equilibrium, with suddenly manifesting symptoms.

Dam Analogy for LGS

Think of a dam holding back calm water. Cracks may spring leaks, but these can be patched to ensure that the dam is as strong and functional as ever. If, however, the water swells and becomes a churning river, a small crack may turn into a gaping hole that cannot be quickly repaired. The hole will leak as long as the water continues to exert pressure on the dam, and the water must become calm again before the dam can be repaired. Similarly, in treating a leaky gut, you must first improve the fundamental facets of health in order to create a balanced state that allows healing.

Gut–Brain Axis

The gut–brain axis refers to the two-way communication that occurs between the brain and the digestive tract. Not only does the brain communicate with and influence the gut, but the gut also influences the activity of the brain. Communication is mainly through the vagus nerve, a cranial nerve that extends down from the brain, through the neck and chest, and into the abdomen and digestive tract. The vagus nerve comprises about 80% to 90% of the nerves that communicate information from the senses (sight, touch, taste, smell and hearing) back to the central nervous system (brain and spinal cord).

Vagus Nerve

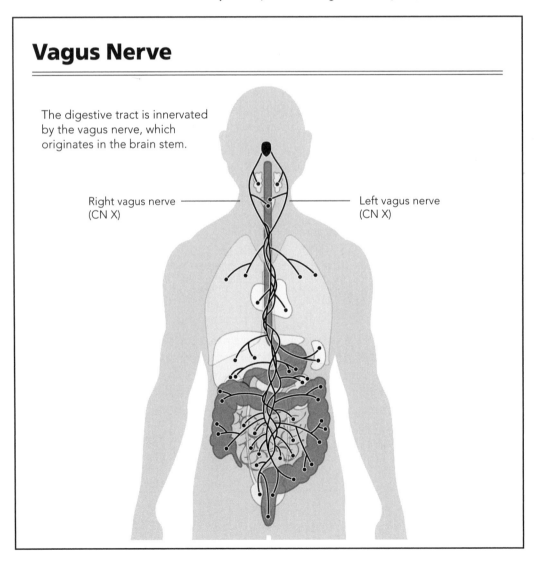

The digestive tract is innervated by the vagus nerve, which originates in the brain stem.

Right vagus nerve (CN X)

Left vagus nerve (CN X)

Where to Find It

A Quick Dewey Reference Guide

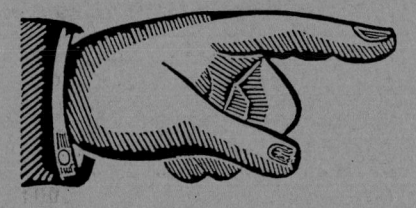

Enteric Nervous System

The gut has its own network of nerves, the enteric nervous system, which controls the gut portion of the gut–brain axis. The enteric nervous system is made up of 100 million neurons, which is more than in either the spinal cord or the peripheral nervous system. This is more proof of the amount and complexity of information that is relayed to and from the digestive tract. Acting independently of the brain, the enteric nervous system communicates with other parts of the body via the hormones, peptides and neurotransmitters it produces.

The enteric nervous system comprises the myenteric plexus and the submucosal plexus. The myenteric plexus is embedded within the musculature of the gut and regulates movement of food through the digestive tract. The submucosal plexus is located just below the mucous membrane lining of the intestines and stimulates the blood supply and the functioning of epithelial cells.

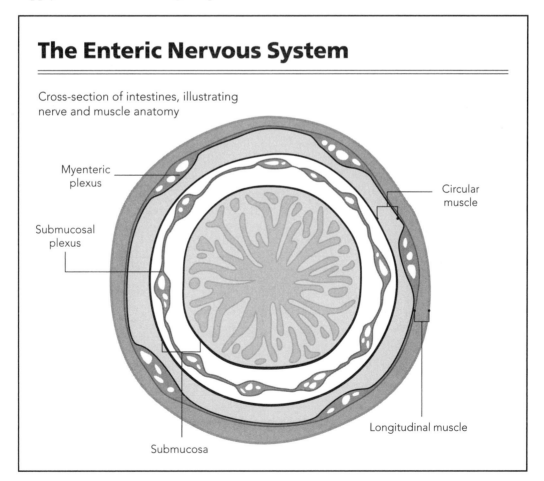

The Enteric Nervous System

Cross-section of intestines, illustrating nerve and muscle anatomy

Myenteric plexus

Circular muscle

Submucosal plexus

Longitudinal muscle

Submucosa

Innervations of the Sympathetic and Parasympathetic Nervous Systems

Sympathetic division

Parasympathetic division

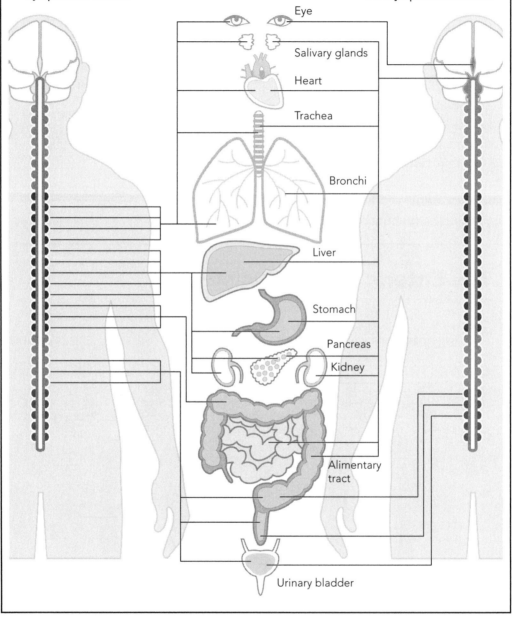

Eye

Salivary glands

Heart

Trachea

Bronchi

Liver

Stomach

Pancreas

Kidney

Alimentary tract

Urinary bladder

The brain is considered to be our command center, overseeing all bodily functions and regulating emotions and mood while processing all of the information coming in from our five senses. Research strongly supports the idea that the gut can do the same: learn, remember, produce emotion-based feelings and perceive sensory information. This is why we often refer to the gut as the "second brain."

Microbiota

Another key player in the gut–brain axis is microbiota, or gut flora, which are beneficial bacteria in the digestive tract that are critical in immune function, digestion, nutrient production and gut health. Recent studies have shown that microbiota influence mental state, psychological and emotional well-being (including outlook and perception of and response to stress) and possibly memory.

It has long been established that the physical health of the brain, as well as your emotional and psychological

Research strongly supports the idea that the gut can learn, remember, produce emotion-based feelings and perceive sensory information.

Second Brain Functional Components

The following components affect the gut, also known as the second brain. There is still much more to discover about how the gut influences emotions and mind–body connections that can help heal a leaky gut.

- **Vagus nerve:** One of the main large nerve bundles, connected to the intestines. While you might assume that neurons (cells that make up a nerve) in the vagus nerve direct signals from the brain to the gut, in fact 90% of the neurons in the vagus nerve direct messages from the gut to the brain. This supports the notion that the gut actually relays important information to the brain and plays an important role in contributing to the brain's functions, rather than the reverse. In essence, the emotions we experience may actually be triggered by messages from our digestive tract.

- **Neurotransmitters:** The brain uses neurotransmitters (brain chemicals) to help regulate mood, energy, sleep and other essential functions. So far, researchers have identified about 100 different neurotransmitters used by the brain. Surprisingly, the gut is not far behind, using about 40 different neurotransmitters to relay messages and support function.

- **Serotonin:** One of the best-known neurotransmitters. Low levels of serotonin contribute to mood disorders, insomnia and fatigue. Such disorders are commonly viewed as disruptions of normal brain function. However, it turns out that more than 90% of the body's serotonin is located in the digestive tract. Researchers continue to research the intimate connections in how our gut health may be influencing our emotions.

state, directly influences the health and function of the gut, including its permeability. Chronic stress can lead to increased gut permeability, increased mucosal inflammation, decreased intestinal blood flow, decreased pancreas and gallbladder activity and many other conditions. Stress can cause changes in intestinal motility (the rate at which food moves along the digestive tract) and imbalances in the healthy microbiota, increasing the risk for unhealthy bacterial or yeast overgrowth. In turn, the health of the gut affects brain activity, including behavior, mood, depression, attention deficit hyperactivity disorder (ADHD) and our general sense of stress.

The dynamic, interconnected relationship between the microbiota, gut and brain cannot be ignored when it comes to overall health.

> *Stress can cause changes in intestinal motility and imbalances in the healthy microbiota, increasing the risk for unhealthy bacterial or yeast overgrowth.*

Doc Talk

Leaky gut syndrome has become the focus of considerable research in the past few years, especially studies of the symptoms and causes of this insidious condition. There is enough research to assess gut hyperpermeability in many disease states, but we need to apply more effort to developing therapies that can heal the gut. When treating a leaky gut, you must first improve the fundamental factors of health in order to create a balanced state that allows for healing.

CHAPTER 2

The Symptoms of Leaky Gut Syndrome

The symptoms of a leaky gut can vary widely from person to person. This is because leaky gut syndrome is not a collection of symptoms but a possible cause of several conditions that affect various systems and organs. Although the "leaky gut" part of the name implies that the symptoms will show in the digestive tract, this is not always the case. Leaky gut syndrome is associated with certain factors that can take a toll on the digestive tract and irritate the intestinal lining, resulting in increased permeability.

The symptoms of leaky gut syndrome can be divided into categories: digestive stress, such as diarrhea and constipation; the presence of associated conditions such as inflammatory bowel disease, irritable bowel syndrome and celiac disease; skin symptoms; and impaired cognition. LGS can also have an impact on other disease states in a number of different systems in your body, such as the reproductive system, central nervous system, immune system and respiratory system.

Leaky gut syndrome is not a collection of symptoms but a possible cause of several conditions that affect various systems and organs.

Predisposing Factors

One or a combination of predisposing factors can play an integral role in initiating leaky gut syndrome and its associated conditions.

- Bacterial/viral/fungal infections and other underlying disease states
- Chronic stress
- Food sensitivities
- Hormone imbalances
- Insufficient physical exercise
- Obesity
- Prescription medication
- Unhealthy diet laden with processed foods and artificial ingredients
- Unhealthy lifestyle choices, such as smoking or excess caffeine or alcohol consumption

Digestive Distress

Did You Know?

Discomfort

LGS symptoms are typically discomforting, like other gastrointestinal (GI) conditions, but a patient with leaky gut syndrome does not always experience digestive discomfort. The intensity of symptoms and the disruption to a person's life have been shown to be associated with increased gut permeability and increased inflammatory markers in irritable bowel syndrome (IBS). A subgroup of IBS patients with increased hyperpermeability reported more significant impact and interference in daily life and experiences of anxiety and depression.

The most direct presentation of leaky gut is digestive distress. Typical early symptoms of leaky gut syndrome are vague, undiagnosed digestive disorders similar to IBS: bloating and gas accompanying constipation and diarrhea.

Bloating and Gas

Bloating or gas can start on its own, even with normal bowel movements, as an annoying symptom. Initially, these symptoms may come and go, but in advanced cases, they can affect daily functioning. Bloating can distend the abdomen to a point where clothing fitted around the waist (for example, skirts or pants) is uncomfortable to wear. People commonly describe the effect as feeling "several months pregnant." Flatus (gas) can be uncontrollable and difficult to hold back, which is embarrassing, particularly in public settings and if accompanied by a foul odor.

Gas or bloating symptoms are often worse after eating, peaking in intensity at the end of the day but calm or even nonexistent in the morning upon waking. This pattern strongly suggests a food sensitivity. Between late evening and morning, when you are asleep and therefore fasting, your digestive tract has a chance to settle down after processing food for the day. Once you begin to add food to your system in the morning, your digestive tract once again begins to react to the trigger food that is aggravating gas and bloating.

Did You Know?

Regularity

Although constipation is medically defined as having fewer than three bowel movements per week, having four or five per week is still far from optimal. Ideally, you should have at least one easy-to-pass solid bowel movement per day, and up to two or three times per day.

Constipation

Constipation can lead to physical discomfort and pain. Trips to the bathroom are often fruitless. Abdominal cramps, bloating and an uncomfortable feeling of fullness are commonplace. When you finally have a bowel movement, you may need to exert a lot of effort to pass stools because of their compactness and lack of moisture. Hard, dry stools rubbing against the soft mucous membranes of the anus can lead to the pain and blood that come with anal fissures. The increase in lower abdominal pressure and strain you need with this type of bowel movement can either cause hemorrhoids or aggravate existing ones.

Diarrhea

The constant unpredictable need to run to the bathroom to pass urgent diarrhea can be both embarrassing and untimely. Going to the bathroom can disrupt important meetings, affect social plans and just leave you feeling lousy, physically and emotionally. Sometimes the accompanying discomfort, bloating and cramps can be tempered only by relieving yourself repeatedly. Explosive bouts of diarrhea drain you of energy and lead to unpleasant bathroom cleanups.

Diarrhea can also leave you with an uncomfortable local irritation of the anus. Long-term chronic diarrhea results in the malabsorption of nutrients. An inadequate supply of nutrients can result in nutrient deficiencies and suboptimal functioning, which can perpetuate leaky gut syndrome. Such deficiencies can also lead to fatigue, malaise, foggy thinking and insomnia.

Malabsorption

With severe chronic diarrhea, the poor absorption of protein, fats and carbohydrates can lead to difficulty in keeping a healthy weight. The malabsorption of vitamins and minerals can disrupt ideal hormone functioning, which can lead to decreased libido, abnormal menstrual cycles or premenstrual symptoms, and disrupted sleep as well as energy and weight problems. It can also affect the strength and luster of your skin, hair and nails. Likely your immune system will not function adequately, which can lead to a higher incidence of infections, colds and flus, particularly when leaky gut syndrome facilitates the passage of more pathogens into the bloodstream.

> **Did You Know?**
>
> **"Leaky Butt" Syndrome**
> One patient jokingly described the condition as "leaky butt syndrome." A leaky gut implies that there is something "leaking," and "gut" implies that it is related to digestion. People put this together intuitively and equate this with diarrhea. Many people have this misconception. Diarrhea may occur in irritable bowel syndrome or inflammatory bowel disease, which may be associated with leaky gut syndrome; however, diarrhea may not occur in the many other permutations of leaky gut syndrome.

Associated Diseases

Leaky gut disease symptoms are typically associated with inflammatory bowel disease (Crohn's disease and ulcerative colitis), irritable bowel syndrome and celiac disease. These are serious digestive conditions that can become life-threatening. They are all triggered by a misdirected immune response that causes the body to attack its own tissues. Celiac disease is an autoimmune disease in which the absorptive surface of the small intestine becomes susceptible to damage by a substance called gluten. People who have celiac disease benefit greatly from strictly avoiding gluten-containing grains such as wheat, rye and barley, and the food products that contain them.

These conditions may severely affect your ability to absorb nutrients, causing deficiencies, malnutrition and drastic weight loss. During a flare-up, your energy will plummet, and your day will revolve around severe digestive upset, including urgent, unrelenting, painful and cramping bowel movements, which are often accompanied by blood loss in IBD. Flare-ups are followed by periods of remission, in a pattern that is frequently unpredictable.

Skin Symptoms

Psoriasis, acne, eczema and other types of dermatitis can be mild localized patches or severe breakouts over your entire body. These skin conditions can show up on your face and hands. They can greatly affect your self-confidence and thus your relationships and your performance at work. The pressure from constantly thinking about your appearance naturally causes further stress, which also contributes to the cycle of inflammation and perpetuates the skin condition.

When these skin conditions cause itchiness, the feeling can range from mildly annoying to an unrelenting, uncontrollable need to scratch your skin raw, until it bleeds. This itch–scratch cycle leads to a continual cycle of skin irritation that can be very difficult to break. In addition, openings in the skin greatly increase the risk of possibly serious secondary infections.

Impaired Cognition

Schizophrenia, mood disorders and autism can present as symptoms of LGS. When foreign molecules enter your bloodstream by way of a compromised gut filter, they can act as chemical triggers that disrupt the brain's normal functioning and lead to episodes of psychological distress or impaired cognition. This can lead to energy and mood swings, depressive episodes, paranoia, anxiety, hyperactivity, foggy-headedness, decreased attention span and inability to concentrate. The attention, communication and hyperactivity of many children with autism spectrum disorder have been found to improve in response to a gluten-free and casein-free diet.

Gluten and Casein Protein

Gluten is found in wheat, barley, rye and, to a lesser extent, spelt and kamut; casein is found in most dairy products. Gluten and casein proteins can trigger LGS by increasing inflammation, thereby irritating the gut. During digestion, these proteins are broken down into smaller components called peptides, which mimic the action of certain brain chemicals in the opioid class (others include heroin and morphine). These peptides can alter moods, disrupt normal speech and hearing pathways in the brain and alter pain perception and cognitive ability. These proteins should be avoided in the presence of leaky gut symptoms.

Impact on Other Disease States

Leaky gut syndrome can have an impact on many systems besides the digestive tract. This impact is a characteristic symptom of LGS. LGS is associated with diseases that can limit or even cripple movement or make movement painful, such as rheumatoid arthritis, multiple sclerosis and fibromyalgia. These conditions drastically affect the quality of life of those who live with them, as well as their families, partners and friends. In advanced cases, such conditions can be debilitating and even life-threatening — for example, death is a potential outcome of multiple sclerosis.

Reproductive System

Leaky gut syndrome can affect the reproductive system and lead to chronic conditions such as polycystic ovarian syndrome, premenstrual syndromes, menstrual irregularities and menopausal symptoms. Drastic mood swings, depression, sleeplessness, pain and anemia (a condition of fatigue caused by low iron and/or low vitamin B_{12} and exacerbated by excessive menstrual bleeding) can result, affecting work performance, quality of life, relationships and fertility.

Central Nervous System

Chronic fatigue syndrome and fibromyalgia, chronic conditions of the central nervous system associated with leaky gut syndrome, are often difficult to diagnose and are challenging to treat with conventional medications. They lead to long-standing fatigue, body pains, headaches and cognitive impairment. This can be debilitating in many cases.

Immune System

If you have a leaky gut, food particles that would normally be filtered out by a healthy digestive tract (because of their size) enter the bloodstream. The immune system treats these food particles in the same way it treats pathogens such as bacteria and viruses. It detects the foreign substances by using antibodies, corrals them and attempts to eliminate them. This process triggers inflammation, which, in the case of unmanaged leaky gut syndrome, may persist as a chronic disease. Leaky gut syndrome is also associated with certain inflammatory diseases in which the increased gut permeability contributes to a dampened ability of the immune system to fight off the infection. No matter what your symptoms, the digestive tract is critical in regulating the immune system and ensuring the proper assimilation of nutrients.

Mimicry

When your immune system is chronically engaged in eliminating food particles, it can overreact, leading to autoimmunity. An autoimmune response may also be triggered when certain food molecules, which a healthy gut would normally filter out, mimic proteins found in our body. Such confused signals can cause the immune system to target your own organs.

Did You Know?

Gut–Brain Axis
We still don't automatically correlate mental illness and mood disorders with nutrition, but the response to a diet that eliminates all processed ingredients and foods that cause sensitivities can be quite dramatic. The gut–brain axis is a concept that is gaining traction as more evidence becomes available to support this connection.

Diabetes and Dysbiosis

Increased gut permeability and intestinal inflammation have been observed in children who have developed type 1 diabetes. Altered gut immunity is the likely culprit. Other autoimmune conditions potentially originate from an altered gut state. Research is also investigating the interrelated issues of dysbiosis (microbial imbalance), intestinal inflammation and leaky gut syndrome.

An example of a food that mimics proteins from our tissues is A1 beta-casein (found in cow's milk), which is similar to proteins in pancreatic tissue. This similarity can lead to mixed signals and an autoimmune reaction that causes your immune system to attack the pancreas, impairing the body's ability to produce insulin. Children with type 1 diabetes often have increased gut permeability and intestinal inflammation.

Respiratory System

People with chronic obstructive pulmonary disease (COPD) and other diseases of the lungs have less oxygen in their bloodstream and tissues. This induces inflammation and decreases functioning throughout their bodies, including in the gut barrier. Research has found that COPD patients experience gut hyperpermeability.

Such associations, in which conditions and diseases in one part of the body affect other parts of the body, support the notion that we should look at inflammation not just where it originates but also in terms of how it affects the whole body.

Did You Know?

Microbial Imbalance
Gut hyperpermeability can be caused by bacterial overgrowth in the small intestine. Researchers are studying several cellular mechanisms that may explain these connections.

Doc Talk

Leaky gut syndrome can affect your body in many different ways. Even within the same affected system or organ, a compromised gut filter can result in a wide range of symptoms. No matter how leaky gut syndrome presents, it will always have a negative impact on your daily life. It can begin as a mild, bothersome transient or episodic issue and progress to an intense, debilitating condition that prevents you from working, maintaining relationships and enjoying life.

With any symptoms, no matter how minor, you should seek help as soon as possible. The longer a problem persists, the more widespread the ramifications can become. This also means that the longer you avoid treating a condition, the longer it will take to heal.

CHAPTER 3

Assessing Leaky Gut Syndrome

Diagnosing leaky gut syndrome is challenging because the symptoms of LGS are not clearly discernable and cannot be readily differentiated from related conditions, such as IBD and IBS. The standard differential diagnosis of symptoms is not effective, and categorizing symptoms by body system is no less illuminating. Arthritis is a disease of the musculoskeletal system, multiple sclerosis is a disease of the central nervous system, eczema is a disease of the integumentary system (meaning that it is related to the enveloping layer, or skin, of an organism), and diabetes is a disease of the endocrine system. Leaky gut syndrome can be involved in any one or more systems. Unfortunately, conventional testing methods do not adequately identify if leaky gut syndrome is a contributing factor in a disease.

Unfortunately, conventional testing methods do not adequately identify if leaky gut syndrome is a contributing factor in a disease.

The first step is finding a doctor who will listen to your concerns, take them seriously and order the appropriate tests to determine a diagnosis. The urine intestinal permeability test, which looks for abnormalities relating to permeability across the intestinal wall, is the most effective of the diagnostic tests. Other tests include the comprehensive stool analysis with parasitology test, the immunoglobulin G (IgG) food sensitivity test, the small intestinal bacterial overgrowth test, the serum IgA test and the hair heavy metal test.

The effects of LGS are many, so determining a prognosis is easier said than done. Whether leaky gut syndrome is the cause or an effect of your condition, improving gut health will certainly improve your symptoms and prognosis.

The Doctor–Patient Relationship

The relationship you create with your health-care professionals is a first step to recovery. Choose your health-care team wisely. When you seek out professional help to assess and treat your health, make sure that you are being heard. Your health-care providers should be your partners in your care, and you should feel comfortable asking them questions about your health.

Unfortunately, leaky gut syndrome often runs concurrently with IBS, and patients may present with overlapping and similar symptoms; neither condition fits nicely into a packaged diagnosis. IBS can affect a patient's quality of life to a high degree: it may be embarrassing and disruptive during social engagements and work commitments. A disparity between the patient's experience of IBS and the doctor's perception of the patient's concerns can develop into patient dissatisfaction with the doctor. Patients feel they have not been adequately heard and that the severity of their condition is not understood.

Although based on science, medicine is an art when put into practice. The doctor collaborates with patients, listening to their story and combining this narrative

---

Research Spotlight
Bedside Manner

Studies show that physicians with better communication skills and a more positive attitude initiate more discussions about the psychosocial aspects of health. This is important not just for the doctor–patient relationship but also to address the mind–body aspect of health.

In a 2009 study, patients addressing digestive symptoms similar to irritable bowel syndrome (IBS) reported on their experiences with their health-care providers. Only 11% were categorized as positive experiences, and 89% were assessed as neutral or negative experiences. Patients may be frustrated with the lack of successful conventional treatment options. Vague digestive symptoms are also often dismissed as something the patient "has to learn to live with."

---

information with objective reports from diagnostic tests and physical assessments. However, some doctors rely solely on test results and cannot see the patient behind the reports. If the test results are negative but you are not feeling well, your doctor should not tell you, "You are fine," or

Patient Bill of Rights

It is your right and responsibility to ask questions of your health-care provider if you are uncertain or confused. You are entitled to ask questions so that you can understand the assessment of your condition, the testing options and the recommended treatment options, as well as any available alternative options. You should understand the answers to all these questions, and your doctor should be willing to make sure you are knowledgeable about your condition and the right treatment for it. It is important for you to be a part of the process, to understand the process and to be proactive in your own healing.

1. If tests are not showing any abnormalities when you know you are not feeling normal, ask for other tests. Tests measure very specific indicators in the body. Since numerous mechanisms trigger disease, a standard panel of tests is only meant to rule out a standard set of diseases.

2. Ask many questions to understand your concerns. The symptoms you are describing are essential to creating a working diagnosis and a treatment plan.

3. Your doctors may not have the perfect answer for your issue at your first or even your second appointment, but they should be monitoring your symptoms on each follow-up visit and taking into account your progress or changes in symptoms to determine whether to modify your treatment plan or leave it unaltered.

4. Two people with the same disease can have vastly different disease triggers, presentations and responses to the same treatment protocol. The important thing is for your doctor to be willing to be flexible with your treatment plan and adjust it according to new information.

5. Because things do not always go smoothly or as expected, ensure that your doctor is persistent and creative in approach. Above all, your health-care provider should have your best interests at heart and be motivated to help you reach a better state of health. Your doctors' goal should be to use their knowledge and skill sets to provide you with the best care that they can. Their priority should be your health.

6. If your doctors have exhausted all their treatment options, ask for a recommendation to another health-care provider who may have additional tests or treatment routes available. Good health-care providers should also have the humility and awareness of their own limitations to know when to refer a patient to another practitioner.

7. Be patient and optimistic that you will find a health-care provider who will want to address your needs and will have the right tools and resources to get you to a state of health. Keep exploring and trust your instincts. You will know when you feel you have the right fit for your needs.

"You are exaggerating." Nor should your doctor say that your symptoms are "all in your head" or "a normal part of aging." You know your body better than anyone, and you know that something is not right. If you feel your doctor is dismissing you too easily or ignoring your symptoms, consider looking for the help of a new doctor.

Diagnostic Tests

Conventional Tests

Conventional means of testing digestive disorders include one or more of the following tests: barium swallow, endoscopy, colonoscopy, stool analysis and blood work. These tests are very useful to rule out any major underlying structural abnormalities, as well as parasites. However, they are not very helpful when assessing and establishing functional pathology.

Complementary Tests

Diagnosing LGS using both conventional and complementary diagnostic tests is much more useful than using conventional tests alone. Many tests are available as a complement to standard medical tests. Some of the tests described here directly measure digestive function, while others are trying to rule out other contributing factors that can initiate or perpetuate leaky gut syndrome. These tests are useful to validate that your symptoms are not just a figment of your imagination and to help determine the best treatment for you.

We have given each test a usefulness rating (scores are out of 5) to help you determine which are most relevant to you and to help you prioritize, particularly when budgetary concerns are an issue. All of these tests help to assess the health of gut function and also help to rule out potential contributing factors.

Urine Intestinal Permeability Test

The urine intestinal permeability test is currently the most directly relevant test for abnormalities that relate to permeability across the intestinal wall. This test measures two different sugars, lactulose and mannitol, in your urine after you have drunk them in solution.

Most Useful Tests
- Urine intestinal permeability test
- Immunoglobulin G (IgG) food sensitivity test
- Comprehensive stool analysis with parasitology test
- Small intestinal bacterial overgrowth test

Usefulness Rating:
★★★★★

In a healthy digestive tract, mannitol is typically readily absorbed from the intestinal lumen into the bloodstream and excreted in the urine. In contrast, lactulose is typically not well absorbed and shows up only in minute amounts in the urine.

In a hyperpermeable or leaky gut state, elevated levels of both mannitol and lactulose may be detected in the urine, indicating an increase in permeability across the intestinal wall. In advanced leaky gut syndrome, you may see elevated levels of lactulose and, paradoxically, decreased levels of mannitol. (The mechanism behind the decrease in mannitol levels is not yet understood.) These changes in sugar levels mean that not only has permeability increased, absorption of smaller particles such as nutrients has also decreased. The ratio of the two sugars in the urine determines whether permeability falls into the normal or hyperpermeable range.

The abnormal result of this test, with elevated levels of lactulose versus mannitol, is analogous to the reversed state of absorption in a leaky gut. In other words, nutrients that should be well absorbed are not, and larger food particles that should not permeate into the bloodstream do. Thus we have an environment with both a state of nutrient deficiency and an excess of problematic molecules that need to be bound and eliminated from the body. This results in tissue inflammation.

FAQ

Q How do I know for sure if I have a leaky gut?

A Some patients who visit our clinic have done a lot of research before they see us and suspect that leaky gut syndrome may be the cause of their health concerns. Other patients may come in simply looking for a new perspective on stubborn health conditions that are not responding to conventional treatment. In any case, if their symptom picture and health assessment point to leaky gut syndrome, we discuss the appropriate testing and treatment options.

The test that actually confirms the presence of leaky gut syndrome is the urine intestinal permeability test. During the early stages of leaky gut syndrome, permeability may wax and wane. Because of this, it is advisable to repeat the test more than once, and to do so when your health condition is in an exacerbated state to ensure that you do not get a false negative result.

The ELISA test is particularly relevant to treating leaky gut syndrome because it helps identify foods that are activating an overeager immune response that starts at the level of the gut.

Immunoglobulin G (IgG) Food Sensitivity Test

A critical first step in the healing process is the identification of any immunoglobulin G (IgG) food sensitivities — foods that cause your immune system to react with delayed and sometimes chronic symptoms. Regularly consuming foods to which you have an IgG sensitivity will make you susceptible to inflammation in your gut and, hence, leaky gut syndrome. The results of an IgG food sensitivity test will help your doctor identify inflammation and evaluate digestive and immune system function.

The IgG antibody levels in your blood sample are quantified using an ELISA test (enzyme-linked immunosorbent assay), a test commonly used in biochemistry labs to measure antibody or antigen levels (antigens trigger antibodies). Because this test is very sensitive, the amount of blood required is minimal. A simple finger-prick blood sample is taken in the office of your health-care provider. Just a few drops of blood are required to measure IgG antibodies for up to 100 common foods (or more if required), which minimizes your discomfort.

The ELISA test is particularly relevant to treating leaky gut syndrome because it helps identify foods that are activating an overeager immune response that starts at the level of the gut. If these foods are not identified and you continue to consume them, your healing will ultimately be delayed or even prevented.

IgG food sensitivities vary from person to person in the degree that they contribute to inflammatory processes.

FAQ

Q I can afford to do only one test. Which one should I do?

A Patients often have a health budget in mind. This is understandable, especially because the tests mentioned in this book may not be covered by insurance plans. If you can choose only one test, we often recommend the IgG food sensitivity test over the urine intestinal permeability test. The pragmatic reason for this is that the output of the food sensitivity test is more practical and useful in customizing an individualized treatment plan. The food sensitivity test helps identify the foods that are likely aggravating your digestive tract. The presence of a large number of positive results (approximately 15% or more) on the food sensitivity test also indicates that leaky gut syndrome is likely present.

The results of this test are very useful because they will tell you which foods are aggravating your immune function. In this way, the test helps you to directly modify your diet by eliminating the offending foods and starting the process of addressing leaky gut syndrome.

Comprehensive Stool Analysis with Parasitology Test

A typical stool ova and parasite test, which your family doctor can perform, measures adult parasites and parasite eggs. It is used to rule out major pathogenic species that can cause overt symptoms, typically in, but not restricted to, the digestive tract, including various parasitic species of bacteria, fungi and protozoa and multicellular parasites such as worms and their eggs. However, this test may provide limited information with respect to leaky gut syndrome.

A comprehensive stool analysis with parasitology test involves a more thorough analysis of the stool than the standard test. It typically involves a 3-day stool collection (versus the standard 1-day stool sample for a conventional stool test). Stool samples collected over 3 consecutive days provide a better representation of the bacterial and yeast colonies present, because these may be missed from one stool sample to the next as a consequence of their clumping growth pattern.

A comprehensive stool analysis with parasitology involves a more thorough analysis of the stool than the standard test.

Unlike the conventional stool ova and parasite test, comprehensive parasite stool testing goes a few steps further by quantifying the levels of symbiotic or beneficial bacteria and yeasts in your stool.

The comprehensive stool analysis also identifies markers that reflect the functional health of your digestive tract. It measures compounds in the stool that correspond to inflammation, digestion and absorptive function of the intestine, as well as stool pH and the presence of white or red blood cells.

This test provides information about the functional health of your gut, along with the health of your gut microbiota (beneficial microorganisms). Both must be healthy to improve gut function and normalize leaky gut syndrome.

Small Intestinal Bacterial Overgrowth (SIBO) Test

Small intestinal bacterial overgrowth is a not uncommon condition linked to the development of gut hyperpermeability. Gut bacteria release methane and hydrogen, which can be detected in the breath after passing from the gut to the blood and being released through the lungs. Measuring these levels and comparing them to a baseline can help determine if bacterial overgrowth in the small intestine is contributing to your health concerns.

The SIBO breath test has two variants: the glucose breath test and the lactulose breath test (both glucose and lactulose are sugars). Both glucose and lactulose are processed by gut bacteria and release methane and hydrogen in the process.

Glucose is absorbed early on in the digestive process in the small intestine. This means that the glucose breath test measures bacterial overgrowth only in the upper region of the small intestine.

Lactulose is not readily absorbed by the small intestine. This means that the lactulose variation of this test measures potential bacterial overgrowth in the lower region of the small intestine, which is more common and therefore may be the more relevant of the two options.

The preparation for both these tests is similar. For a short time, you follow a diet devoid of foods that would feed bacteria and lead to artificial positives. After this fasting period, you ingest either of the corresponding sugar solutions to provide a food source for the bacteria. After the right amount of time has elapsed for gases to be absorbed and then released into the lungs, the breath test is performed to measure methane and hydrogen levels.

Did You Know?

Flora Balance

In addition to ruling out disease-causing species, the comprehensive stool analysis with parasitology test helps to determine the balance of healthy gut flora ("good" microorganisms), dysbiotic flora ("bad" microorganisms) and opportunistic microorganisms (microorganisms that are benign as long as they remain below an acceptable level).

Serum IgA Test

Immunoglobulin A (IgA) is a particular class of antibody that is secreted by mucous membranes (such as the intestines) to tell the immune system that resources are needed to heal and repair the membrane. Serum IgA levels may be elevated when intestines are inflamed. The test for serum IgA levels confirms inflammation in the digestive tract and indicates that there is the potential for an autoimmune response to be triggered by the immune system.

This test can be performed by a family doctor, but because it is not a routine test, you may have to specifically ask your doctor to administer it. It does not give much information about the cause of inflammation or even if it specifically presents in the gut, but it can help to confirm a diagnosis if other tests are pointing in the direction of leaky gut syndrome.

Hair Heavy Metal Test

Hair testing is a useful way to measure tissue stores and the excretion of heavy metals. The hair test usually involves sampling 3 months' hair growth closest to the scalp, or about a tablespoon of hair that is one inch (2.5 cm) long, to measure the heavy metals being gradually eliminated from tissue stores. This test typically measures at least 20 different heavy or toxic metals (for example, aluminum, lead, mercury and cadmium), often along with nutritional elements (for example, iron, potassium, selenium and boron). Most heavy metals at toxic elevated levels can depress the immune system, aggravate digestive function and increase inflammatory processes, all of which contribute to leaky gut syndrome.

Furthermore, several metals (for example, copper) can induce a zinc–deficient state when they are at high levels. Zinc supports the health of the intestinal mucous membrane. Lack of zinc will contribute to and maintain a leaky gut syndrome state.

Usefulness Rating:
★★

Most heavy metals at toxic elevated levels can depress the immune system, aggravate digestive function and increase inflammatory processes, all of which contribute to leaky gut syndrome.

Ratings Review

Although these tests can confirm individual reactions to suspect foods, they can be expensive and time-consuming, and many tests are not definitive, with false positives or false negatives. In addition, not enough tests are available to comprehensively measure every possible food reaction.

If you don't have the resources to do the tests that determine your gut hyperpermeability, you can always support your digestion by following the calming anti-inflammatory dietary approaches we recommend in this book and by monitoring your health for improvements.

Prognosis

The relationship between various systemic or organ-specific inflammatory diseases, gut inflammation and leaky gut syndrome is nonlinear. What we do know is that a vicious cycle exists that is associated with leaky gut syndrome. This means that intestinal disorders and diseases can develop elsewhere in the body. What's more, symptoms usually manifest after the downward spiral of inflammation has already started.

Symptoms usually manifest after the downward spiral of inflammation has already started.

The variables that affect prognosis are complex and include the following four criteria:

- Type of disease(s)
- Severity of the disease(s)
- Degree of dysfunction in the gut
- Overall health of the individual

Leaky Gut Syndrome Cycle

Vicious cycle: An inflammatory response in the body leads to inflammation at the level of the gut. This initiates a leaky gut, causing an influx into the bloodstream of inflammatory particles that trigger an immune response. Over time, this leads to the development of a disease state. This disease state subsequently aggravates inflammation elsewhere in the body, which perpetuates the cycle and can lead to a worsening of health or the multiplication of disease states.

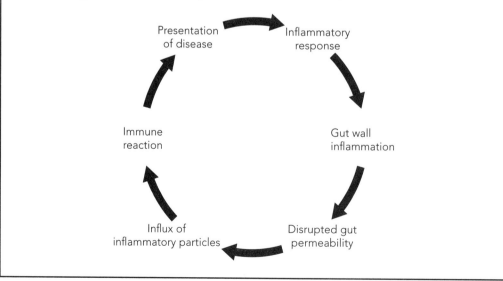

All of these considerations are relevant in establishing a prognosis.

Because the effects of leaky gut syndrome can be so broad and varied, a clear prognosis based on statistical analysis may be impossible. However, whether leaky gut syndrome is the origin of disease or a state that results from disease, treating the gut will help to break the cycle of inflammation, strengthen the digestive tract and normalize immunity.

If leaky gut syndrome is left untreated, your inflammatory state and clinical presentation may continue on the same trajectory and become more severe. With a hyperpermeable gut, other conditions can also propagate because of the continued exposure to trigger molecules (pathogens as well as molecules of food or waste by-products) in the bloodstream.

> ### Did You Know?
>
> **No Chronology**
> There is no distinct chronology of events that always occurs in leaky gut syndrome. Symptoms occur in series or concurrently, with variable overlap at different stages. In some cases, digestive problems may lead to inflammation in other body systems, and in other cases, systemic problems may show first and digestive problems later.

Long-Term Outcomes

In general, whether leaky gut syndrome causes or is associated with your condition, addressing the hyperpermeability of your gut and supporting your gut mucosa and gut immunity result in more optimistic long-term outcomes. Since drug therapies that address gut permeability at a cellular level are only now being investigated, the safest and most rational approach is to work with our bodies to encourage healing. Medication may improve symptoms but does not necessarily address the root of the problem. Treating the cause of leaky gut syndrome involves improving the underlying susceptibility. The ideal approach to treating leaky gut syndrome is to follow an appropriate low–inflammatory diet full of naturally occurring nutrients that strengthen the mucosa and encourage the normalization of function. Not only is this a more balanced approach, but the end result of using a non–pharmaceutical whole-body treatment is that potential adverse effects are negligible.

Treating the cause of leaky gut syndrome is important for two reasons:

> ### Did You Know?
>
> **Neglecting Healing**
> The importance of treating a leaky gut in any of its insidious manifestations cannot be overemphasized. Neglecting to heal the gut when it is part of or the cause of the problem will lead to continued inflammation and the potential to trigger other diseases.

- Strengthening your body's immunity and improving gut permeability through proper treatment prevents new diseases. If left untreated, the effects of leaky gut syndrome can worsen as foreign substances continue to permeate the bloodstream and the cycle of inflammation and decreased immunity continues.

- Healing the intestinal mucosa allows the body to recalibrate its resources and focus on healing the primary disease rather than trying to manage the consequences of the leaky gut. This is analogous to emergency crews (your immune system) trying to track down and capture a criminal on the loose (active disease state) while their surroundings are being flooded by heavy rains (concurrent leaky gut syndrome). The flooding and its resulting damage have to be stemmed before forces can be effectively mobilized to work toward finding the perpetrator.

Treating leaky gut will halt the spiral of inflammation, preventing exacerbation and letting true healing begin.

In essence, treating leaky gut (as either the source of or an accessory to your condition) will halt the spiral of inflammation, preventing exacerbation and letting true healing begin. Permeability at the gut level should always be normalized as part of the treatment plan.

Doc Talk

Leaky gut syndrome can present in many different forms and in many places throughout the body, which makes it difficult to rule out or rule in a diagnosis. However, differential diagnosis with related intestinal diseases and disorders, such as IBD and IBS, can reveal LGS. Conventional medicine uses endoscopy, colonoscopy, imaging studies and blood tests to measure the health of the gut, but conducting both conventional and complementary diagnostic tests can make it easier to reach a diagnosis of leaky gut syndrome.

CHAPTER 4

The Causes of Leaky Gut Syndrome

A leaky gut is caused by chronic irritation of the intestinal lining. This irritation can have many origins. Even low-level irritation over a long period of time can cause chronic inflammation. Think of a new pair of shoes. You try on the shoes at the store and notice a bit of rubbing, but nothing uncomfortable or painful — and you love them. You bring them home, wear them to go out a couple of times, and after each time, you notice a bit of redness on your heels. You even notice that your heels are blistering after longer stretches of walking in the shoes. Your body develops inflammation as a naturally adaptive protective measure. Blisters form to cushion the impact of repeated rubbing. You have to stop wearing the shoes for a long time to allow your skin to recover. The ointment you apply soothes the discomfort for a very short period but does not provide long-term relief.

> *Even low-level irritation over a long period of time can cause chronic inflammation.*

Research Spotlight
Mucosal Mast Cells

Over time, chronic stressors cause inflammation to become a chronic condition, a state of hyperpermeability, or leaky gut syndrome, where the intestinal wall is compromised enough to manifest symptoms throughout the body. Research has demonstrated that mucosal mast cells mediate the inflammation involved in initiating leaky gut syndrome. Mast cells are messengers of the immune system and they signal the start of an inflammatory cascade that readies the immune system to act on the targeted tissue. At the level of the gut mucosa, mast cells serve to modulate intestinal motility and increase permeability. Research has identified mast cells as important components of the pathogenesis, or origin, of irritable bowel syndrome (IBS) and inflammatory bowel disease (IBD). This emphasizes the interconnectedness between the immune system and inflammation and gut dysfunction.

Common Stressors

- Physical: poor posture, inadequate chewing, underlying inflammatory conditions, infectious gastroenteritis, parasites
- Chemical: environmental pollutants, occupational toxin exposure, cigarette smoke, pro-inflammatory diet, chemical food additives, antibiotics, oral contraceptives, anti-inflammatory medication, immunosuppressive medication, proliferative medication to increase cell turnover
- Mental–Emotional: chronic stress, anxiety, depression

Did You Know?

Tolerance Threshold

Leaky gut syndrome often starts insidiously. Something is not quite right, but you continue with your daily routine, diet and lifestyle and mostly feel fine. But then your condition worsens. Eventually you exceed your tolerance threshold, you feel bothered and frustrated, and you look to your physician for help.

Similarly, when overstimulated by certain aggravating factors, the digestive tract triggers the immune system to initiate an inflammatory response. This inflammation exerts pressure that pushes apart the cells of the gastric lining. Eventually, with continued inflammation, the integrity of the gut filter is affected. The price you pay for style over comfort in shoes can be analogous to eating an extremely tasty but poor-quality diet, or having an unhealthy lifestyle over a long period of time.

Stressors

Leaky gut syndrome sets the stage for inflammation in other tissues and organs. But what triggers initiate the process that causes a leaky gut in the first place? Potential stressors that initiate the process of gut hyperpermeability are ubiquitous and all too common. Stressors can be classified into three general categories: physical, chemical and mental–emotional.

Physical Stressors

You may know that feeling: you've never felt quite well since that last infection — that cold, gastrointestinal parasite or bout of food poisoning, or acute bacterial or viral gastroenteritis. Onset of a condition and a particular physical stressor often correlate. Despite the fact that the initial stimulus has been resolved or the pathogen eliminated, your body still malfunctions.

An example of an intestinal disorder brought on by a physical stressor is post-infectious IBS. This variation of IBS occurs in about 1 in 10 IBS cases. The symptoms, most commonly diarrhea, are present only after an acute bout of bacterial gastroenteritis and last for an average of about 6 years. Post-infectious IBS involves chronic gut inflammation, altered gut immune regulation and increased permeability of the gut barrier.

In addition, chronic poor posture or gross physical trauma (from a motor vehicle accident or sports injury, for example) can trigger symptoms that affect the body systemically by interrupting proper neural function, preventing those nerves from regulating organ function. This type of disruption is common with misalignment of the spine.

Research Spotlight
Air Pollution

Air pollution can have an effect on the gut, playing a role in the ability of your immune system to function properly. The quality of our air — outside and inside — has deteriorated. Inside air is contaminated with dust, debris, mold, fungi, bacteria and viruses — the very substances that the gut tries to filter out. Recent research suggests that air pollution, quantified by measuring particulate matter in air samples in various Bulgarian cities, affects the modulators of our immune system function. Increased pollutants in the air shift the balance of the immune system's chemical messengers from a state of anti-inflammation to pro-inflammation. This shift creates an environment that promotes the development of autoimmune diseases and allergies.

Air pollution in large cities was found to influence respiratory dysfunction and, to an even more pronounced degree, the prevalence of immune, cardiovascular and blood abnormalities. With levels of immune cells changed, the ability to heal damaged tissues also changed. Although air pollution may not be the main trigger for gut hyperpermeability, it can be one of the many variables that prevent tissues from healing.

Chemical Stressors

Chemical stressors trigger inflammation at a molecular level. Chemical stressors may include prescription medications (in particular, antibiotics and oral contraceptives disrupt healthy levels of gut bacteria), artificial ingredients in processed foods, pro-inflammatory foods (such as sugars and refined carbohydrates), toxins, excess caffeine, alcohol and cigarette smoke. Included in this list are the foods to which you are sensitive. This is because your body treats the results of breakdown of these products as foreign compounds.

If there is sustained exposure to any of these chemical stimuli, your immune system will trigger chronic inflammation, which increases the likelihood of developing leaky gut syndrome.

Antibiotics

Antibiotics are predictable in their effect on the body. Antibiotics are primarily taken orally to address a localized infection in the throat, ear or urinary tract, for example. The antibiotics are given at a dose high enough to be effective after permeating the bloodstream and reaching the location of the infection.

> **Did You Know?**
>
> **Stress-Induced**
> Acute and chronic stress can alter the integrity of the mucosal barrier, increasing intestinal permeability and worsening symptoms of both IBS and IBD. Stressful situations at early developmental stages can be implicated in gut pathologies in adulthood.

However, antibiotics can disturb the delicate balance of gut flora and bacterial colonies that have been established from birth. These bacteria colonies, known as microbiota, are depleted when you take a course of broad–spectrum antibiotics to treat an infection. Good bacteria are a critical component of your immune system and work as a first-line defense system to protect against pathogens and toxic materials before they come in contact with the intestinal wall. The continual administration of antibiotics for recurrent infections (commonly, ear or throat infections) in childhood can drastically damage the protective gut flora, which sets the stage for more infections and compromised integrity of the gut filter.

> *Good bacteria are a critical component of your immune system and work as a first-line defense system to protect against pathogens and toxic materials.*

Mental–Emotional Stressors

The gut has its own independent nervous system, called the enteric nervous system. Often referred to as the second brain, the enteric nervous system contains more neurotransmitters than does the actual brain. We use the phrases "I had a gut feeling," "butterflies in my stomach" and "a gut response" because our digestive tracts may experience emotions before we are consciously aware of

Research Spotlight
Early Exposure to Antibiotics

Childhood use of antibiotics is common but can lead to adverse effects down the road. Several studies have indicated a significant relationship between antibiotic exposure in children and the development of inflammatory bowel disease (Crohn's or ulcerative colitis). In these conditions, the likely association is compromised intestinal permeability. Whether causal or secondary, it is important to address.

Adult patients with a digestive disorder or other leaky gut symptoms often recall frequent use of antibiotics for recurrent childhood infections. Eczema and asthma have a direct dose-dependent relationship based on the cumulative effect and frequency of antibiotic use before 2 years of age. At 7.5 years of age, eczema, asthma and hay fever incidence were all increased based on antibiotic use. Even with just one round of antibiotic use before 2 years of age, the increase was significant, and it continued to increase with each subsequent use of antibiotics in infancy. Interestingly, the eczema was not related to an atopic effect (related to genetically associated allergic triggers), and so it may plausibly be connected to gut hyperpermeability. This merits further investigation.

them. This also means our digestive tracts are extremely sensitive to mental–emotional stressors and trauma. Over time, multiple daily pressures and demands wear us down in ways that can have physical ramifications.

Psychological trauma occurs when mental–emotional stressors surpass your threshold for stress tolerance and begin to affect your day-to-day functioning and enjoyment of life. In many cases, the onset of certain physical ailments can be traced back to a certain stressful traumatic experience. Your mind can suppress stressors to cope with expectations. However, when such stressors are not properly processed and resolved, your body may initiate an inflammatory cascade that can develop into leaky gut syndrome.

Food Allergies, Sensitivities and Intolerances

Food allergies are one of the most overlooked aspects of physical or chemical stress on your digestion. When you ingest an allergen every day, it acts as a constant aggravating factor that disrupts your digestive system and prevents it from functioning properly. It is critical that you reduce and/or eliminate stressors that strain your digestive tract and prevent you from achieving your optimal health.

By definition, a food allergy is an immune system reaction that takes place after consuming a certain food, and it involves the activation of immune system cells and antibodies whose goal is to rid the body of the food it considers to be an unwanted foreign substance. Generally speaking, this activation leads to the classic immunoglobulin E (IgE) allergy response of immediate symptoms — hives, redness, tongue or throat swelling, and severe anaphylactic reactions. This is one particular type of food allergy mediated by IgE antibodies. Most often, it is an obvious trigger because of the quick onset of symptoms. For example, if you eat peanuts and notice an itchy throat within a few minutes, you can link that reaction to the peanuts as the food allergy trigger. However, other forms of food allergies present differently.

A food sensitivity can describe vague, insidious symptoms that may appear after you eat a trigger food. Immunoglobulin G (IgG) food allergies, which have a more delayed, slow-building reaction, are called sensitivities so as not to be confused with the typical IgE food allergies.

"Sensitivity" and "intolerance" are used to describe an aggravation that does not involve the immune system and one that presents differently than the classic allergy. In the case of common lactose intolerance, for example, lactose (a milk sugar) cannot be properly broken down by the body

Research Spotlight
IgG Food Sensitivities and Leaky Gut Syndrome

Food sensitivities can occur because of a hypersensitive reaction to foods by IgG antibodies in the blood. This class of food sensitivities has shown higher positives in patients with irritable bowel syndrome (IBS) compared to a healthy population. In one study, when trigger foods were eliminated from the diet of patients with IBS, digestive health improved significantly after 8 weeks. In 34% of cases, symptoms improved remarkably based on a quality-of-life analysis, and in 31% of cases, symptoms completely resolved. These results emphasize the importance of controlling food aggravators in the diet as a critical part of the recovery plan to treat and heal a damaged gut.

In another study, 77 patients with IBS-D (IBS with a tendency toward diarrhea) all showed significant relief from abdominal pain, abdominal distention, diarrhea frequency, stool quality and feelings of distress when they excluded IgG food intolerances from their diet for a 12-week period.

The prevalence of food intolerances is based on disease manifestation. In children, food intolerances are more prevalent among those with immune system disorders and developmental abnormalities. Children with multiple-system disease also showed higher rates of intolerances when compared with those with a single-system disease. This epidemiological data is in line with what happens when a leaky gut co-occurs with a condition. The condition will worsen and affect other systems if hyperpermeability is not addressed, and food intolerances will also increase as a consequence.

The food categories that most commonly cause inflammation are dairy, egg and gluten-containing grains. Food sensitivities, allergic reactions and intolerances are also often instigated by alcohol, beef, caffeine, chocolate, cruciferous vegetables, garlic, legumes, onion, peanuts, pork, shellfish, soy and tomato. Restricting all these foods is important to improve gut immunity, hyperpermeability and inflammation, which are all part and parcel of leaky gut syndrome and feed off one another to allow the disease to persist.

Aggravating BRAT and CRAM Diets

To treat diarrhea, dyspepsia (indigestion) and gastroenteritis, medical doctors and gastroenterologists have often recommended the BRAT diet (banana, rice, applesauce and toast), the extended BRATTY diet (BRAT + tea and yogurt) or the CRAM diet (cereal, rice, applesauce and milk). Although some studies showed that these diets caused a minor decrease in digestive disorder symptoms, they are overly simplistic treatments. They also contain some of the foods many people cannot tolerate, which is likely to aggravate inflammatory processes in a large percentage of the population.

While studies have observed some improvements with the BRAT diet, this diet can aggravate diarrhea over the long term. Consuming high amounts of fruit sugar (bananas, applesauce) and simple starches (white rice, toasted white bread) — to the exclusion of everything else — can further aggravate and inflame the digestive tract. The BRAT diet is also full of gluten-containing products, which is one of the more common food sensitivities. Over the long term, because this diet does not provide a complete nutrient spectrum, it can lead to macronutrient, mineral and vitamin deficiencies. In addition, the BRAT diet may not provide adequate amounts of energy, fat, protein, fiber, vitamin A, vitamin B_{12} and calcium.

---

because of a lack of the enzyme lactase. This leads to loose stools and bloating shortly after consuming milk.

Conventional Allergy Testing

The standard allergy test that your allergist performs, the IgE test, checks for the type of antibodies (immunoglobulins) that initiate the immune response. By scratching your skin and applying a series of potential allergens in liquid drops to the scratch marks, the allergist can identify which substances cause a response on the skin. This test also determines seasonal and environmental allergens that can cause symptoms such as runny nose, watery and red eyes, and sneezing.

An IgG food reaction does not follow the classic allergy response. Its response to the trigger food is delayed by as much as a few hours or even days, and it presents in a more insidious manner. Because of the delayed and subtle symptoms, these allergens are difficult to identify even when you strictly monitor food consumption. Because we generally understand IgE allergic responses to be actual food *allergies*, IgG food responses are easier to think of as food *sensitivities*.

> ### Did You Know?
>
> **Mutual Aggravation**
> Food sensitivities and hyperpermeability go hand in hand and aggravate one another. With such a chicken-and-egg cycle, we may not know which factor first triggered the other, since they coexist.

Triggers

One of the theories for the development of food sensitivities is opportunistic overcolonization by *Candida albicans* yeast in the digestive tract. Research has shown that candida promotes the infiltration and activation of certain immune cells called mast cells at the intestinal wall in mice. Genetically altered mice that were deficient in these mast cells did not develop gut hyperpermeability until they had mast cells re-established in their systems via bone marrow transplant. This implies that candida overpopulation initiates a mast cell response that disrupts the gut filter, triggering the development of food sensitivities.

Some of the other plausible triggers of food intolerances or sensitivities are gastrointestinal bacterial or viral infections, parasites, genetics, overexposure to particular food groups, and overexposure to processed and concentrated proteins from certain food groups (for example, casein from dairy, albumin from egg, or hydrolyzed protein from soy). Keep in mind that the many instigators of leaky gut syndrome listed above may also initiate the development of new food sensitivities.

Doc Talk

Human beings are highly adaptable. Adaptability allows us to continue functioning and focus on more pressing matters. Unfortunately, the downside to adaptability is that it makes it easier to normalize our symptoms and ignore the importance of taking action to understand why they are there and how to properly treat them. We typically ignore a health concern until it intensifies to a degree where it affects and interrupts our day-to-day lives, affecting work performance, relationships with romantic partners and our socialization with friends or family. By this point, the health concern has become quite entrenched because the pathology has progressed and persisted to the point where it is a chronic condition affecting other systems.

Be aware that it is normal for the majority of us to wait longer than we should to address our health concerns. That being said, use this experience to become more in tune with your body's needs and imbalances so that you can fix problems at an earlier time — and at a more readily treatable state — in the future.

PART 2

Managing Leaky Gut Syndrome

CASE HISTORY

Avoiding Surgery

Royce is a 16-year-old male with ulcerative colitis. He is enrolled in high school but does most of his course work at home because of the severity and unrelenting presentation of his ulcerative colitis symptoms, which started at the age of 11. The disease significantly upsets his daily life and his ability to function and socialize normally.

For 2 years, his gastroenterologist has been urging Royce to have his colon surgically removed, to which Royce is strongly opposed. From the gastroenterologist's perspective, all the criteria for surgery have been met. Royce is currently taking monthly injections of Remicade, which suppresses his immune system in order to control the autoimmune aspect of his condition. This provides only limited relief.

His bowel movements are urgent, mushy to liquid in consistency, with weekly episodes of bleeding and cramping. Almost every second day he has severe bloating and gas. Royce also suffers from insomnia, waking frequently, and has low back pain and eczema, which started 3 years after the onset of colitis. He is underweight and fatigued as a result of long-term disrupted absorptive function and a hyperpermeable gut.

Upon reviewing his diet, I noticed a moderately high intake of dairy and gluten products, including a commercially available high-calorie canned "nutrition" drink. He had consumed this drink daily for over a year to increase his calorie count and improve his weight (this was obviously not successful). This product is full of refined sugar, high-fructose corn syrup, artificial flavors and a concentrated milk protein.

Based on his severely compromised state, we recommended that he immediately eliminate these packaged drinks and stick to a whole foods diet with no processed or artificial ingredients. We recommended that he adhere as best as possible to the Calming Diet (see page 126) to dampen his inflammatory state. We also recommended probiotics and L-glutamine to support healing of the intestinal epithelium.

At the second visit, about 1 month later, Royce showed that he had been more compliant than we ever would have expected from a teenager. He had followed the recommended diet plan religiously. As a result, he had seen vast improvements, more than he had experienced in years of conventional treatment. I reviewed the results from his IgG food sensitivity test, which confirmed strong sensitivities to gluten, dairy, egg and garlic, and recommended that he continue to avoid these foods.

Royce's gut symptoms had abated to the point that he was confident enough to transition back to school rather than study via distance education. His energy and vitality had improved so much that he could confidently leave the house for an entire day, which had not been possible previously. His severe and constant low back pain had improved significantly, and his eczema had decreased to about half of its original intensity. There was still a lot of work to do to ensure that he gained weight and continued along the same path. With his gut functioning at this enhanced level in such a short time, no competent gastroenterologist could persuade Royce to undergo a colectomy.

CHAPTER 5

Conventional Drug and Surgical Treatments

Because leaky gut syndrome can produce a variety of symptoms throughout the body, there are several ways to assess its impact on each of the affected systems and organs. Conventional allopathic medicine views the symptoms in the affected systems and organs as distinct from one another, whereas complementary naturopathic medicine sees all body systems functioning as a whole.

In conventional medicine, symptoms are monitored and their effects are treated independently of each other. A patient with eczema, for example, would be referred to a dermatologist, who would first assess the skin, primarily by examining it closely. Just to be certain, a biopsy might be ordered to rule out any serious dermatological conditions (such as cancer), or a skin scrape might be used to rule out fungus as a causative agent. Digestive function and food sensitivities are not considered as possible culprits.

Likewise, IBS is diagnosed only if tests rule out structural disease. In other words, it is a "diagnosis of exclusion." In the absence of other pathologies of the digestive tract, the remaining collection of symptoms is labeled irritable bowel syndrome (IBS). IBS explains the intricate connection between systems that seem not to be associated. It may be caused by a food sensitivity, dysbiosis (microbial imbalance), stress or a combination of these and other contributing factors.

Since leaky gut syndrome is also a functional syndrome, standard diagnostic tests provide little insight into the permeability of your gut and its relation to your health and symptoms. Because allopathic medicine uses tests to rule out specific pathologies and physical disease, patients with leaky gut syndrome may be told that their test results are "normal" despite the fact that they don't feel normal. Standard diagnostic testing does not assess any functional compromise, the hallmark of leaky gut, and symptoms will persist.

Because allopathic medicine uses tests to rule out specific pathologies and physical disease, patients with leaky gut syndrome may be told that their test results are "normal" despite the fact that they don't feel normal.

Alternatively, leaky gut syndrome may be associated with pathology, either as a cause or as a result. Standard diagnostic testing will fall short again. For example, ulcerative colitis is diagnosed using a colonoscopy, whereas the assessment of leaky gut syndrome is not that straightforward. Whether leaky gut contributed to the development of ulcerative colitis or was brought on by ulcerative colitis, the diagnosis and therefore the treatment will focus on ulcerative colitis. A more holistic approach of treating both would be critical for proper long-term healing.

Allopathic medicine generally treats symptoms, and the allopathic toolbox consists of drugs and surgery. This would apply for digestive issues and other manifestations of leaky gut syndrome. Prescription medication can be miraculous at preventing undue suffering in severe situations and in treating serious infections. Likewise, in the case of structural and anatomical abnormalities, surgery to remove diseased tissue or obstructions may be warranted and even lifesaving in extreme cases. However, each of these powerful treatment strategies has side effects. They should be used responsibly and only when they are absolutely indicated.

Unfortunately, because allopathic medicine considers that there are no other options for the many manifestations of leaky gut syndrome, prescription medications or

When Are Drugs or Surgery Warranted?

1. When the condition is life-threatening.
2. When, if the condition is left untreated, it will cause organ or system damage.
3. When the symptoms are debilitating.
4. When the structural abnormalities are affecting normal functioning.
5. When diseased tissue is beyond repair and needs removal.
6. When nonsurgical non-pharmaceutical treatment options have been explored and exhausted without success.

Keep in mind that if drugs or surgery were deemed necessary, supporting your body through diet and lifestyle changes would be important for recovery, to lessen side effects, prevent relapse and improve your state of health. In certain cases, if you are successful in proactively treating your health state with diet and lifestyle changes or in other ways, you may be able to decrease your medication dose or wean yourself entirely off medication, under the supervision of your physician.

surgery is usually the only available treatment choice. Conventional medicine rarely considers diet as a treatment option, or leaky gut as a plausible contributor to digestive disorders and other symptoms linked to leaky gut syndrome. Essentially, allopathic medicine is quite limited in effectively healing a leaky gut.

Medications

Prescription or over-the-counter medication can be effective in the short term for an acute illness, to dampen a flare-up of an existing condition or for the long-term control of symptoms. While prudent use of medications is often warranted for both acute and chronic conditions, some medications can worsen inflammation.

While prudent use of medications is often warranted for both acute and chronic conditions, some medications can worsen inflammation.

Medications for digestive disorders include prednisone, a strong anti-inflammatory for controlling flare-ups in inflammatory bowel disease (IBD); immune-suppressing medication to control autoimmune conditions (such as ulcerative colitis); and anti-motility drugs to slow down bowel function in IBS. These medications control symptoms but do not address the cause of the problem. They also frequently have side effects and should be recommended only if the severity of your disease outweighs the severity and risk of the potential side effects.

Treating with or without Medication?

If leaky gut is determined to be a potential causative or associated aggravating factor of an inflammatory disease (ulcerative colitis or rheumatoid arthritis, for example), it opens up the possibility of avoiding the use of medication and/or surgery. Treating leaky gut with dietary changes, lifestyle modifications and natural complementary therapies is safer than using medications, and such a treatment plan works with and supports your body's natural immune response. This gentler approach can be explored, with the guidance of a health professional, in mild to moderate cases (where symptoms may be annoying or bothersome but are not life-threatening or intolerable), and cautiously implemented in severe cases.

However, if your symptoms are greatly affecting your daily functioning and inflammation is severe, medication is likely warranted, though the treatment plan for leaky gut syndrome can be concurrently implemented. Again, consult with a health-care professional to discuss and assess your individual health concerns, potential medication interactions and treatment options.

Chronic Medication Use

Long-term medication use may cause chronic adverse effects that you experience initially but that your body gradually dampens over time. This is similar to the sometimes severe adverse symptoms you experience with your first cigarette. After only a short period of smoking regularly, you stop experiencing these symptoms. However, this does not mean that the body is no longer under stress. Rather, it means that your homeostasis and metabolism have compensated by adapting to tolerate toxins from the stressor (cigarette smoke) more efficiently.

Our bodies adapt and adjust. This has helped the human species to survive but has not helped with the prevalence of chronic disease and quality of life. From a leaky gut perspective, some unnecessary long-term medications can obstruct proper healing because they can alter normal

> *Long-term medication use may cause chronic adverse effects that you experience initially but that your body gradually dampens over time.*

Medication Questions

Physicians should be able and willing to answer the following questions about any medications they prescribe. Be certain you know the answers to the questions. Otherwise, request clarification from your doctor.

1. Have you done all the available tests to determine the cause of my symptoms?
2. Should I expect to experience any side effects from the medication you are prescribing?
3. What should I do if I experience side effects?
4. How long do I have to use this medication?
5. What will happen once I stop taking this medication?
6. Why are you recommending this particular medication (the rationale)?
7. What is the prognosis for my condition and the expected timeline for your treatment?
8. What are the next steps after completing this course of medication?
9. What are the alternatives to this treatment plan?

Research Spotlight
NSAID Dangers

Nonsteroidal anti-inflammatory drugs (NSAIDs), such as ibuprofen, can relieve some symptoms of LGS, providing comfort in acute situations. But prolonged use of NSAIDs can exacerbate the condition. Recent studies have shown that after 1 week of use, NSAIDs were shown to cause not just visible damage to small intestinal mucosa but also dysfunctional permeability. After a 4-week washout period, the damage was not visible. However, the increased permeability continued. This provides evidence to support the concept of leaky gut syndrome as a mechanistic pathology of a disease, even if a structural abnormality is not seen. In other words, leaky gut syndrome can exist without a diagnosed gastrointestinal condition presenting concurrently.

Athletes commonly take NSAIDs prior to intense exercise to mitigate pain and, in theory, improve their performance by allowing them to push themselves harder. One study demonstrated that cyclists who took ibuprofen before exercising induced an intestinal barrier dysfunction as well as intestinal damage. With an acutely induced response such as this, we can extrapolate that NSAID use could contribute to longer-term sustained permeability alterations. It goes without saying that medication should be recommended and used responsibly and only in circumstances that truly warrant its use.

metabolic pathways, disrupt gut flora (as do antibiotics and oral contraceptives), suppress the immune system, initiate cycles of inflammation as a result, and deplete the body of nutrients. (For example, cholesterol-lowering medication blocks the production of the coenzyme Q10, oral contraceptives are linked to B-vitamin deficiencies, and anti-inflammatories deplete us of folic acid.)

Surgical Procedures

Occasionally, surgery is an option for managing leaky gut syndrome symptoms associated with IBD (Crohn's disease and ulcerative colitis). The most common surgeries for intestinal disease are resections and ostomies. Resections involve removing diseased portions of the small intestine or colon and essentially reattaching the healthy ends. Ostomies, such as colostomies and ileostomies, involve extending portions of the intestines through the

The most common surgeries for intestinal disease are resections and ostomies.

Small and Large Intestine Resection

Small intestine resection

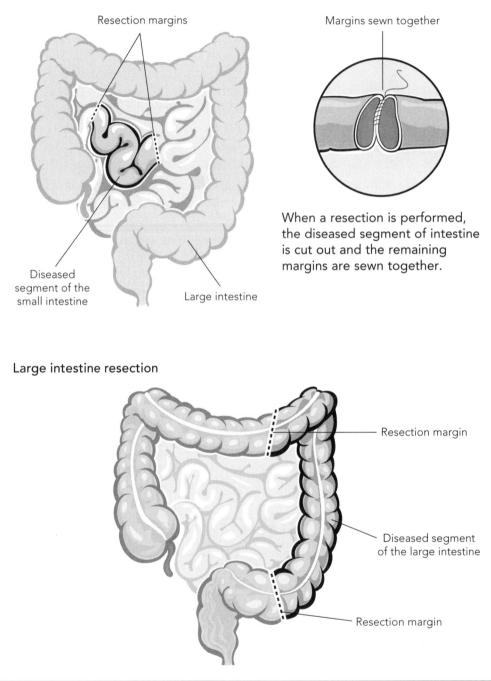

Resection margins

Margins sewn together

Diseased segment of the small intestine

Large intestine

When a resection is performed, the diseased segment of intestine is cut out and the remaining margins are sewn together.

Large intestine resection

Resection margin

Diseased segment of the large intestine

Resection margin

Closed Ileostomy

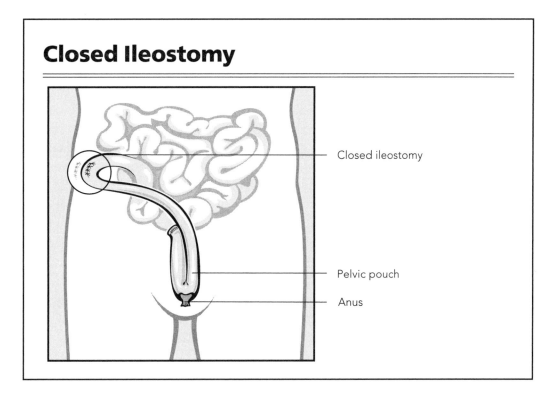

Closed ileostomy

Pelvic pouch

Anus

abdominal wall and out through the skin (this opening is called a stoma). An external pouch apparatus is usually attached to the stoma to collect the intestinal waste. Discuss all the options, risks and outcomes of surgery with a surgeon.

Doc Talk

Address your regular medication regimen with your doctor. Certain medication is necessary and lifesaving, as is the case with supplementing deficiencies (for example, insulin for diabetics). Other medication may not be necessary in situations where lifestyle changes or diet therapies can address the cause of the problem effectively and with less risk (as may be the case with cholesterol- or blood-pressure-lowering medication, for example).

It is essential that you discuss any possible changes in medication with the doctor who prescribed your medication. All changes in medication should be assessed carefully and rationally within the context of your overall health, and with safety being the chief consideration. Alterations to your medication regime should be considered only if alternative treatment options (such as improvements in lifestyle, diet and exercise) are concurrently recommended by a naturopathic doctor or registered dietitian, and implemented with careful monitoring to ensure that your health targets are achieved.

CHAPTER 6

Lifestyle Modifications

The first step to treating leaky gut syndrome is to ensure that you are not causing any additional aggravation or damage because of your lifestyle choices. You need to remove any factors that may be aggravating inflammation and perpetuating hyperpermeability in your gut. These variables include uncontrolled stress, poor sleep habits, lack of exercise and a negative attitude. In the same way that a wound must remain uninfected and must be protected from further physical trauma to begin repairing, your gut must be free of aggravating factors in order to heal. The goal here is to allow the immune system to work unobstructed by removing any barriers and then to support the process by natural means.

First, you must eliminate stressors that exacerbate inflammation of the gut and increase hyperpermeability of the intestinal mucosa (gut lining), and there are many different ways to do this. Be prepared to face some challenges in this process; some stressors are more easily tackled than others — some can be addressed on your own and others may require the help of a professional, such as a counselor or psychologist. Having a positive attitude can affect the success of your health goals, so try to view your condition and treatment regimen as an opportunity to improve your overall wellness.

Lifestyle Modifications
• Reducing stress
• Improving sleep
• Getting enough exercise
• Adjusting your attitude

Reducing Stress

Stress will affect your body's ability to repair itself and will suppress immune function. We often overlook chronic emotional stressors as contributing to physical symptoms because our adaptable bodies are able to manage short-term stresses. When you are under stress, your body reallocates resources to neutralize the stressor. The endocrine and nervous systems secrete hormones and neurotransmitters that assist you in coping. For example, cortisol is a stress hormone that triggers a signal to release sugar into the bloodstream to provide muscles with the energy needed to escape a potential threat. The problem arises when stresses become a chronic, constant presence. In these cases, stress hormones are depleted and our immune system becomes suppressed, wounds heal more slowly and inflammation increases.

Chronic stress is often the primary source of inflammatory conditions, and it can be detrimental to digestive health. Psychological stress has been shown to disrupt the interaction between our brain and our gut (the gut–brain axis), which increases intestinal permeability and is linked to the development of irritable bowel syndrome (IBS), inflammatory bowel disease (IBD) and other disorders of the gut. In addition, psychological stress, even under acute situations, prompts the stimulation of cortisol release and has been shown to increase the permeability of the gut barrier.

Potential Stressors

We live in a more socially complex age than even just 100 years ago, with work, family, relationships and personal expectations compounding to increase stress levels. A century ago, our extended families helped with child and elder care, work involved more physical activity and we did not need to be constantly connected (pre-Internet). Today, we are more sedentary, get less sleep and feel perpetually rushed. This equates with ongoing chronic stress, to which our evolution has not caught up.

The multiple stimuli to which we are exposed are not drastic or overt. Neither are the resulting slow-building,

Stressed Out

- Do you pride yourself on being constantly busy?
- Do you commonly find yourself multitasking?
- Do you feel that you have very little "me time"?
- Do you consider yourself stressed out?
- Would people close to you (family, friends and colleagues) describe you as stressed out?

Answering yes to even one of these questions means you are likely under a considerable amount of stress, which can impact your gut health.

insidious health consequences. But be aware of these stressors and your responses to them. It is important to keep these potentially health-exacerbating factors in check. By slowly letting these stressors trickle into your life, you introduce a pro-inflammatory state in your body, one that can readily turn into leaky gut syndrome when other triggers are added to the mix.

Warning Signs

If multiple chronic stressors continue to exist and keep your body in an inflammatory state, true healing cannot occur. Leaky gut syndrome may start with minimal digestive symptoms and escalate insidiously. For example, you could develop a skin rash, which you ignore as just one more bothersome stress in your life. But eventually you may develop systemic autoimmune disease, which becomes a much bigger and potentially life-altering issue, one that will actually force you to take a break from your stressors. This is the point where your body screams at you that it is time to slow down.

Logically, it is better to identify the path you are heading down before it is too late, and to take preventive steps to correct your trajectory. A place of health and wellness is the goal. Watch for warning signs and listen to your body. Keep in mind that a leaky gut is a mechanical malfunction instigated and promoted by certain triggers. If left — unidentified and uncorrected — to persist and worsen over time, the health ramifications can snowball and severity can increase exponentially.

Mental–Emotional Stressors

Mental–emotional stress can affect the permeability of the intestinal wall. For true, permanent healing to occur, make sure that you address your emotional stressors and do not internalize them. Experiencing a stressful emotion triggers the release of certain brain chemicals that can temporarily disrupt the immune system. This link between our psychological state, nervous system and immune system is termed psychoneuroimmunology. Dealing with emotions to address physical disease in our body is not some ethereal or esoteric practice — it is simply how we are wired. Properly treating physical illness should involve self-reflection, which may, in certain cases, benefit

How Your Second Brain Copes with Stress

Your gut experiences mental–emotional stressors as physical manifestations. In some cases, it may experience or manifest stress before your brain has acknowledged the issue. The gut really does act as your second brain in this way. When your gut is not functioning optimally, it may be processing stress that your mind is not ready to handle. Your second brain addresses stress consciously by venting the trigger, and subconsciously by buffering stressful situations.

1. **Stressed Out:** In this case, you are very aware of your stress level, feeling overwhelmed, anxious or angry, and you notice that your digestive function is acting "stressed out" by being upset. In this situation, your gut is reflecting the stress you are consciously experiencing.
2. **Buffering Your Stress:** In this case, you feel that you should be more stressed out than you are, and wonder how you are coping so well. However, you notice that your digestive function has noticeably worsened. In this situation, your brain subconsciously chooses not to deal with this stress but your digestive tract still experiences and expresses the stress.

In both situations, digestive stress can present with symptoms of pain, bloating, discomfort, indigestion, diarrhea and constipation. Over time, this stress may lead to chronic inflammation and gut hyperpermeability.

Listen to the messages your body is trying to communicate. Don't use medication to suppress the symptoms without taking a pause to examine the potential stress triggers that may be leading to your disrupted digestive function.

---

from professional guidance. Professional guidance can help you determine the source of emotional stagnation and work with you toward resolving it.

You need to support and strengthen your emotional health to relieve stress and inflammation in the digestive tract. The gut is particularly vulnerable to emotional stressors, and it can be affected before you are consciously aware that you are in distress. When you resolve to handle chronic psychological stressors, only then can true healing and a normalization of permeability occur.

The gut is particularly vulnerable to emotional stressors, and it can be affected before you are consciously aware that you are in distress.

Trauma

Part of a physician's job is detective work. Doctors enter into a dialogue with their patients to determine when the illness first occurred and investigate if there were any mental, emotional or physical triggers that might have coincided with the onset of the disease. They also investigate the impact of any current trauma, such as:

- The end of a long-term relationship
- Death of a friend or family member
- A new job or the loss of a job
- Conflict with a friend or family member
- Uprooting or moving
- Emotional, physical or sexual abuse
- Living in a war-torn environment
- Major financial loss

Bathroom Stress Questionnaire

Stress that affects digestive function can be the result of long-standing patterns related to fears about using the bathroom. Your bowel habits and your conscious control of these habits can establish unhealthy rhythms in your intestinal function.

Consider your answers to the following questions:

1. Do you have any unusual behavior(s) related to bowel movements? Yes/No
2. Do you have fears or anxiety about using bathrooms in public places? Yes/No
3. Do you hold in your bowel movements because you would rather wait to go at home? Yes/No
4. What do you fear when using a public bathroom?
   Germs Yes/No
   Lack of privacy Yes/No
   Non-familiarity Yes/No
   Strangers hearing you use the toilet Yes/No
5. Was there a traumatic event that triggered these fears? Yes/No
6. Did you have any difficulties using the potty when you were a child? Yes/No
7. Did you experience any fears in childhood related to using the bathroom? Yes/No

If you answered yes to any of these questions, try to understand how these fears may be interfering with your normal bowel urges. Your intestines relay messages to your brain when your body is ready to have a bowel movement. Consciously superseding these signals consciously prevents your bowels from working normally. This may decrease your brain's ability to recognize these signals, by essentially training it to stop listening. Holding in stool may lead to the reabsorption of toxins and increased inflammation.

Try to work out where these fears originated and be aware of how they are altering your bowel habits. Understand and confront your fears, so that you can eventually overcome them and reset your bathroom patterns. Learn to pay close attention to your gut's messages and prioritize them to help you change your behavior.

In many cases, the timing of these types of psychological stressors coincides closely with the onset of an illness in the gut. If you are in survival mode, reacting to the trauma, you need to address these stressful situations.

You may be able to do this on your own through journaling, writing an unsent letter to someone you need to communicate with, or opening up to a trusted friend or family member. This may be enough to work through your suppressed feelings.

If the life event was particularly traumatic, consult a trained professional to help you deal with your emotions. Talk to a licensed psychologist, counselor or psychotherapist.

Improving Sleep

Sleep is such an important component of health, but one of the easiest to overlook. According to Gallup poll data, the average American today gets approximately 1 hour less sleep per night than in 1942. The proportion of the population that gets 6 hours of sleep or less per night went from 11% in 1942 to a whopping 40% in 2013. Furthermore, 65% of the population does not get the standard 8-hour restorative sleep. This means that more than half of Americans are experiencing chronic mild to moderate sleep insufficiency.

More than half of Americans are experiencing chronic mild to moderate sleep insufficiency.

Getting enough restorative sleep — typically one-third of every day — is critical to our normal functioning. We have a natural biological rhythm, the circadian rhythm, which repeats every 24 hours and fluctuates slightly with changing seasonal light patterns.

An example of how we experience a disruption in this pattern occurs when we travel across time zones and experience jet lag. Even in the short term of jet lag, travelers experience decreased motivation, mood changes, malaise and fatigue, and are susceptible to illness. Insufficient sleep over an extended period of time is similar to prolonged jet lag.

The cortisol hormone is secreted if we stay awake too long. Cortisol levels are normally highest in the morning upon waking and gradually decline through the course of the day. When you have mild to moderate chronic sleep deprivation, cortisol can essentially flatline throughout the day. This has an impact on melatonin, another hormone, which is secreted in response to light exposure during the day.

Gut–Brain Functionality

Diurnal rhythms, governed by our innate biological clocks, have also been linked to intestinal mucosal function, growth and repair. A recent review investigated the connections between the role of circadian rhythm and gut membrane functionality. Although the exact mechanisms have not been fully explained, proliferation of the gut membrane cells (enterocytes) has been connected to the day–night cycle. In addition, the actual function of the digestive tract, including the secretion of enzymes and the absorption of nutrients and electrolytes, is also governed by a biological clock. In essence, this means that even our internal parts, including our gut, respond to changes in the light–dark cycle, even though they are obviously not exposed to the changing light in our environment.

When cortisol levels bottom out because of inadequate sleep, our ability to tolerate negative stimuli and our tissues' ability to heal become compromised. Lack of sleep will also limit the rate at which the gut mucosa can heal. So what is the best way to improve long-term cortisol function? Sleep well, exercise and reduce your stress — although this may be much easier said than done. Yet it is a critical component of healing the gut in many situations, so it is well worth exploring the many natural ways to support the stress response and enhance your natural sleep cycle.

Did You Know?

A Vicious Cycle

Levels of melatonin are inversely related to cortisol levels. Melatonin normally increases in the evening and peaks during normal sleeping hours. When cortisol levels are compromised, our quality of sleep is affected, and when sleep is compromised, our cortisol levels are affected. In a vicious cycle, lack of sleep affects our ability to sleep effectively over time. Lack of sleep also diminishes the body's ability to tolerate stress with declining cortisol levels.

Research Spotlight
Circadian Rhythm Disruptions in Mice

Research has shown that inducing various disruptions of the circadian rhythms of mice affects the integrity of the mice's gut mucosa and increases the state of gut permeability, particularly when combined with alcohol consumption. Maintaining a healthy circadian rhythm is a key to — though an often overlooked component of — maintaining a healthy gut filter. Though disruptions in sleep patterns are likely not a direct trigger of leaky gut syndrome, they can accentuate the effects of agents that can trigger the disrupted condition.

Sleeping Tips

- Unplug: Do not use electronic devices, particularly those that emit light, within 90 minutes of bedtime, and do not keep them in your bedroom.
- Improve your sleep times: Work on getting to bed earlier by half an hour per week, until you are able to get 8 hours of rest.
- Ditch the snooze button: Snoozing is wasted sleep time. Set your alarm for the time you actually should get up and put it on the other side of your room so that you need to get up to turn off the ringer.
- Drink your fluids earlier: If you keep hydrating yourself right before bed, you will have to interrupt your sleep to urinate. Stop all fluids 90 minutes before bed — except for sips if your throat is dry.
- Avoid alcohol and recreational drugs to help with sleep: Although you may fool yourself into thinking these crutches help you to sleep, they affect your quality of sleep in the long term.
- Write to-do lists: Clear your mind of the clutter and anxiety of tomorrow's tasks by writing them down so you can fall asleep more easily.
- Practice a calming bedtime routine: Just like a baby, you need a routine that helps prepare you physically and psychologically for sleep. Choose something that is relaxing for you (for example, reading a book, taking a bath, meditating or praying).
- Dim the lights: Keep the lights in your house on a lower setting or turn off lights that shine in your eyes, as these can stimulate your brain into thinking it is daytime.

Getting Enough Exercise

Exercise is a natural way to enhance your immune system and to help manage daily stresses, in addition to directly improving an abnormal intestinal barrier function.

Just as you need to get enough sleep to help your gut to heal, so too do you need to get enough exercise. Exercise is a natural way to enhance your immune system and to help manage daily stresses, in addition to directly improving an abnormal intestinal barrier function.

Exercise needs to be enjoyable. If going to the gym and lifting weights in a crowded environment bothers you, doing so will not have the intended effect, because exercise ends up becoming just another counterproductive

Research Spotlight
Aerobic Exercise

Studies show that regular aerobic exercise improves natural metabolic processes and reduces systemic inflammation. Even white blood cell counts and immune function are enhanced through moderate regular exercise. These improvements are very important in normalizing a hyperpermeable gut.

In one study, rats with chronic stress-induced gut hyperpermeability demonstrated improvements in gut function with exercise, even just 30 minutes of swimming per day. The recovery was postulated to be related to the antimicrobial effects of exercising, meaning that exercise inhibits the growth of microorganisms and prevents pathogens from penetrating the gut mucosa.

stress. Implement a form of physical exercise that gives you pleasure. Whether this is dancing to music in the comfort of your home, going out for a brisk walk, playing sports, attending aerobic classes or going to the gym to lift weights or use the treadmill, do it regularly and as often as your health allows.

Consult your doctor and determine if exercising regularly is safe and beneficial for your state of health. If you are not physically or psychologically prepared for exercise, seek the guidance of a certified personal trainer to show you the proper techniques and how to exercise at an appropriate pace for you.

If you have been inactive for a long time, start off slowly, with light exercise twice a week for 20 to 30 minutes, to avoid overstraining yourself. Gradually increase the duration, frequency and intensity of exercise over 3 months, aiming to exercise regularly at a moderate to high intensity for 45 to 60 minutes, 3 or 4 days per week.

If you are not physically or psychologically prepared for exercise, seek the guidance of a certified personal trainer to show you the proper techniques and how to exercise at an appropriate pace for you.

Exercise Tips
- Make time for your exercise routine.
- Choose physical activities that you enjoy.
- Start slowly.
- Work up to a moderate pace.
- Partner with a friend to make it more enjoyable and to keep each other accountable.
- Consult your doctor and physiotherapist if you have questions about your physical limitations.

- Drink 30 ounces (1 L) of water or electrolyte fluid (free of additives and artificial ingredients) for every 1 hour of moderate exercise.
- If you plan to incorporate body weight, free weights or weight machines into your routine, consult a licensed personal trainer for assistance with safe, effective techniques and to help you create an exercise program appropriate to your goals.

Adjusting Your Attitude

Your attitude toward your health plays a central role in your treatment and recovery. You can give up or give in — or you can face the challenge of poor health head-on, fully aware. Accepting these challenges allows us to find meaning in an illness rather than viewing it as a random misfortune. An optimistic point of view rather than a pessimistic one reduces your experience of stress, supports your immune system and promotes your natural capacity to heal.

An optimistic point of view rather than a pessimistic one reduces your experience of stress, supports your immune system and promotes your natural capacity to heal.

Quitting Smoking

Smoking is known to be a risk factor in lung cancer, heart disease and many other diseases. It is also known to be an agent that promotes inflammation in gut disorders. In other words, leaky gut syndrome is yet another condition we can add to the long list of diseases induced and/or aggravated by smoking. No matter the case, we are all very aware that smoking is not good for our health.

Smoking Cessation Tips
- Pick a realistic quit date.
- Let your friends and family know that you are quitting on that date.
- Remind yourself of all the reasons why you decided to quit.
- Embrace the fact that quitting is mind over matter.
- Understand your smoking patterns and triggers.
- Discover new, healthy habits to take the place of smoking.
- Breathe through cravings and know that they are transient.
- Start a savings account with the money you would spend on cigarettes.
- Drink plenty of water.
- Take a break from friends who smoke.

Learning to face poor health directly is essential for resolving hyperpermeability in your gut. Consider the gut–brain axis, the bidirectional communication between the brain and the digestive tract. If you work to correct the function of the gut, you can help to heal the psyche by restoring the correct balance of brain chemicals.

Did You Know?

Bidirectional Healing
Because the gut–brain connection is bidirectional, we can help to heal the digestive tract by healing the mind. In essence, the most comprehensive approach to optimizing function of the gut is to address not only the gut itself but also our mental and emotional states.

Metaphysical Parallels

Illness can be assigned metaphysical meanings in relation to emotional and spiritual experiences. Consider these metaphysical parallels that can present as a result of leaky gut syndrome:

- Gastroesophageal reflux disease may mean that you are hesitant to swallow and digest new ideas.
- Constipation may reflect that you are not processing emotions efficiently and tend to hold on to emotions for longer than you should.
- Diarrhea may mean that your gut is purging feelings that you want to avoid.

Body-Mind-Spirit

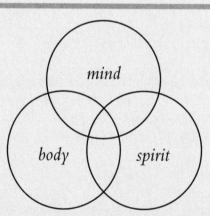

Your body, mind and spirit, although commonly viewed as distinct entities, fall on an overlapping continuum. A deviation or disturbance in any of these spheres has a ripple effect of symptoms that manifest in the other spheres.

Your emotions and spirit are forms of energy, as is your physical body. Although emotions and spirit appear to be less tangible, we know that emotions and spiritual experiences are catalyzed by neurotransmitters and involve neurons stimulating activity in certain parts of the brain. How exactly these physical mechanisms translate into powerful emotions, psychic phenomena and life-changing spiritual experiences is still unknown.

FAQ

Q What is meant by "metaphysical"?

A Metaphysics is a form of philosophy that attempts to provide a meaning for our existence. It assists us in becoming more in tune with our own body, mind and spirit. It also helps us to understand how our life fits within the context of the universe and the existence of all other beings. Metaphysics overlaps with the spiritual realm, which also provides us with meaning. In this case, we are exploring the metaphysical nature of disease; that is, we are looking for meaning in physical illness from an emotional-spiritual perspective.

- Eczema may be a sign of unexpressed agitation and anger coming out on your skin.
- Autoimmune diseases may indicate a state of extreme pressure on yourself and excessive self-analysis and self-criticism.
- Leaky gut syndrome may mean that you are not establishing adequate healthy boundaries in your life and in your relationships, which is manifesting as multiple stressors.

Improving aspects of your life by using insights from your illness not only helps to make your life happier and more enjoyable but also works to achieve true healing of your state of "dis-ease."

Whatever your individual symptoms, try to understand the message your body is trying to convey. Improving aspects of your life by using insights from your illness not only helps to make your life happier and more enjoyable but also works to achieve true healing of your state of "dis-ease."

It can be challenging to acknowledge potential gaps in your ability to understand your emotions and express them in a healthy way, but doing so makes you healthier. It takes courage to do so, but when you are able to rewire your thought processes to react to negative emotional stimuli in a more positive, constructive manner, it not only improves your human experience but also helps your physical health.

Being Proactive

When you are proactive about making positive decisions for your health, you can help direct the outcome. In fact, illness can provide you with permission to rest and to reset your routine. You sometimes get stuck in unhealthy patterns of behavior, and despite knowing this, you do not act to recalibrate your life. Being physically unable to carry out your day-to-day tasks may be the only way to get you to slow down, take a breath and reexamine your situation from a different perspective. We may take our health for granted and indulge in unhealthy behaviors because we don't see the negative ramifications. An illness or another physical setback may be what is necessary to make us more appreciative of our health and more aware of the repercussions of neglecting it.

Benefiting from Ill Health

The notion that a bothersome or life-changing health issue can improve your life may sound counterintuitive, but when you look closely at how your ill health is affecting your life, you may observe ways in which it is helping you.

Your behavior is affected when you are suffering from any type of disease, sometimes mildly and other times drastically. It may throw you off your day-to-day routine, alter your interactions with others and isolate you. However, if you change your perspective and your initial negative knee-jerk reaction to these unplanned disruptions, you may find that your ill health is teaching and challenging you and allowing you room to change.

Examining Your Relationships

Everyone is made up of many unique interwoven relationships. You have a relationship with your family, your romantic partner, your children, your friends, your colleagues, your mentors, your health-care provider and even your pets. You have essential relationships with other,

> *An illness or another physical setback may be what is necessary to make us more appreciative of our health and more aware of the repercussions of neglecting it.*

How Illness Can Be Healthy

- It may be the only way that we get a chance to rest from our daily stressors.
- It may allow us to have loved ones around to support us and express their love for us, whether directly with words or indirectly through care.
- It may be a way to get attention from our loved ones that we are not able to ask for.
- It may be the only way we allow ourselves time to be present with just ourselves and to focus within ourselves. This can provide us with insight and self-reflection. We often fill up our social and work schedules to the point where we lose touch with ourselves and our identity.
- It may help us prioritize what is most important in life and put trivial matters or conflict into perspective.

less tangible things or even inanimate objects: your house, your car, your career, your health, the Internet, celebrities, hobbies, your body, food and eating, exercise, appearance and countless others. You also have important spiritual relationships, with your ancestors or other important deceased figures in your life, or with your spiritual guides — deities, religious leaders, heroes. Spiritual relationships also consist of times when you self-reflect and contemplate your existence.

One of the most important relationships, one that is often neglected, is your relationship with yourself. You may be confused about your identity; you may be conflicted; you may be delusional; or you may have an unhealthy self-image, low self-esteem or even self-hatred.

Ask yourself right now: "Who am I?" You will likely describe yourself based on your external relationships: "I am a divorced real estate agent and mother of two children." "I am a single, 25-year-old student aspiring to be a leader in business." "I am a devout Buddhist and I live to help others in need." Without these descriptors, do you know who you truly are?

Many of our relationships will be reexamined or reconfigured in times of ill health. Ill health is by far the primary reason why people unexpectedly put their careers on hold. It is often the only way we will pause in our hectic lives to allow our bodies and minds to slow down, recuperate and reset. In essence, our bodies are giving us permission to take a break.

Procrastination

When you are ill, you may create excuses to justify why you cannot commit to a healing plan. This is the response to anything in life that we don't feel ready to take on. If this is the case, it may be time to reexamine your attitude.

Take note of the obstacles to healing, the excuses that you make. Examine how you feel about the changes that are recommended to help you to heal and your motivation to go ahead with them. Be comfortable with acknowledging that you may not be prepared to make a lifestyle overhaul (if need be) right now.

Maybe what you mean to express is: "I feel that my health is a problem, it is getting worse, but it is still something that I can cope with. I am just not ready to let

Snowball Effect

Underlying anxiety can create a snowball effect: your physical symptoms trigger anxiety, which exacerbates your physical symptoms, which exacerbates your anxiety, and so on in a downward spiral. Address and treat all contributing factors to halt this negative process and redirect it toward a more positive direction of healing.

Lighting the Way to Wellness

Recognizing your idiosyncrasies is just another step forward on your journey to healing. Each of us has an individual path, and you have to light the way before you are able to see where you are going. Following your path blindly can be done only with great difficulty and limited success. All you need is enough light shed on the path to take one step forward in the right direction.

go of my routine or comfort foods right now. Maybe when it gets worse, or gets to a point where I feel that I have to reexamine my lifestyle, I will take this on." Accept this. It is okay to just listen to advice for now and store it for future reference, when you feel ready to act on it.

Letting Go of Illness

Some people don't want to heal. Part of the healing process involves letting go of health problems and everything that accompanies them. For most people, this would be a dream come true. But for those who define themselves by their health problems, the healing process can be more complicated.

In some cases, a health challenge may provide something that you feel helps or comforts you. For example, people may react to your ill health with attention, concern or love, and you may fear (consciously or unconsciously) that this support will no longer be available once the health problem has resolved. This fear is nothing to be ashamed of, but you do need to identify it in yourself if it is impeding your path to healing. If you have deep-rooted emotional issues, realize that it may take time and an objective third party, such as a counselor, to help you to understand and overcome these challenges.

Behavioral Thresholds

Everyone has behavioral thresholds. For instance, you have your own physical and emotional tolerance for pain and suffering. What you may perceive as "annoying" or "distracting" might be a life-altering physical handicap to someone else. Some challenges can be accommodated within the context of your day-to-day responsibilities or because of flexibility in your schedule and environment. For example, someone with chronic diarrhea who works at home may find it to be merely bothersome, whereas for someone in back-to-back meetings at the office all day, it is intolerable.

You also have your own threshold for change. Sometimes it is only when your tolerance threshold has been exceeded that you become comfortable with making the necessary changes and are ready to incorporate lifestyle modifications to manifest positive change in your health. We are creatures of habit, and we like our routines. Some of us enjoy episodes of spontaneity and change, but we often later resort to the routines that provide comfort and familiarity.

Ingrained Patterns of Behavior

Ingrained patterns of behavior can be seen both in repetitive physical activities, such as your dietary habits, and in your emotional response to stimuli. We each tend to cope in our own way and fall back on particular reactions to a specific situation. Different people, with different life experiences and personalities, react completely differently to the same stimuli.

Ingrained patterns can be very challenging to address. They take time and introspection to resolve. Have patience. Certain behaviors can take a lifetime to overcome.

Healthy Anger

Being ill can elicit anger, which can have an effect on your healing pathway. Think about how you normally respond to situations that make you feel irritated or angry. Do you suppress your anger and bottle it up inside, or do you rage out loud? How do you manage anger? How can you make it a healthy experience? Anger is one of the most difficult patterns of behavior to change and control.

Step back for a moment and visualize a situation that provoked a feeling of anger within you. Now replace yourself with a stranger. Would you, as an outsider, feel that the anger was warranted in this situation? Would you expect someone else to be equally angry? If not, think about why you experience anger when someone else would not. Does the situation remind you of previous traumatic experiences? Do you feel it reveals weaknesses within yourself? Do you feel exposed, embarrassed or ashamed? Or do you feel mistreated, disrespected and offended?

If you do think that you rightfully should feel angry, that your anger is justified, then it may be a healthy, normal response to the situation. Anger is a reasonable human response to triggers that affect us negatively. Feeling angry helps us find ways to establish boundaries for ourselves so that we can permit ourselves to live comfortably. If we do not understand this and we express our anger unhealthily — by either over- or under-communicating our emotion — we are sabotaging the

> **Did You Know?**
>
> **Positive Outcomes**
> When you change your deep-seated negative patterns of behavior to more productive, positive ones, your physical health becomes more stable and tolerant to flux in your environment. The improvements in your psychological state are reflected in your physical state.

opportunity to create a healthy space for ourselves. Anger is an opening for you to teach others about your comfort zone. Be sure to make good use of this opportunity.

Think now about that stranger experiencing a trigger that would normally set you off. Consider a variety of ways in which the stranger could react. Picture how he might overreact by shouting, yelling and causing a scene. Then visualize the opposite response, where he under-communicates his emotion: he might grumble to himself, curse under his breath — all the while putting on a forced show of pleasantness. Is either of these reactions typical of your own anger response?

Now picture the stranger reacting in a way in which he communicates his dissatisfaction effectively while keeping his composure. What sorts of words would he use? Can you imagine yourself doing this?

Resolving Anger

We tend to focus on the negative manifestations of anger, but there are positive responses that can be used instead. A healthy expression of anger has these qualities:

- It is direct and clear.
- It is communicated in a composed manner.
- It uses words intended to communicate your concern rather than to insult, belittle or offend the listener.

This turns expressions of dissatisfaction away from a potentially toxic experience into one that is helpful and positive. It reverses the outcome from destructive to constructive.

Anger needs to be used positively to reinforce your emotional boundaries, to ensure that you are protected from negative external stimuli. Doing so in a constructive manner will prevent you from being influenced negatively by your emotional environment and will allow you to live a happier and healthier life. Remind yourself that feeling angry is not a bad thing; it is merely a chance to establish your identity. Express anger in a calm, clear and composed manner, and your life will be a lot less stressful. This is an important key to resolving your digestive health.

Confrontation

Every day, you face new challenges and tests. Don't run from them. Instead, embrace them as invitations to help you nurture your emotional and spiritual health. Remember: confrontation is not necessarily negative and does not always turn into conflict; confrontation is necessary to resolve conflict and miscommunication. If your mindset expects conflict, you will manifest this outcome and it will become a self-fulfilling prophecy. Try to be flexible and pliable and to find common ground. This will become a reality for you.

Overexpressing and speaking from a place of hostility to deliberately hurt whoever confronted you is as equally unhealthy a manner of communication as suppressing your feelings. It jeopardizes establishing healthy boundaries because you have also overstepped boundaries by using offensive words.

If your mindset expects conflict, you will manifest this outcome and it will become a self-fulfilling prophecy.

Conscious Breathing Exercise

Although this exercise can be done at home, it is also useful to calm your mind in the midst of a hectic environment — at work, at school or even while commuting on a busy subway or bus. Doing the full routine for five full cycles takes only $2\frac{1}{2}$ minutes, which means there are no excuses not to implement this routine at least once per day if you are under siege from stress. Because it is inconspicuous, you can even incorporate this technique into the middle of a stressful business meeting or to calm yourself if you are feeling overwhelmed or anxious.

1. Sit comfortably in your chair (at work or school) or cross-legged on the floor.
2. Ensure that you sit up straight, keeping your chest elevated and your shoulders and arms relaxed.
3. Take a deep, slow, conscious breath in through your nose.
4. Start by filling the lower part of your lungs slowly for 5 seconds, by pushing your abdomen and ribs out.
5. Slowly continue filling the upper part of your lungs for another 5 seconds, which fills your chest and tightens your abdomen.
6. Hold this position with filled lungs for 1 to 5 seconds (working up to 5 seconds, if it is difficult at first).
7. Slowly release your breath and exhale over 10 seconds until your lungs empty.
8. Hold this position with emptied lungs for 1 to 5 seconds.
9. Repeat steps 3 to 8 for up to five full cycles (or longer if needed)

Relaxation

Give yourself permission to relax. Many people place value on how busy they are, how many tasks they can accomplish, how little sleep they are getting, how many activities they enroll their children in and how many hours they work in a week. In doing so, they are not making time to look after themselves. Yes, they have a busy life, but they need to ensure that they schedule time to focus on their own health. For many people, this sounds unattainable, since they barely have the time to get all of their daily tasks completed. But if they keep up this constant frenetic pace, they will eventually hit a wall where the body shuts down and forces them to rest, through ill health.

Relaxing the mind does not have to be a large commitment. It can take just a few minutes every day. This can be as simple as doing some breathing exercises for 5 minutes every night while you are settling down in bed. It can mean 10 minutes of gentle stretching in the morning or 30 minutes of yoga or meditation. If you need a creative outlet, maybe you can do some personal expressive writing or painting twice a week. An evening walk every second day can help clear your mind and move your body. Maybe you would be best able to relax in a calming bath with essential oils every Saturday night. When did you last take a holiday? If it has been a long time, schedule a vacation to recharge your batteries and recuperate from your daily stresses.

Doc Talk

Understand that your pathway to healing will be challenging. It will involve introspection and addressing stressors that are not exclusively physical. This could mean that you may need to address an emotional or situational stressor that is the underlying cause of your digestive challenges. Your path to healing will involve examining yourself, your habits and your patterns of thought. Sometimes you do not like to admit that you have flaws or weaknesses in any aspect of your life. Other times you are not ready to commit to lifestyle changes that could affect schedules, grocery shopping, cooking, the foods you eat or the vices from which you derive pleasure — smoking, drinking or recreational drugs. Trust what your gut tells you — there is a reason why it is called your gut instinct. A negative response in the gut can be a reaction to a poor food choice, but it may also be a response to an emotional stress in your life that your conscious mind is choosing to ignore.

CHAPTER 7

Natural Complementary Therapies

Once you have eliminated (or at the very least reduced) stressors, the body starts the healing process. However, with compromised immunity and a long-standing dysfunctional gut state, you likely need additional support to encourage rebalancing to a healthy state. The next step is to support your body in its natural physiological response to heal itself and achieve healthy homeostasis. You can help the healing process by providing adequate nutrients through diet and supplementation with nutraceuticals and medicinal herbs and spices. Other natural therapies, such as acupuncture, homeopathy, biomechanics and chiropractic, can also accelerate the body's healing process.

Nutraceuticals and Medicinal Herbs and Spices

Taking therapeutic nutrients and medicinal herbs and spices can support the restoration of gut integrity and healthy functioning. Certain nutrients and herbs help mitigate intestinal hyperpermeability. Demulcent herbs, fish oils, L-glutamine, probiotics, prebiotics, 5-HTP, turmeric and zinc — or a combination of these — should be part of a treatment regimen for leaky gut syndrome.

Demulcent Herbs

A demulcent is a substance that helps to soothe irritated mucous membranes. By virtue of their high polysaccharide content, demulcent herbs produce a watery, sticky coating that calms inflamed mucous membranes by creating a

Natural Complementary Therapies
- Nutraceuticals and medicinal herbs and spices
- Acupuncture
- Homeopathy
- Biomechanics
- Chiropractic

✳ Caution
Nutritional and herbal remedies should be taken with caution, under the supervision of a health-care professional. Although natural health products generally have a much better safety profile than prescription medication, they can still cause side effects. Find out if the natural health products you want to use are appropriate and safe for your specific health status and whether they interact with the medications you are already taking.

protective film. These herbs are all useful in cases of leaky gut syndrome, where the gut mucosa is inflamed:

- Licorice root
- Slippery elm bark
- Aloe vera gel
- Marshmallow root

You can purchase many of these demulcent herbs in prepackaged lozenges at health food stores. The lozenges dissolve in your mouth to form the mucilage, which you swallow to coat your digestive tract. Alternatively, you can find many of these demulcent herbs in powdered form, which you mix with hot water and drink. Aloe vera gel can be found in an edible form that can be consumed every day (look for products that don't contain additional additives or preservatives).

Essential Fatty Acids

Essential fatty acids (EFAs) include omega-3 fats that are high in EPA (eicosapentaenoic acid) and DHA (docosahexaenoic acid). They help increase the production of anti-inflammatory cytokines (messenger chemicals). Cytokines shift the body away from a state of inflammation and promote the normalization of gut function. These EFAs are readily found in fish.

DHA has been shown to protect the intestinal wall from inflammatory stimuli and to help maintain the integrity of the tight junctions ("spot welds") to support gut barrier function. EPA has also demonstrated positive effects in mitigating gut hyperpermeability under stress-induced triggers that would normally lead to intestinal wall dysfunction. In line with these findings, fish oil supplementation has been shown to support and protect the function and integrity of the intestinal wall.

Dosage: 1,000–4,000 mg total EPA plus DHA per day.

L-glutamine

Glutamine is an amino acid that is concentrated in skeletal muscle tissues. L-glutamine, the form of glutamine used by the body, is best known as a post-workout supplement that helps with muscle recovery and prevents the delayed onset of muscle soreness.

In critically ill patients, glutamine has been shown to improve prognosis and reduce the incidence of systemic infection by normalizing the permeability at the level of the gut. In patients who had undergone abdominal surgery, glutamine lessened the systemic inflammatory response, decreased hyperpermeability and maintained the gut barrier. In premature infants, oral glutamine supplements given after birth reduced gut hyperpermeability and improved susceptibility to infection. Glutamine has also been shown to improve diarrhea and even assist in the recovery from acute bacterial gastroenteritis — which is perpetuated by the hyperpermeable gut state that it triggers.

L-glutamine is also used to support and strengthen digestive health and as a primary fuel source for enterocytes (the cells lining your intestines). Using glutamine as a complementary nutrient therapy in leaky gut syndrome assists with strengthening and improving the integrity of the gut filter.

Dosage: Take glutamine in its L-glutamine form, as a powder rather than in capsules, to ease digestion. Typical doses for L-glutamine range from 2 to 10 g per day.

Probiotics

Your gut microbiota (the symbiotic "good" bacteria) are an integral component of the immune barrier function of the gut. Trillions of bacteria reside on the large surface area that makes up your intestinal lining. This gut microbiome (the community of naturally occurring microorganisms) is a layer of protection, the first line of defense for your gut epithelium (the thin outer tissue lining the alimentary canal). It is extremely important that probiotics are in the right balance to maintain healthy gut permeability. In fact, one theory suggests that disruptions in these normal colonies of probiotics trigger the development of irritable bowel syndrome (IBS) and inflammatory bowel disease (IBD).

Microbiota help with the breakdown of foods into more manageable particles through hormone and neurotransmitter metabolism, and with the synthesis of nutrients. Disruption of these functions is detrimental to

It is extremely important that probiotics are in the right balance to maintain healthy gut permeability.

preexisting inflammation in the gut and can also initiate inflammation that can lead to leaky gut syndrome. Microbiota have also been shown to improve the integrity of the digestive barrier and control the immune system, mitigating excessive gut permeability.

Many factors can negatively affect our microbiota. Oral contraceptives and anti-inflammatories disrupt gut bacteria. The consumption of processed foods and refined carbohydrates feeds opportunistic organisms that may multiply and disrupt the balance of gut microorganisms. Stress, lack of sleep and underlying disease also contribute negatively.

Probiotics are essential to helping heal digestive disorders and gut hyperpermeability. Restoration of the appropriate balance of beneficial gut flora is necessary to improve immunity and reduce inflammation.

Dosage: Dosing for probiotics can vary depending on the brand, format, concentration and composition.

- Choose a good-quality, high-potency probiotic supplement with a minimum of 10 billion CFUs (colony-forming units).
- Choose a probiotic containing at least 8 mixed species, including *Lactobacillus* and *Bifidobacterium*.
- Use enteric-coated capsules, which are durable enough to survive your stomach's acidic environment so that the probiotics are released in your small intestine.
- Choose a probiotic that also contains prebiotics. Prebiotics provide a food source for the probiotic bacteria (fructo-oligosaccharides) so that they can multiply and reproduce once they are established in the gut.

It would be helpful if health-care providers recommended appropriate probiotic supplement regimens with each prescribed round of antibiotics, to prevent issues with disrupted immunity and inflammation. Consider taking a high-potency probiotic supplement any time you require antibiotics. Take the probiotic as directed, and at least 2 hours before or after your dose of antibiotics. Continue taking the probiotics for 2 weeks after you have completed the antibiotic schedule.

Probiotic Foods

Probiotic foods are naturally fermented and preserved by the *Lactobacillus* strain of bacteria, which is also a critical component of your microbiome. Kefir, kimchi, kombucha tea, miso soup, natto, pickles, sauerkraut and tempeh are all examples of foods that contain good bacteria that help to colonize your gut and support its function.

Look for naturally lacto-fermented forms of these foods rather than commercial varieties where vinegar, sugar and preservatives are added to alter the flavor and shelf life at the cost of their health benefits. Lacto-fermenting vegetables, herbs and even fruit at home is quite a simple process (see page 120). Lacto-fermentation often uses whey (a derivative of milk) to accelerate the fermentation process. However, this ingredient is not necessary and is best to leave out, particularly if you have a potential dairy sensitivity. Home lacto-fermentation is as simple as chopping up the vegetables and fruits you want to preserve, adding some herbs and submerging them in brine in a jar for a few days (up to a week) to allow the naturally occurring bacteria to ferment the vegetables.

Serotonin

About 90% of serotonin is synthesized in the lining of the digestive tract, in specialized cells called enterochromaffin cells. Serotonin metabolism and responses to serotonin may both be modified in digestive disorders, so it is important to ensure that adequate serotonin is available for normalizing function. Serotonin helps direct the function of the digestive tract by regulating perception of pain, fluid secretion and motility. However, the role of serotonin at the level of the gut has recently been shown to be less direct than previously thought. The connection between serotonin in the gut and in the brain is still not fully understood, but we do know that serotonin plays a very important role in supporting both physical and mental health. This underlines the importance of normalizing serotonin levels in leaky gut syndrome.

5-HTP (5-hydroxytryptophan) is the direct precursor of serotonin. To make sure your body can synthesize the serotonin required to manage the inflammatory state and assist with normalizing gut function, supplements of 5-HTP are recommended.

Dosage: 50–200 mg per day.

> **Did You Know?**
>
> **Prebiotics**
> Prebiotics are a food source for your gut flora. The more of these foods you eat, the more you support the growth of your microbiota and thereby restore the integrity of your gut immunity. Foods high in prebiotic inulin and fructo-oligosaccharides include asparagus, burdock, chicory, dandelion greens, garlic, Jerusalem artichoke, jicama, leeks and onions.

Turmeric

Also known as curcumin, turmeric is both a culinary and a medicinal spice. It is a powerful antioxidant, scavenging free radicals that cause damage at a cellular level and supporting detoxification pathways in the liver. Turmeric is also considered to have anti-inflammatory effects that have general systemic health benefits and the potential to treat inflammation at the level of the gut.

In patients with IBD, turmeric not only decreased inflammation but also prevented relapses. In a study on albino rats, turmeric normalized intestinal motility (the rate at which food moves along the digestive tract), which improved gut function. In addition, turmeric was shown to reduce pro-inflammatory signals in several diseases, including digestive disorders.

Turmeric is useful in dampening systemic and gut-level inflammation and normalizing gut function. In leaky gut syndrome, these abnormalities need to be addressed with targeted therapeutics. Turmeric should be part of a complete treatment strategy to improve gut hyperpermeability.

Turmeric should be part of a complete treatment strategy to improve gut hyperpermeability.

Dosage: 300–1,200 mg per day.

Health Benefits of Honey

Honey has numerous properties that make it a useful complement to treat and heal leaky gut syndrome. Many studies have demonstrated that honey has wound-healing properties. It provides antibacterial support, wound protection, immune cell stimulation and soothing attributes to help repair tissue. In the same way, ingesting honey coats the mucous membrane lining of your digestive tract when it comes in contact with it.

Honey also encourages antimicrobial activity, a result of the hydrogen peroxide and methylglyoxal compounds in it, along with other, as yet, unidentified constituents. Honey has been shown to effectively treat even antibiotic-resistant strains of bacteria, such as MRSA (methicillin-resistant *Staphylococcus aureus*) and VRE (vancomycin-resistant *Enterococci*).

Use raw, unprocessed honey — ideally manuka honey from New Zealand. Manuka honey has a property called Unique Manuka Factor (UMF), which provides it with additional antimicrobial activity. Look for a UMF rating of 10 or higher to maximize therapeutic benefit.

Caution: *Do not give honey to infants under 1 year old. There is a risk of botulism because of the underdeveloped immune system of children.*

Zinc

Zinc is a mineral cofactor that supports the integrity of the cells lining the intestines, which is very important in resolving a leaky gut. Zinc also encourages normal immunity and supports energy production and hormone metabolism. Regular zinc supplementation helps to slowly displace any heavy metals that have accumulated in tissues, so that they can be eliminated.

Zinc deficiency has been associated with intestinal wall damage and an increase in the ability of inflammatory cells to migrate across the gut barrier.

Zinc should be incorporated as part of a supplementary regimen to help rebuild the gut lining and restore its integrity in cases of leaky gut syndrome.

Dosage: Best taken as zinc citrate, 15–50 mg per day. Be sure to take zinc with a large meal to prevent nausea.

Acupuncture

Acupuncture is a system of medicine that has been used traditionally in China for thousands of years. It is based on the principle of energy balance within the body and among organs; the diagnosis from a traditional Chinese medicine perspective involves a whole-body approach. To determine a treatment protocol, acupuncturists assess the totality of your symptoms as well as specific characteristics — for example, asking, "Is the abdominal pain better or worse with pressure?" "Did it start suddenly or gradually?" and "What time does it occur?" — and gather information about your personality as well as your tongue and pulse.

Rebalancing energy helps to trigger the body into reaching a new, healthier homeostasis (internal physiological balance).

The actual process of acupuncture involves inserting very fine-gauge sterile needles into specific points on the body to help increase the available energy or to sedate disrupted energy meridians (channels of energy flow that travel through the body). For leaky gut syndrome, the acupuncturist will likely select acupuncture points that regulate digestion along with associated diseases. Rebalancing energy helps to trigger the body into reaching a new, healthier homeostasis (internal physiological balance).

Be sure to consult a naturopathic doctor or acupuncturist who is licensed in traditional Chinese medicine for a comprehensive assessment and acupuncture treatment plan for leaky gut syndrome and its associated manifestations.

Homeopathy

Homeopathy is a gentle but profound system of medicine that has been used the world over for more than two centuries. The remedies are based on very dilute amounts of substances derived from plants, minerals or organisms. The theory behind homeopathy is "like cures like," meaning that a substance that normally elicits a certain response and triggers a certain set of symptoms in you can be used to treat and resolve those same symptoms if administered in diluted doses.

Consider integrating homeopathy into your treatment plan when your body is not responding well to various other treatments. This system of medicine can help trigger a shift in your body's homeostasis to move toward a direction of healing. Some people seem to get stuck in a stagnant state where their body stubbornly refuses to react to treatments. If this happens to you, consult a licensed homeopath or naturopathic doctor specializing in homeopathy for assessment and treatment to support your body's natural healing process.

Homeopathic Remedies for Leaky Gut Syndrome

- Arsenicum album
- Baryta carbonica
- Bryonia album
- Carbo vegetabilis
- China officinalis
- Lycopodium clavatum
- Morgan pure
- Natrum carbonicum
- Nux vomica
- Sulfur

Biomechanics

The biomechanics of the body can affect the functioning of the digestive tract if pressure or abnormal forces are placed on the intestines. Any unnatural twisting or torsion applied to the intestines can affect how they function and can aggravate leaky gut syndrome.

Incorrect biomechanics can be the result of poor posture, chronically tense muscles because of stress, or compensation after trauma such as an injury or surgery. If these factors sound like they may play a role in preventing your digestive tract from healing, consider contacting a bodywork practitioner, such as a doctor of osteopathy or a registered massage therapist, for a complete assessment and treatment plan.

Incorrect biomechanics can be the result of poor posture, chronically tense muscles because of stress, or compensation after trauma such as an injury or surgery.

Chiropractic

The nervous system is an integral part of the body, acting as the wiring that activates the function of all our systems and organs. Our digestive tract is controlled by a complex set of nerves called the enteric nervous system. If the nerves supplying the gut are compromised, gut function will also be affected.

The spinal cord runs through the vertebrae in your spine, and nerves diverge from it to support various organs. Even a small amount of pressure on the nerves that supply your intestines, which can happen if your vertebrae are misaligned, can dampen their ability to properly conduct signals.

Consult a licensed chiropractor for a full spinal assessment to determine if subluxations (displacement of vertebrae that may lead to reduced nerve function) are present at the level of the nerves affecting your gut. Chiropractic treatment may help to correct the problem and optimize your intestinal function.

Doc Talk

Unfortunately, we live in an artificial world with unavoidable chronic aggravators of inflammation, such as environmental pollutants, a contaminated food supply (since the plants and animals that make up our diet are exposed to the same toxins), medications and chronic stress. As a result, we need more nutrients to boost our body's metabolic processes to compensate, particularly when our health is compromised. Nutritional and herbal supplements are a good option because they help hasten the healing process, using concentrated extracts of foods to achieve therapeutic outcomes more efficiently.

In addition, complementary therapies such as acupuncture, homeopathy, biomechanics and chiropractic can help to support, strengthen and correct potential imbalances that contribute to leaky gut syndrome. You may achieve complete resolution with the treatments recommended here, or you may see only partial improvements. In the latter case, other variables may be preventing you from reaching optimum health. Be open-minded and persistent as you try different supportive therapies. Keep in mind that not every treatment works for every person or every underlying health issue. You may need to experiment to some degree to determine what works best for you.

PART 3

The Leaky Gut Syndrome Diet Plan

Calming Diet

Pat was 42 when he first visited our clinic suffering from acute ulcerative colitis, which first occurred while he was on holiday in a rural area. The chief symptom was the sudden onset of severe, unremitting chronic diarrhea. Bowel movements were urgent and up to 12 times over the course of day and night, with cramping and back pain. The consistency of stool was unformed, ranging from mushy to watery, with mucus present. Pat was hospitalized for 4 days as an inpatient with intravenous antibiotics and oral anti-inflammatories. Stool tests were negative for parasites. A serum inflammatory marker and liver enzymes were elevated significantly past the upper end of the normal ranges (3 to 12 times the normal ranges). The diarrhea continued for 3 weeks with only minor notable improvements. When Pat ate a hamburger, the acute, severe onset of symptoms returned suddenly. When he came to us, it was about 7 weeks following the first presentation of symptoms. There had been no relief and no sign of improvement.

We implemented the Calming Diet immediately. Pat's diet was already very low in allergens. He had eliminated caffeine, dairy, eggs, alcohol, processed foods and practically all gluten-containing foods before seeing us. In addition to his already healthy hypoallergenic diet, we recommended that all foods should be cooked (no raw salads or leafy greens), and we suggested that he consume congee with seaweed every day and drink only warm beverages. We also recommended gastrointestinal support through supplements: L-glutamine, enteric-coated probiotics, chewable licorice root capsules (deglycyrrhizinated) and a non-psyllium-based bulking fiber. The goal was to focus on repairing the integrity of the gut mucosa to settle inflammation, improve immunity and treat gut hyperpermeability.

Pat was highly compliant and incorporated changes the next morning. Remarkably, within 48 hours of applying the recommended diet changes and gut support, his bowel movements normalized to twice daily and were formed and nonurgent. Now, 2 months since his first appointment, he reports that all his blood work is within normal range and his bowel movements have continued to be within the normal range. With his improved digestive function and tolerance, Pat has expanded his diet without consequence.

CHAPTER 8

Eliminating Inflammatory Foods

The Leaky Gut Syndrome Diet Plan is a modified elimination diet that avoids foods that trigger allergic reactions, sensitivities and intolerances. This chapter outlines the most common food triggers that aggravate the gut. The aim of the diet plan is to reduce problematic inflammation and support healthy digestion by eliminating the foods that most commonly aggravate the gut.

Identifying your food triggers enables you to adjust your diet to begin the healing process. A diet diary can help you track symptoms and severities, and learning to read ingredient labels can help ensure that you don't mistakenly ingest one of your trigger foods. If certain foods you commonly eat trigger an adverse response, remove them from your diet.

It would be best to eliminate foods with the support of a qualified health professional who knows the severity of your condition and can monitor you for improvements and adjust the treatment plan accordingly.

> **Did You Know?**
>
> **Dietary Approach**
> A dietary approach will settle inflammation, improve nutrition and reduce potential food aggravators. Targeting your diet in a safe and comprehensive manner will not only avoid causing harm but will improve your health and start the process of healing your gut and your body.

Determining Your Food Triggers

The first step, of course, is to determine which foods are aggravating your gut so that you can eliminate them from your diet. You can do this by taking an IgG food sensitivity test and/or by keeping a diet diary.

IgG Food Sensitivity Test

Although no available test can measure every possible reaction to foods (because there exist so many mechanisms that can lead to different sensitivities and intolerances), the IgG food sensitivity test (described in detail on page 44) can measure a particular type of food sensitivity that can commonly affect gut inflammation, immunity and permeability, so the results are relevant and important to treating leaky gut syndrome.

These results will indicate the foods that may cause a strong, moderate or mild reaction when you consume them. Eliminate those foods that test positive on the IgG food sensitivity test according to the following criteria:

- Avoid foods that may cause a strong reaction for at least 3 months.
- Eliminate foods that may cause a moderate reaction for 1 month.
- Reduce the consumption of foods that may cause a mild reaction to once every 1 to 2 weeks.

These foods can often be reintroduced once gut hyperpermeability has settled, although you should continue to consume them infrequently in the long term. The goal is to strengthen your immunity and gut state so that occasional doses of trigger foods do not surpass the threshold to chronic inflammation. This process is about moderating the frequency and the amount of aggravating foods in the long term, rather than implementing an unrealistic lifetime of avoidance.

Diet Diary

A more immediate way to determine what foods are not gut-friendly is to keep a diet diary, recording what you eat and how you respond to the food item or ingredients. Use this diary to track your diet and digestive patterns, as well as your stress levels, sleep habits and all your symptoms throughout each day for at least a 2-week period. Include bowel movements (indicate with an asterisk★) and qualifiers, if applicable.

Guidelines for Completing a Diet Diary

1. Establish a timeline and make a firm commitment to tracking your daily intake of all foods, beverages (including coffee and alcohol), cigarettes, recreational drugs, supplements and medications — essentially anything you are putting into your mouth. Write these down in the order that you consume them throughout the course of the day.

Sample Diet Diary

	Day 1	Day #
Breakfast	2 fried eggs, whole wheat toast, banana, glass of orange juice	
Symptoms:	Felt tired 1 hour after eating ($^3/_{10}$) * UL	
Snack	Salt and vinegar chips	
Symptoms:	None	
Lunch	Mixed spring greens salad with grilled chicken breast, ranch dressing, 1 can of cola	
Symptoms:	Bloated, gassy ($^4/_{10}$)	
Snack	Carrot sticks and hummus, medium cup of coffee (2 cream, 1 sugar)	
Symptoms:	Feeling foggy-headed, hard to concentrate on work ($^5/_{10}$)	
Dinner	Roast beef with baked potatoes and corn on the cob with butter	
Symptoms:	Headache started shortly after dinner ($^3/_{10}$)	
Snack	$^1/_2$ cup (125 mL) of vanilla ice cream topped with blueberries	
Symptoms:	None * IFG	
Sleep time and quality:	60 minutes to fall asleep, woke one time for 15 minutes; total = 6 hours	
Stress rating (0–4):	3	
Additional notes:	Stressful day at work	

Bowel movement qualifiers:
B = blood, F = undigested food, G = gas, H = hard, I = incomplete, L = loose, M = mucus, P = pain, S = straining, U = urgent

Stress: 0 = nonexistent, 1 = mild, 2 = moderate, 3 = high, 4 = overwhelming

2. Also note down on the same timeline all the symptoms that occur over the course of the day. A symptom would be any sensation that makes you feel less than 100%. This can include such occurrences as fatigue, headaches, moodiness, anxiety, bloating, itchiness from eczema, or joint pain, to name a few. If possible, indicate the severity of the symptom on a scale of 1 to 10, with 10 being the most severe presentation possible.

3. In addition, because digestion is the cornerstone of the body's overall health and it's necessary to optimize the health of the gut to treat cases of leaky gut syndrome, be sure to track all your bowel movements and when they occur during the day. Unless it is a perfect, easy-to-pass, well-formed stool, make notes about anything that varies from this norm. For example, you can note that your bowel movement 1 hour after lunch was unformed, black and mushy and it irritated you as it was coming out, if that applies.

4. Because sleep is so essential for tissue repair and immune regulation, also note your sleep duration and quality. We tend to underestimate our sleep needs. Record how much you sleep and determine if you are sleeping enough or if lack of sleep is impacting your health.

5. Finally, make a note of stress levels on each given day. You can rate your levels of stress on a scale of 0 to 4.

Record your symptoms, bowel movements, stress levels, sleep patterns and diet for at least 2 weeks to observe and track patterns. Ideally, follow your normal diet with its usual variations (for example, eating out or missing meals) so that you have a true baseline measure of your symptoms and patterns.

Functions of the Diet Diary

1. To be aware of — and provide a visual reference of — what foods you are sensitive to and how often you are consuming them, contributing to gut inflammation.

2. To be aware of the severity of your symptoms and how often you experience them. Some people downplay their symptoms while others may overestimate them. Track honestly for a more objective assessment.

3. To determine if the diet provides adequate nutrition and appropriate calories and whether it is balanced across food categories.

> We tend to underestimate our sleep needs. Record how much you sleep and determine if you are sleeping enough or if lack of sleep is impacting your health.

4. To monitor potential hidden triggers, such as processed chemical ingredients in prepared or prepackaged foods.

5. To provide a visual reference for your health-care provider. This reference will help your doctor or dietitian assess your nutrient levels and note any relationship between foods and systemic reactions that you may not be able to recognize on your own.

Analyzing Your Diet Diary

Once you have completed your diet diary, check it over to see if you can identify correlations between particular foods and symptoms. You may notice some obvious patterns, but others may be more difficult to interpret.

Using a couple of highlighter pens, try color-coding certain suspect meals or ingredients, along with symptoms, to make it easier to visualize potential negative responses.

If you find that your diary is too difficult to interpret, don't give up. It is still a useful practice to make you more aware of your diet and other health-related habits, and you will also be helping your health-care providers by giving them information about your level of nutrition and how it may be connected to the onset of your symptoms.

Foods to Avoid

There are several foods that should be strictly avoided while recovering from leaky diet syndrome. Dairy, egg and gluten-containing grains are the most common IgG classes of foods. Other common food sensitivities and intolerances include alcohol, artificial ingredients, beef, caffeine, chocolate, cruciferous vegetables, garlic, legumes, onions, peanuts, pork, tomatoes, shellfish and soy. All of these foods are eliminated in the LGS Diet Plan.

There are several foods that should be strictly avoided while recovering from leaky diet syndrome. Dairy, egg and gluten-containing grains are the most common IgG classes of foods.

The Big Three: Dairy, Eggs and Gluten

The general first reaction when you find out that you may have sensitivities to common food categories is one of shock or disbelief, especially if the foods are one of the Big Three groups (dairy, eggs and gluten). These most commonly elicit sensitivities. Dairy, eggs and gluten are part of a vast array of food products, either in their whole form or as a hidden ingredient. It is exactly because of this overprocessing that, as a society, we are consuming too many of these foods and have instigated an increase in sensitivities toward them. You have eaten all these food types, in one form or another, consistently and possibly even multiple times every day since infancy. If you are sensitive to one or more of these foods, you are, in essence, regularly dosing yourself with a toxin.

Many patients claim to eat a dairy-free, gluten-free or egg-free diet, but upon investigating their diet records, it is apparent that they still regularly consume foods they think they are avoiding. Dairy, eggs and gluten have become so pervasive in our food supply that we often ingest them without even realizing it.

Many variants and much confusion exists about which foods fall into these categories. The most effective way to avoid foods with these culprits is to follow a meal plan that involves only whole foods (no processed or packaged foods) so you actually know what is going into what you are preparing. If it becomes too difficult to manage yourself, consult a physician, doctor or dietitian versed in dealing with food sensitivities to assist you with your meal planning.

> *Dairy, eggs and gluten have become so pervasive in our food supply that we often ingest them without even realizing it.*

Cruciferous Vegetables

Cruciferous vegetables contain sulfur-containing compounds that can instigate gas, bloating and flatus, which is why they are included on the elimination list. While broccoli and cauliflower are the best known in this family, cruciferous vegetables also include arugula, bok choy, Brussels sprouts, collard greens, kale, mustard

---

Hidden Ingredients

These ingredients are hidden in many processed foods. Read food labels very carefully.

- Eggs: albumin, binder, coagulant, emulsifier, globulin, lecithin, lysozyme, ovalbumin, ovomucin, ovomucoid, ovovitellin, vitellin
- Dairy: casein, lactalbumin, lactalbumin phosphate, lactose, modified milk ingredients, potassium caseinate, sodium caseinate, whey
- Gluten: barley, couscous, durum, Kamut, malt, oats, rye, spelt, triticale, wheat, wheat berries, white flour, whole wheat flour

---

greens, radish, rutabaga, Swiss chard, turnip, watercress — a large cross-section of vegetables. Because heating these vegetables can help to break down some of their sulfur-containing compounds, they are allowed in Phase 2 of the diet if they are cooked.

Raw Fruits and Vegetables

Fruits and vegetables contain beneficial medicinal compounds called phenols. However, sensitive digestive tracts can find phenols difficult to process. Raw fruits and vegetables are known to aggravate the symptoms of inflammatory bowel diseases (Crohn's disease and ulcerative colitis). Cooking helps reduce the phenol content of fruits and vegetables, making them safer to consume in inflammatory states, including leaky gut syndrome.

Fruit and Vegetable Peels and Nut Skins

Peels and skins are the protective coatings of fruits, vegetables and nuts. They are tough and thick, to protect their contents, and so are more difficult to digest. They also contain more insoluble fiber, which can act as an irritant to an inflamed gut lining. Consequently, it is best to avoid peels of produce and the skins of nuts when addressing a compromised gut.

Onion Family

Garlic, onions, shallots, chives and leeks, from the *Allium* genus, all contain a potent compound called allicin, which provides them with their powerful medicinal properties.

> ### Did You Know?
>
> **Tomato Sauce**
> Barring any individual intolerance to fresh tomatoes, sensitivities to tomato sauces are more common than sensitivities to fresh tomatoes because of the additives, spices, sugars and processing. Tomato sauce is often mistakenly believed to be a safe food, but because of its concentrated, acidic and processed nature, it is best to avoid it.

However, allicin also contains sulfur, which is difficult to digest, particularly when these foods are raw. Allicin is broken down in the cooking process, so you can eat cooked allium plants in Phase 2 of the LGS Diet Plan.

Black Pepper and Other Seasonings

When your gut is in a non-inflamed state, black pepper can be beneficial since it increases blood flow. However, when your gut is in a severely inflamed state, black pepper will act as a local irritant, worsening inflammation of the gut mucosa. Because of this stimulating nature, avoid black pepper in Phase 1 of the LGS Diet Plan.

Avoid all hot spices and spice blends (seasonings made from or with hot peppers, such as cayenne pepper, chili powder and hot pepper flakes) for the same reason — they are irritants to the digestive lining. In addition, herbs, spices and spice blends with especially pungent flavors (particularly Chinese five-spice powder, curry powder, mustard and oregano) tend to act as irritants in their raw form, even if they are not "hot." For this reason, use only cooked non-spicy herbs and spices in Phase 1 of the LGS Diet Plan. Safe choices include basil, bay leaves, cilantro, coriander, cumin, fennel, mint, parsley, rosemary, sage, tarragon, thyme and turmeric.

Cold Foods and Beverages

Cold foods shock the compromised digestive system and make it more difficult for your body to tolerate them. Cold foods and beverages are not recommended in leaky gut syndrome because:

- They cause vasoconstriction, or a narrowing of the blood vessels, thereby depressing peristalsis (the rhythmic wavelike action of the smooth muscles that line the digestive tract) and reducing gastric secretions, which leads to suboptimal digestive function, particularly in a compromised state.
- They require a substantial amount of additional metabolic energy to become warmed up to body temperature.
- Enzymes have a particular range of pH and temperature in which they function most effectively, and it is best to encourage their optimal performance in a state of intestinal hyperpermeability.

Traditional Chinese medicine (as well as Ayurvedic medicine) recommends that cold foods and beverages always be avoided, because cold depresses the "spleen function" (this differs from the spleen organ in Western medicine), which governs digestion.

In essence, cold food slows digestion. Consume only foods and drinks that are heated or at room temperature when you are in a highly inflamed state.

Refined Sugar

Refined sugar is a confirmed detriment to our health, particularly in the way that it quickly spikes our blood sugars, making our body scramble to compensate. Artificial sweeteners are not good alternatives. Regular consumption of refined sugar will prevent the immune system from functioning optimally, compromise hormone metabolism and increase inflammation. All of these disruptions will prevent the body from healing from leaky gut syndrome. Other high-glycemic variants of refined sugar linked to dysfunction and worsened inflammatory state include cane sugar (and evaporated cane sugar), cane syrup, Demerara sugar, dextrose, fructose, glucose, high-fructose corn syrup, maltodextrin and muscovado and turbinado sugars. Keep these sugars and sugar variants out of your diet when starting an anti-inflammatory diet, and minimize exposure to all of these high-glycemic substances in general.

Artificial Ingredients

Artificial ingredients are food additives that are synthetic or chemically extracted in a laboratory. While many artificial ingredients used by the food industry are "generally recognized as safe" (GRAS, a designation given by the American Food and Drug Administration), their impact on chronic disease has not been comprehensively studied. Nevertheless, we don't consider artificial additives to be intended for human consumption. Nor do they have any beneficial health effects. In fact, after having been commercially available for decades, many artificial food additives have now been shown to have adverse effects or to impact health in the long term. Their sole purpose is to preserve, sweeten, texturize, bind or color our foods, or to artificially enhance their flavor.

Did You Know?

Caffeine Withdrawal
Eliminating caffeine is often the most difficult restriction to implement, for a few reasons. Caffeine is physically addictive, and the withdrawal symptoms can include rebound headaches, fatigue, major cravings, moodiness and restlessness. Keep in mind that these symptoms typically last only 2 to 3 days, although in some cases they can be nonexistent or last just for the first day, and in others they can last for a week or longer. The withdrawal period depends on your caffeine tolerance, your psychological dependency and how much caffeine you were previously consuming.

Common Artificial Ingredients to Avoid

Ingredient	Where It's Found	What It Does
Preservatives		
Butylated hydroxyanisole (BHA) and butylated hydroxytoluene (BHT)	Cereals, gum, butter, shortening, beer, snack foods	Used to prevent rancidity of fats in food; may have carcinogenic/teratogenic (developmental) effects
Nitrites	Processed meats, deli meats, hot dogs, sausages	Produces a known carcinogen, nitrosamine, in stomach acid and with cooking
Sodium/potassium benzoate	Acidic foods such as pickles	Slows down fungal and bacterial activity; links to cancers and attention deficit hyperactivity disorder (ADHD)
Sulfites	Dried fruit, wine	Elicits allergic responses; worsens asthma symptoms
Colorings		
Listed as "FD&C" followed by the color name and number (for example, FD&C Blue No. 1)	Candy, drinks, cereals, pastries, water flavor enhancers, medicines, chips, yogurt, cheese, sauces	Linked to tumors in animal studies and behavioral changes in children
Flavor enhancers		
Hydrolyzed vegetable protein (HVP)	Dips, hot dogs, gravy, chips, vegetarian products, dressings	Contains MSG
Monosodium glutamate (MSG)	Chips, fast food, soups, dressings, Parmesan cheese, dips, instant noodles	Leads to neurotoxic effects
Fats		
Trans fats	Hydrogenated/partially hydrogenated oils	Strong link to heart disease
Artificial sweeteners		
Acesulfame potassium (Acesulfame-K)	Sunett, Sweet One, Sweet & Safe	Produces cancer in animals
Aspartame	NutraSweet, Equal, Sugar Twin	Produces formaldehyde metabolite; possible link to neurologic/immunologic toxicity, cancer, behavior-adverse effects; similar chemical structure to chlorinated pesticides

Ingredient	Where It's Found	What It Does
Neotame	Neotame	Similar to aspartame but possibly more toxic; carcinogenic effects
Saccharin	Sweet'N Low, Sweet Twin, Necta Sweet	Has been linked to cancer, especially bladder cancer
Sugar alcohols: sorbitol, mannitol, erythritol, xylitol	Nectresse	Main effects are mild digestive disruptions and laxative effects
Sucralose	Splenda	May be linked to neurologic/immunologic toxicity; long-term health studies not available; similar chemical structure to chlorinated pesticides

Research Spotlight
The Long-Term Health Effects of Food Additives

Many food additives have been shown to have long-term effects on health. Monosodium glutamate (MSG), a flavor enhancer, has been associated with adverse impacts on fibromyalgia and irritable bowel syndrome. Aspartame, an artificial sweetener, has been linked to adverse neurologic effects. A recent study showed that one of its metabolites, diketopiperazine, leads to the growth of tumors — including gliomas, medulloblastomas and meningiomas — in the central nervous system. Safety concerns suggest that its use needs to be urgently reevaluated. It has been recommended that foods in the GRAS category should be renamed "generally recommended to avoid," particularly when disease and underlying inflammatory processes are present. Treat artificial ingredients as guilty until proven innocent, because they are not required by your body for your survival and they may be detrimental to your health outcomes.

For this reason, avoid all artificial ingredients while following the LGS Diet Plan. Stick to eating foods as they exist in their natural form. Humans have been consuming food additives for less than a century, which means that they are new to metabolism and digestion.

Caffeine
Caffeine is a nervous system stimulant and diuretic (stimulates the voiding of fluids via urination). Coffee, as well as black, white and green tea, pop, energy

Did You Know?

Natural Decaffeination

For the longest time, caffeine used to be extracted primarily through chemical separation via methylene chloride. Although the methylene chloride remains in only trace amounts in coffee decaffeinated by this method, it is always preferable to avoid chemicals, particularly with something that we consume regularly. Look for a non-chemically decaffeinated coffee. These are labeled with descriptions of the natural decaffeination methods they use — for example, "Swiss water process," "mountain water process" or "carbon dioxide process."

Did You Know?

Alcohol Restraint

Alcohol can affect inflammation or aggravate the function of the digestive tract, which is why we suggest that you eliminate alcohol from your diet. At higher doses, depending on your body's tolerance and metabolic efficiency, alcohol causes toxic effects.

drinks, chocolate and caffeine pills can all increase contraction of the gut's nervous system. This effect will worsen diarrhea, constipation, cramping, nausea and — consequently — gut permeability. It is best to completely avoid all sources of caffeine to ensure that it is not aggravating gut dysfunction.

The other issue related to caffeine is that we typically consume it every day and sometimes in quantities that exceed individual tolerance. For example, excessive caffeine use can affect sleep quality and energy levels, overstimulate the adrenal glands (which regulate hormones and the stress response), aggravate anxiety and, as a result, promote inflammation and deregulate the immune system. Because of how it directly stimulates the gut and its systemic effects, caffeine should be avoided while you are trying to normalize intestinal function. The majority of people experience some adverse effects after just one cup of coffee per day or two cups of tea per day.

If you experience a return of symptoms after reintroducing caffeine following the LGS Diet Plan, be wary of consuming it regularly. If you miss caffeine solely for the boost of energy, other lifestyle factors usually need to be corrected to improve your well-being. If you just miss the taste, ritual and social aspects, consider enjoying a naturally decaffeinated coffee or tea, which has all of the taste and health benefits and none of the caffeine.

How to Wean Yourself Off Coffee

Depending on how ingrained your dependency is, or if you are averse to a cold-turkey method of caffeine cessation, you can use a wean-down method to minimize withdrawal symptoms before starting the leaky gut diet.

To minimize withdrawal effects, gradually reduce from full-strength coffee to decaf coffee in the following manner:

Day 1: regular caffeinated coffee
Day 2: $\frac{2}{3}$ caffeinated + $\frac{1}{3}$ decaffeinated coffee
Day 3: $\frac{1}{2}$ caffeinated + $\frac{1}{2}$ decaffeinated coffee
Day 4: $\frac{1}{3}$ caffeinated + $\frac{2}{3}$ decaffeinated coffee
Day 5: decaffeinated coffee
Day 6: no coffee

Alcohol

Alcohol depresses the nervous and immune systems. It also depresses reabsorption of water from the kidneys — thereby leading to dehydration — and irritates the digestive tract. Since intestinal function is governed by nerve function, and stool quality is greatly affected by disrupted fluid balances in the body, you need to eliminate alcohol consumption while you are trying to correct leaky gut syndrome.

Degrees of sensitivity to alcohol vary, from obvious to insidious, so it is best to just avoid it altogether in the restrictive phase of the LGS Diet Plan. The other issue is that many people tend to consume alcohol either habitually in moderate amounts or occasionally in a binge pattern. Neither of these patterns of alcohol consumption is beneficial to chronic inflammation in the digestive tract. Alcoholic drinks take many different forms, making them difficult to compare and assess, and they may also be mixed with beverages that contain sweeteners and artificial flavors and colors.

After the normalization of your gut function and systemic symptoms, you can cautiously reintroduce alcohol in minimal amounts, if it is medically safe for you, with careful monitoring of adverse responses. Alcohol in moderation, defined as a maximum of one drink per day for women and two drinks per day for men, is associated with cardiovascular health benefits.

Doc Talk

Sometimes patients are overwhelmed by the leaky gut syndrome treatment plan and may not be ready to give up attachments to favorite foods and other unhealthy habits. They often ask half-jokingly (but with some optimism) for a quick fix, because they may be resistant to making changes to their diet and lifestyle. A person in a drastic state of ill health is often more ready to take drastic measures. Some patients may require more coaching than others to understand this connection before they are prepared to embark on their treatment plan.

There are natural supplements (as discussed on page 87) that assist with normalizing a leaky gut, and these may lead to benefits if implemented on their own. This may be the only realistic treatment plan for some patients to start with, which is fine, as it may be a starting point for them to notice improvements and gain motivation to gradually build upon their progress with stepwise recommendations. However, in the majority of cases, diet combined with added nutritional or herbal support is recommended to achieve the best results in the long term.

CHAPTER 9

Choosing Gut-Friendly Foods

From the psychological point of view, it is usually easier to focus on what you *can* have in your diet rather than what you are eliminating. Many meal combinations in the Leaky Gut Syndrome Diet Plan are not only easy to prepare but also taste great. All of the foods in the LGS Diet Plan are natural whole foods. These are the foods to which our bodies have adapted throughout our evolution. We can process them and they can properly fuel us. They contain the nutrients that promote a healthy, functioning digestive tract and so prevent and treat inflammation in the body.

Preparing gut-friendly snacks for when you're on the go is just as important as preparing LGS-healing meals at home. Incorporating superfoods into your diet is one way to improve the health of your gut lining, as is ensuring that your eating ritual isn't rushed, stressed or characterized by inadequate chewing.

Incorporating superfoods into your diet is one way to improve the health of your gut lining, as is ensuring that your eating ritual isn't rushed, stressed or characterized by inadequate chewing.

Safe Foods

A leaky-gut-friendly diet consists of the following categories of foods:

- Quality protein
- Gluten-free whole grains
- Vegetables and fruits
- Nuts and seeds
- Healthy oils
- Hydrating fluids
- Natural flavorings and sweeteners

Choose foods from each category to ensure proper nutrition. If you note that any of the foods aggravates your health condition, be sure to modify the selection accordingly. Keep in mind that altering how you cook or how long you cook foods can alter their composition to improve how you digest them.

FAQ

Q Will this diet lead to nutrient deficiencies while my leaky gut is healing?

A If you choose a variety of foods from each category, this diet will provide you with adequate protein, carbohydrates, fat and essential nutrients. Note that a lack of variety may lead to nutrient deficiencies in the long term. Initially, the focus is to heal a hyperpermeable gut state to ensure adequate nutrient absorption. This should be discussed with a qualified health practitioner.

Quality Protein

- **Fish:** cod, haddock, herring, mackerel, salmon, sardines, tilapia, trout — but not marlin, shellfish, swordfish or tuna, because of mercury contamination
- **Pulses:** adzuki beans, black beans, black-eyed peas, chickpeas, lentils, lima beans, pinto beans
- **Meat:** bison, buffalo, chicken, elk, lamb, turkey, venison — but no beef or pork

Gluten-Free Whole Grains

You may have been advised to avoid all grains because they are high in a protein called lectin. However, in my experience, the following gluten-free whole grains will not hamper your progress to good health as long as they are prepared appropriately to maximize their benefits and prevent any adverse effects. For more information, see page 115.

- Amaranth
- Brown or white rice
- Buckwheat
- Millet
- Quinoa
- Teff

Vegetables and Fruits

- Apples
- Apricots
- Asparagus
- Bananas
- Beets
- Berries
- Carrots
- Cassava
- Cucumbers
- Leafy greens
- Lettuce
- Nectarines
- Papaya
- Parsnips
- Peaches
- Pears

✱ Caution
Pulses can cause gas and irritate gut mucosa. They should not be consumed unless they are well-cooked. You can add a piece of kombu (kelp, a type of seaweed) while cooking to break down the raffinose, which is responsible for causing gas when you eat pulses. Unless you follow a vegan or vegetarian diet, it may be safer to exclude pulses from your diet. If you do include pulses in your diet, see page 116 for more information on preparing them.

- Peas
- Pineapple
- Plums
- Red and green bell peppers

- Seaweed
- Spinach
- Sweet potatoes
- Zucchini

Nuts and Seeds

Nuts can be raw or roasted, but not salted. Avoid peanuts. Choose only skin-free nuts.

- Almonds and almond butter
- Cashews and cashew butter
- Macadamia nuts and macadamia nut butter

- Pine nuts
- Green pumpkin seeds (pepitas)
- Hemp seeds
- Sesame seeds
- Sunflower seeds

Healthy Oils

- Avocado oil
- Extra virgin olive oil
- Grapeseed oil

- Macadamia nut oil
- Sesame oil
- Virgin coconut oil

Hydrating Fluids

Avoid alcohol, caffeinated beverages, dairy, fruit juices, pop and other carbonated drinks in favor of the following hydrating fluids:

- Additive-free coconut water
- Herbal teas
- Milk alternatives (such as almond, coconut, hempseed or rice milk); ensure that they are carrageenan-free, as this derivative of seaweed can exacerbate digestive inflammation
- Water (not cold), with added lemon or lime slices, if desired

Natural Flavorings and Sweeteners

In addition to the flavorings and sweeteners listed below, basil, bay leaves, cilantro, coriander, cumin, fennel, mint, parsley, rosemary, sage, tarragon, thyme and turmeric are acceptable when cooked in Phase 1 recipes and are permitted uncooked in Phase 2, as long as you have no known sensitivities.

Natural Flavorings

- Balsamic vinegar with no added color or sulfites, in small amounts
- Cider vinegar, in small amounts
- Cinnamon
- Ginger
- Lemon or lime juice
- Rice vinegar, in small amounts
- Sea salt

Natural Sweeteners (acceptable in small amounts)

- Agave nectar
- Amasake
- Barley malt
- Brown rice syrup
- Coconut sugar
- Date sugar
- Honey
- Maple syrup
- Pure fruit juice
- Whole-leaf stevia
- Yacon syrup

Why Pulses and Whole Grains Are Included in the LGS Diet Plan

Pulses and grains are high in lectin, a naturally occurring protein that deters pests from consuming the plants by acting as a weak toxin. Studies have shown that, when we eat lectin, it acts as a digestive irritant, leading to functional and structural changes in the colon, and prevents the assimilation of nutrients into the body. It is often viewed as an "anti-nutrient," and some health authorities speculate that it may exacerbate leaky gut syndrome.

Because pulses and grains are higher in lectin than other plant products, the theory is that they may irritate our digestive tract, impair our digestive function, weaken our immune system and decrease our energy. Some groups (such as paleo diet proponents) argue that they should therefore be excluded completely from the diet. But in practice, when pulses and gluten-free whole grains are consumed in small to moderate amounts and are properly prepared in a balanced, varied diet, the anti-nutrient and gut-aggravating effects are negligible.

Did You Know?

Dairy Dilemma

The classically recommended requirement of including dairy products in the diet to ensure comprehensive nutrition is flawed. Dairy products do supplement a diet with more protein, calcium, B vitamins and so on, but they are definitely not essential — other categories of foods will provide the same nutrients. The issue is that dairy products, along with eggs, are the most common instigators of food sensitivities, which can aggravate leaky gut syndrome and its associated constellation of health problems.

FAQ

Q What is the difference between a legume and a pulse?

A "Legume" is an umbrella term that covers all foods that form seeds in pods. Legumes include beans, lentils, peas, soybeans and peanuts. A pulse is the dried seed of various legumes, including chickpeas, beans (kidney, lima, navy, pinto) and lentils.

Did You Know?

Grains Normalize Stools

Grains "fluff up" hard, small or infrequent stools, making them softer, easier to pass and more frequent. But grains also help give bulk to loose, overly frequent or urgent stools, slowing their frequency and making them more formed.

When it comes to restoring and maintaining a healthy gut, which can take six months or more, an attainable diet plan that can be followed for a long time is much more practical than a strict plan that few people will be able to maintain for more than a short period. The exclusion of grains is a restriction many people would struggle with.

In addition, people who avoid consuming grains often have incomplete, infrequent, hard or even loose stools. Adding even a minimal amount of gluten-free whole grains to their diet can improve their bowel movements and stool consistency, which will reduce gut irritation. So eating grains can actually improve gut function.

Keeping all this in mind, the most sensible approach is to maintain a moderate, varied diet and prepare pulses and gluten-free whole grains properly to ensure that they only improve your health.

Preparing Pulses and Grains

Proper preparation, which can involve soaking, sprouting or cooking over high heat for $1\frac{1}{2}$ to 2 hours, can dramatically reduce lectin levels in pulses and grains so that they will not aggravate your gut lining. A combination of two or more of these methods is even more effective. Soaking is particularly effective, so do get in the habit of soaking pulses and grains for several hours or overnight before cooking them. You can then cook them as you normally would, but for greater effect, use more water than you normally would and simmer for $1\frac{1}{2}$ to 2 hours to maximize the breakdown of lectins, some of which may be resistant to lower-heat cooking.

The process of sprouting grains releases enzymes from the seed that readily break down the lectins and other anti-nutrients (such as trypsin inhibitors, amylase inhibitors and tannins) found in pulses or grains. A brief online search will lead you to sites that teach do-it-yourself pulse or grain sprouting; alternatively, sprouting kits are available at health food stores.

Snacking

Ensure that you pack snacks before you leave the house. It is difficult to stay disciplined and stick with your diet if you are hypoglycemic due to hunger. An ounce of prevention, as they say, is worth a pound of cure, and packing the kind of snack that we recommend is less time-consuming than stepping into a store to purchase a processed, unhealthy snack. Keep snacks top-of-mind before you actually need to eat one (and before you leave the house), and make this a new habit.

Keeping your digestive tract engaged with meals and healthy snacks that keep you satiated (but not stuffed) is essential. Eating regular, adequate portions and avoiding excessive eating is the best way to minimize stress on your digestive tract.

* Caution
Remember that pulses are recommended *only* for strict vegetarians and vegans, because there are so few options for vegetarian proteins. If you eat meat and/or fish, it is better to avoid pulses. However, if you are a vegetarian, be reassured that properly prepared pulses will not hinder your progress toward a normalized gut state.

Quick, Healthy, Gut-Friendly Snacks

- Nuts (skin-free during Phase 1 of the diet)
- Fruit or vegetable (peeled and cooked in Phase 1 of the diet)
- Garlic-free hummus with peeled carrots
- Steamed asparagus with garlic-free guacamole
- Steamed peeled cucumber slices with lime juice
- Rice crackers with cashew butter
- Baked yam with olive oil
- Macadamia nuts with cinnamon
- Blue corn chips with garlic- and onion-free salsa
- Roasted seaweed–wrapped sticky rice balls with cashew centers

Mucilaginous and demulcent foods and teas support the protective mucous membrane layer of the digestive tract as a result of their high water content and coating effects.

Superfoods for LGS

Mucilaginous and demulcent foods and teas support the protective mucous membrane layer of the digestive tract as a result of their high water content and coating effects. Chia seeds, manuka honey, marshmallow root tea, okra, seaweed and slippery elm tea are examples of these foods.

Superfoods high in L–glutamine (an amino acid that fuels the cells lining your digestive tract) include beets, chicken, fish, legumes and turkey.

Vitamin A is an important cofactor in rebuilding and strengthening mucous membranes. Butternut squash, cod liver oil, fish, mullein tea, nettle tea, pumpkin, red palm oil and spinach are examples of foods high in both carotenoids (precursors to vitamin A) and preformed vitamin A.

Congee

Congee is a rice-based "porridge" that has been used in traditional Chinese medicine for millennia because of its healing properties for the gut and immune system. The ingredients are suited to work within the parameters of the LGS Diet Plan. They exclude all major food sensitivities and meet the criteria of being well-cooked and easily digestible.

A bonus is that congee is easy to prepare in large batches, particularly if you use a slow cooker. It also provides complete nutrition, supplying adequate complex carbohydrates, fats, protein and vegetables. Use this frequently as a base while you are following the LGS Diet Plan.

Congee Recipe for Gut Health and Immune Support

Makes 12 to 13 cups (3 to 3.25 L)

Enjoy three to four bowls per day at any meal of the day, including breakfast!

Tip

Store individual portions of congee in airtight containers in the refrigerator for up to 4 days or in the freezer for 2 months.

8 oz	bison or chicken bones	250 g
8 oz	boneless bison (leg, chuck or flank), skinless chicken legs or breast, or fish, cut into chunks	250 g
1½ cups	roughly chopped carrots, winter squash, pumpkin, onions and/or garlic (permitted in Phases 2 and 3 only)	375 mL
1 cup	well-rinsed short- or long-grain rice (preferably brown)	250 mL
1 tbsp	sliced gingerroot	15 mL
2 tsp	cider vinegar	10 mL
	Water	
	Nori (optional)	

1. In a slow cooker or large pot, combine bison bones, bison, vegetables of choice (if using), rice, ginger and vinegar. Add water to 1 inch (2.5 cm) below top of cooker or pot. Slow-cook on Low for 8 to 10 hours, or bring to a simmer over high heat on the stovetop, then reduce heat and simmer for 3 to 4 hours.

2. If desired, cut or rip strips of nori and add to bowl before eating for additional mucous membrane support.

Lacto-fermented Foods

Lacto-fermented foods are fermented with naturally occurring bacteria that are beneficial to your gut microbiome. The prefix "lacto" means that the fermentation process involves a species of bacteria, *Lactobacillus*, that creates lactic acid as a by-product.

Foods made using this technique can be found at health food stores. They commonly include kimchi, sauerkraut and pickles. Ensure that these products are made via lacto-fermentation rather than pickled in vinegar, which is the more common process.

Lacto-fermenting Vegetables

Tips

Plastic lids for canning jars can be found at food or hardware stores or ordered online.

Make sure to purchase sea salt that is unadulterated by additives, such as anti-caking agents.

For the vegetables, try carrots, mini cucumbers, cabbage, bell peppers, beets, green beans or cauliflower, alone or in combination.

For the herbs, try basil, dill, bay leaves, rosemary, tarragon, sage, thyme or mint, alone or in combination.

As the vegetables ferment, check carefully each day and discard if any sign of mold appears or there are any off aromas.

- **1-quart (1 L) Mason jar with plastic lid (see tip, at left)**

3 tbsp	sea salt (see tip, at left)	45 mL
4 cups	boiling filtered water	1 L
	Vegetables (see tip, at left), cut into strips, chunks or sticks	
	Fresh herbs (see tip, at left), torn	

1. Dissolve sea salt in boiling filtered water to make brine. Let cool to room temperature.

2. Pack vegetables and herbs into jar, leaving 1½ inches (4 cm) headspace. Fill with brine so that vegetables and herbs are fully submerged. Insert a narrow plastic utensil into the jar in several places to remove any air bubbles. If vegetables float above the surface of the brine, wedge a piece of cabbage leaf into the jar to hold them down. Cover the jar with the plastic lid.

3. Place the jar in a baking dish (in case of spills or leaks) and let stand at room temperature for 3 to 7 days. Starting on Day 2, burp the lid (i.e., open it to allow gases to escape) at least once a day to prevent gas buildup (otherwise, the jar could potentially burst).

4. When the vegetables smell and taste fermented (pungent and sour, not moldy), transfer the jar to the refrigerator to slow the fermentation process. Continue to open the jar periodically to release any accumulated gas. Store in the refrigerator for up to 3 months.

You can eat these fermented foods as an accompaniment to your main dish or even as a topping. If you are interested in lacto-fermenting vegetables at home, it is actually quite easy.

How to Eat Well

Knowing *how* to eat is as important as knowing *what* to eat. When people say that they eat well, they are typically referring to their food choices. Poor eating habits, such as rushed eating and inadequate chewing, affect the mechanical breakdown of food and decrease its exposure to the first digestive enzymes in saliva: salivary amylase (which targets carbohydrate breakdown) and lingual lipase (which targets fat). Consequently, inadequately chewed foods may not be as optimally digested and accessible for further digestion by the stomach and intestines. Also, chewing very quickly or while talking can cause air to be swallowed, which can cause bloating and discomfort further along your digestive tract. Either way, improper chewing may affect the processing and assimilation of nutrients and cause inflammation of the intestinal mucosa, which initiates the process of leaky gut syndrome.

Improper chewing may affect the processing and assimilation of nutrients and cause inflammation of the intestinal mucosa.

The process of eating well requires you to be calm and to have correct posture. You also need to chew your food adequately. No matter how healthy your menu might be, you need to physically help your digestive tract perform at its best. Not eating well in this sense can be an obstacle to curing your leaky gut. Allow yourself at least 15 to 20 minutes to properly enjoy a meal, to actually "eat well"!

1. The digestive tract is served by the parasympathetic nervous system, which is diametrically opposed to the sympathetic nervous system (our go-go-go, flight-or-fight, stress-managing system). If you are eating on the go, in a rush or at your desk while continuing to work because of stressful deadlines, you are preventing your digestive tract from performing at its best.

Chewing effectively eases the workload on the rest of your digestive tract.

2. If you eat while slouching, your spine is bent forward, putting increased pressure on your abdomen and its contents. Ensure that you eat sitting upright in a chair or in a position that allows your torso to be erect. Think of your gut health, and do what it takes to keep your intestines decompressed and relaxed.

3. Digestion starts in your mouth with the mechanical mastication of food and the secretion of salivary enzymes, both of which initiate the process of breaking down food. Chewing effectively eases the workload on the rest of your digestive tract. Be aware of how much you are chewing before swallowing, and don't rush. If you need to, count out 20 to 30 chews with each mouthful of food.

Doc Talk

If you choose a variety of foods from each of the categories in the "Safe Foods" list (page 112), you will consume adequate amounts of protein, carbohydrate, fat and essential nutrients, even in the most restrictive phase of the LGS Diet Plan. The problem with certain historical diets for conditions such as irritable bowel syndrome, like the BRAT (banana, rice, applesauce, toast) diet, is that they are devoid of many nutrients. The BRAT diet does not include vegetables, protein or fats. This kind of narrow diet can lead to nutrient deficiencies if maintained over an extended period of time.

CHAPTER 10

Implementing the LGS Diet Plan

The Leaky Gut Syndrome Diet Plan is a three-stage program designed to lessen inflammation and repair hyperpermeability in your gut. Each phase is based on the degree or severity of inflammation in your body. If your inflammation is severe and unrelenting, you will start with Phase 1: Calming Diet, the most restrictive phase. If your inflammation is mild to moderate, you will start with Phase 2: Restoring Diet (those who start with Phase 1 will progress to Phase 2 as their inflammation improves). Whether you begin with Phase 1 or Phase 2, when you are ready to proceed with Phase 3: Maintenance Diet, you will gradually reintroduce foods in a plan individually tailored to you.

Before you start addressing leaky gut syndrome through diet, the first step is to prepare a game plan that will help you follow the program.

This diet plan is not only restorative to the digestive tract but it provides a balanced, low-inflammatory diet that will prevent chronic disease in the long term. But before you start addressing leaky gut syndrome through diet, the first step is to prepare a game plan that will help you follow the program and ensure that you have the right foods on hand. This takes effort, but you know it is worth it because your condition is affecting your quality of life.

Getting Started

To see measurable improvements in your symptoms, you will need to be disciplined. Start by removing from your cupboards and refrigerator all foods that aggravate your leaky gut syndrome symptoms. This includes all the foods for which you know you have a weakness. The most common food culprits to cause allergies, sensitivities and intolerances are alcohol, beef, caffeine, chocolate, cruciferous vegetables, dairy, eggs, garlic, gluten, legumes, onion, peanuts, pork, shellfish, soy and tomato. Be ruthless as you:

- Get rid of processed boxed foods.
- Dump the juice and pop.
- Toss out added sugars (including refined sugar and all sugar cane derivatives).
- Throw away caffeinated beverages.
- Ban the Big Three: dairy, eggs and gluten-containing grains.
- Cut out flour-based foods (bread, pasta, baked goods).
- Remove artificial ingredients: colors, preservatives, sweeteners, flavorings.
- Ditch the junk food and fried foods: cookies, chips, brownies, chocolate bars, ice cream, french fries and more.
- Hide the alcoholic beverages until the diet plan reaches the maintenance phase.

Make Plans and Stock Up

Write a detailed shopping list and plan for a comprehensive grocery store trip to stock up on foods to use in preparing meals for the LGS Diet Plan. If you use the lists of gut-friendly foods on pages 112–15 as your guide, you will find grocery shopping, stocking your kitchen and food preparation that much easier. Take a balanced approach, choosing a variety of foods from the allowable options at each phase of healing. And make sure to stock up on plenty of nonperishable and accessible snacks.

Follow the meal plans presented in this book or create your own plans ahead of time, choosing recipes that you know you will enjoy and can prepare. If you are in charge of meal preparation in your family, you can incorporate your gut-friendly foods as a main dish and serve side dishes that may be less restrictive and more pleasing to other family members. Alternatively, they can eat the same meal as you but add toppings, such as grated cheese, or serve the dish over pasta. This is easier to manage than preparing two completely separate meals.

If your family is willing, they may be interested in experimenting with the same main dishes and supporting you during the process. Make sure to have this discussion with them first. Their decision may depend on the ages of your children and the flexibility of everyone's palates.

Finally, plan for occasions when you may be on the road without packed food. Research restaurants with healthy options that meet the criteria of the LGS Diet Plan. Otherwise, bring leftovers from the previous night's dinner with you. This ensures that you have healthy, allowable foods readily available to prevent deviations and also saves you a lot of money on eating out.

Cook Ahead

To make following the diet easier, try cooking ahead or cooking in batches. Enjoy a portion for dinner, pack extras for lunch and freeze the surplus. If you do not like eating the same meal over and over, after a few rounds of bulk cooking and freezing, you will have many frozen ready-made and diet-plan-safe options available to choose from.

If you do not already have many reusable containers in which to pack lunches and leftovers, stock up. Glass, stainless steel and ceramic resealable containers are better than plastic. Plastic will never be entirely inert when heated, even when labeled "heat-safe" or "microwave-safe." Volatile compounds (polyvinyl chloride, polycarbonate and plasticizers) may be released in the heating process, potentially increasing the risk of cancer, affecting fertility and mimicking the hormones in your body.

Prevent Self-Sabotage

Family, work and social events are the most likely occasions where you may feel pressured, self-conscious or uncomfortable with your new diet program and menu. If you know there is a wedding, a work function or a special celebration coming up soon, postpone the diet plan until after this event. Make sure you don't have any social commitments or prior engagements that interfere with your new diet plan.

However, if your state of health is severe enough to be compromising your quality of life right now, make this health program your immediate priority. If that is the case, focus on your health first and cancel or postpone social and work plans until a time when you are feeling better.

> ### Did You Know?
>
> **Slow Cooking**
> Because much of the food in the LGS Diet Plan is well cooked, we highly recommend using a slow cooker. These inexpensive small appliances cook foods over a long period of time, helping to break down fibers and other food compounds into more easily digestible components. Stews, roasts and congee (see page 119) are very easy for anyone to prepare in a slow cooker.

Nothing can be more frustrating than self-sabotage. It can impede your progress and set you back to a point where it is difficult to motivate yourself and recover. Have the foresight to plan and prioritize accordingly.

Phase 1: Calming Diet

This gentle, calming phase is the most restrictive phase of diet modification, but it is necessary to dampen the inflammatory response.

The first phase of the diet is intended for severe, unrelenting states of inflammation with a very low threshold of aggravation and increasing gut hyperpermeability. Examples of this state are eczema, psoriasis, irritable bowel syndrome, inflammatory bowel disease and other inflammatory conditions affecting various components of the body. All of these can stem from leaky gut syndrome. This gentle, calming phase is the most restrictive phase of diet modification — permitted foods are typically hypoallergenic and easier to digest — but it is necessary to dampen the inflammatory response. Remember, this phase does not last forever. You will be able to expand your diet once your digestive tract starts healing.

FAQ

Q How do I know if I need to begin with Phase 1?

A You will know that Phase 1 is a necessary stage for you if:

- You are at your wit's end with your current health.
- Your symptoms are dramatically impacting your work, home and social life and causing much distress.
- You can feel quite depressed and you often feel overwhelming anxiety as a direct result of your physical health.

Phase 1 Restrictions

This phase is the only part of the overall diet in which we recommend eating only cooked foods. Cooking food does some of the work of the digestive tract. A compromised, stressed gut has less energy to do all the tasks it normally should, namely breaking down foods into more manageable components to process and absorb. Cooked foods are softer and easier to digest, and many of the macromolecules are broken down by the cooking process, making them easier to assimilate. An added calming measure is that cooked food has fewer large particles available to cross the gut–blood barrier to further aggravate the diseased state. Cooking also helps to break down insoluble fiber, which can be difficult for a dysfunctional gut to handle.

In addition to avoiding raw and cold foods, take the following steps to eliminate troublesome foods from your diet during this phase:

- Avoid all products containing gluten, eggs, dairy, shellfish, soy, beef, pork, peanuts, chocolate, tomatoes, caffeine and alcohol.
- Avoid cruciferous vegetables (arugula, bok choy, broccoli, Brussels sprouts, cauliflower, collard greens, kale, mustard greens, radish, rutabaga, Swiss chard, turnip, watercress).
- Eliminate onions, garlic, shallots, chives and leeks from your diet.
- Avoid fruit, vegetable and nut skins (because of their insoluble fiber).
- Stick to whole foods.
- Eliminate all processed, artificial, additive-laden foods from your diet.
- Omit black pepper and spices (besides those listed on pages 114–115) from your recipes.

This list may seem extensive, but focus on what you *can* eat, as many satisfying and interesting options are still available to you.

> **Food Prep Tips for Phase 1**
> - Remove skins from all fruits, vegetables and nuts.
> - Bake, lightly steam or lightly stir-fry all fruits and vegetables, or add them to soups and stews.
> - Prepare congee (see page 119) as a dietary base to settle your gut.
> - Stick to fluids that are at room temperature or warmer.

Phase 2: Restoring Diet

The second phase is intended for moderately bothersome conditions related to a leaky gut. This restoring phase follows the slightly more restrictive calming phase, which is designed to settle down severe inflammation. Some previously excluded food groups can now be reintroduced. Foods don't all have to be cooked, which makes this phase a little easier to manage. Fruit, vegetable and nut skins are allowed. The restoring phase is designed for mild to moderate instances of inflammation. People with mild to moderate inflammatory states can skip the calming phase to go straight to this phase.

FAQ

Q How do I know if I am ready for Phase 2 or can begin with Phase 2?

A You will know you are ready to implement Phase 2 when:

- Your health problems are annoying or bothersome, but you are still functional.
- Your moods can be affected when symptoms act up, but you are still rational.
- You are frustrated with your health state and want things to improve.
- Your daily life is thrown off from time to time, but you can still manage.

Phase 2 Adjustments

For the most part, the Phase 2 diet is similar to that of Phase 1, with some foods reintroduced and with less strict guidelines on food preparation and temperature. Allowed foods now include:

- Black pepper
- Cooked chives, garlic, leeks, onion and shallots
- Cooked cruciferous vegetables (arugula, bok choy, broccoli, Brussels sprouts, cauliflower, collard greens, kale, mustard greens, radish, rutabaga, Swiss chard, turnip, watercress)

- Cooler foods and fluids
- Nuts (for example, almonds, pecans, walnuts) with their skins
- Raw fresh culinary herbs
- Raw fruits and vegetables, including smoothies
- Tomatoes (but not tomato sauce)
- Unpeeled fruits and vegetables

Phase 3: Maintenance Diet

The third phase is an individually tailored plan to expand your diet to make it more enjoyable and realistic for you to implement and manage in the long term. The diet is designed to allow you to gradually introduce restricted foods, carefully monitoring for reactions to ensure that they don't cause chronic problems down the road. This phase of the diet plan is more fluid, fluctuating over time based on individual responses and your own interest in reintroducing foods.

FAQ

Q When should I start Phase 3?

A When inflammation is normalized, you can carefully reintroduce foods and expand your menu for long-term maintenance. Implement this phase when:

- Your symptoms and digestion have been normalized for 1 month.
- You feel in control of your health and are symptom-free or have minimal and tolerable symptoms.
- You feel confident in your physical health and are mentally ready to start adding foods to your diet.
- You are optimistic and feel ready for the challenge but will diligently monitor reactions as you reintroduce foods.

Guidelines for Reintroducing Foods

1. Reintroduce foods in any order you choose.

2. Eat a moderate portion of each newly reintroduced food at two meals each day for no less than 3 consecutive days.

3. If you want to be very cautious, or if it is not a food you would eat regularly, you can start with a small portion at one meal each day over the 3 days (or longer if you prefer to be extremely cautious).

4. If your symptoms return after you reintroduce a food, exclude it from your diet and categorize it as one to which you are sensitive. Wait for your symptoms to settle down, and only then introduce the next new food, so that you are able to properly track your response from your baseline.

5. If your symptoms do not change over the 3-day introduction, add that food to your list of allowable foods and introduce the next food to your diet.

6. Be sure to track your diet, noting the introduced food, the portions and any symptoms. (You can use the diet diary on page 101.)

Foods to Reintroduce

Here is a list of foods to introduce in Phase 3. Many of these foods were banned in Phase 1 and Phase 2. Reintroducing eliminated foods should be an enjoyable process. Look at it as a chance to expand your diet, and start with the foods you miss the most. Introduce them gradually as part of your regular diet. You do not need to introduce all of these foods.

Introducing them safely allows for a larger variety of food options over the long term. If you do not like some of these foods, if you are certain that they will aggravate your condition, or if you prefer to avoid them for other reasons, skip that food category altogether. Caffeine and alcohol are optional and recommended only in moderation. Be very careful to monitor any aggravation of symptoms with these substances.

- Alcohol: if introduced, drink only moderate amounts, at a maximum frequency of one drink per day for women and two drinks per day for men
- Beef: grass-fed and preferably naturally raised

- Caffeine: if introduced, drink only in moderation (one 8 oz/250 mL cup of drip coffee per day, with milk alternative, or two 8 oz/250 mL cups of quality loose-leaf green or black tea, steeped for 2 minutes or less)
- Chocolate: dairy-free, preferably dark (70% plus), with minimal or natural sweetening
- Dairy (grass-fed dairy products are preferred, if available): aged hard cow's-milk cheeses, such as Parmesan or aged Cheddar; goat's-milk or sheep's-milk cheeses; organic butter
- Eggs: free-range organic; start with hard-cooked or scrambled eggs and work up slowly to soft-boiled or fried eggs while monitoring carefully for adverse reactions
- Gluten-containing products: start with dry pasta as a gluten trial, since it is typically egg-free and dairy-free; limit to two times per week, even for the long term
- Peanuts
- Pork: free-range and naturally raised
- Raw cruciferous vegetables
- Raw onion and garlic as ingredients (for example, in hummus, guacamole, salsa)
- Shellfish
- Soy: reintroduce non-GMO organic tofu and tempeh
- Tomato sauce: preservative-free, preferably organic

Possible Reactions to Reintroduced Foods

Reintroducing a food after a period of avoidance can lead to one of two possible outcomes. You may find that you are now able to tolerate the food and enjoy eating it in moderation. Or the food may trigger a reaction that is even more severe than your previous symptoms after eating that food.

Increased Tolerance

After following these diet modifications and recovering your good health, you may find that your tolerance to certain reintroduced foods is better than it was before, when you were unhealthy. This is not because you weren't sensitive to these foods. Rather, your previous, more extreme reaction was a by-product of a hyperpermeable gut; now, after a period of restriction, the food elicits no response or a much lesser response. In these situations, an

> **Did You Know?**
>
> **Multiple Ingredients**
> Reintroduce products containing multiple ingredients only after you have proved to yourself that the individual ingredients do not aggravate you. For example, pizza commonly contains dairy, gluten, eggs and tomato sauce, each of which is a common allergen.

elimination period reduces inflammation and improves the tolerance of the gut to negative stressors as it recuperates.

Think of a full glass of water spilling over (symptom presentation). Once you empty the glass and start slowly adding drops of water, it does not spill over. Similarly, settling inflammation at the level of the gut mucosa by avoiding trigger foods for long enough is like emptying the glass. After you reintroduce the previously aggravating foods, the symptoms do not manifest as long as you consume the food only occasionally. In essence, certain foods have a cumulative response. After clearing inflammation and keeping your intake minimal, these foods will not produce the same symptoms.

> *Certain foods have a cumulative response. After clearing inflammation and keeping your intake minimal, these foods will not produce the same symptoms.*

Amplified Reaction

When you reintroduce certain other trigger foods, you may find that they aggravate you more than they did before, although you may otherwise feel much improved or even symptom-free. Even a one-time reintroduction can elicit noticeable and sometimes severe symptoms. This is not because your system has weakened but because you are more aware of how that sensitivity manifests when you are in a healthy state.

A good analogy for this is smoking: a two-pack-a-day smoker will always remember how awful he felt when smoking his first cigarette. Our bodies adapt to chronic negative stimuli in such a way that our response diminishes and we can continue to function.

This type of sensitivity occurs because your body adapted to the negative stressor while you were consuming it regularly. Once you eliminate the stressors for an appropriate length of time, your body calms and heals in the absence of the stimulus. When you reintroduce the food, your body's seemingly more severe reaction is its actual, true response to the negative stimulus.

FAQ

Q When can I expect to feel better?

A This can vary dramatically from person to person, and unfortunately the honest answer I have to give patients is: "It depends." There are so many and highly variable presentations of leaky gut syndrome that there is not a linear equation for determining prognosis (as compared to determining the prognosis for one specific medication given to treat one specific condition).

The equation is complicated by a multipronged treatment plan that incorporates several different angles and that may include a diet and lifestyle overhaul. This adds huge variables to the plan, such as the following: patient compliance, to what degree a patient decides to incorporate the recommendations, preexisting health state, preexisting diet and lifestyle, medication regime, how long a patient has had leaky gut syndrome, the severity of the presentation and to what degree a patient's health state is affecting the ability to digest, assimilate and metabolize nutrients.

The list of variables is endless; however, a rough prognosis can be determined by your health practitioner after a full health history has been assessed, along with a physical exam. With proper education, coaching and monitoring, an estimate can be given, assuming full compliance with the plan. As examples of what I have seen in practice, some groups of patients start to notice improvements within just a few days. Other patients may actually worsen initially before getting better (particularly when they make a drastic change from a previously unhealthy diet and lifestyle to the leaky gut plan). Other patients may notice improvements after the plan has been followed for 1 month or more. Generally speaking, I would expect to observe some noticeable improvements within 2 to 3 months of fully implementing the leaky gut syndrome plan. Tweaks and modifications are often implemented during follow-ups and monitoring, based on how the patient's health is progressing. Some patients may have complete resolution in a month, whereas others may take a full year to experience major improvements in functioning.

Doc Talk

As you begin to follow the Leaky Gut Syndrome Diet Plan, be sure that you are under the care of a health-care professional who is monitoring your health and supporting you with an appropriate treatment plan. Be open with your doctor about your intention to implement diet changes to both reduce inflammation and target leaky gut syndrome. Share your motivation and goals, and request a professional opinion.

If your symptoms are in a severe flared-up state, do not use this plan as a substitute for professional assistance. Explore all your treatment options and ensure that you are fully informed. This diet plan may be used as a complement to other treatments that are targeting reduced inflammation. The most critical goal in a severely inflamed state is to get your health to a more manageable level. Try your best to stay even-keeled mentally and emotionally while on the diet plan.

PART 4

Meal Plans for the LGS Diet Plan

Restoring Diet

Tamiko is an outgoing patient who presented with the chief complaint of foggy-headedness and fatigue for 2 years, along with eczema. Upon further querying during her assessment, Tamiko complained of constant low-level gastrointestinal bloating that worsened through the course of the day. Bowel movements were normal for the majority of the time, but episodes of constipation or diarrhea occurred every 2 weeks, with severe, worsening bloating. This condition had preceded her main concerns by 2 years.

The onset of the bloating occurred after an acute episode of bacterial pharyngitis (inflammation of the pharynx, an area at the back of the throat), which was treated with rounds of two different antibiotics because of its persistence. The bloating gradually worsened over a couple of years to the point where it became a daily occurrence. Tamiko had abdominal discomfort but no pain. The foggy-headedness affected her ability to work at her management position and caused her a great deal of stress as a result. Eventually, it led to a chronic lack of energy, and she became dependent on caffeine to get through her days and accomplish her tasks. She had also developed eczema for the first time, within the last year. It was mild but presented on Tamiko's hands, and it sometimes cracked in the winter months, which made it painful to move her fingers. She worked long hours and ate most of her meals at food courts or in restaurants, or by ordering takeout.

The gut hyperpermeability test showed a slightly elevated lactulose-to-mannitol ratio, which confirmed leaky gut syndrome. We also ran a comprehensive stool test, which determined that her levels of *Lactobacillus* and *Bifidobacterium* strains were almost undetectable, indicating she needed a probiotic supplement. Her IgG food sensitivity test showed multiple positives for dietary aggravators (a common occurrence in leaky gut syndrome).

We recommended overhauling Tamiko's diet and put her on the Restoring Diet, and outlined that she had to focus on home cooking and sourcing healthier takeout options if she was pressed for time. This was a huge change for her, but she was willing to commit because of her poor quality of life and decreased work performance. We also recommended that she incorporate into her health routine an easily absorbed multivitamin, probiotics, L-glutamine, high-potency fish oils and rhodiola (a herb for assisting with managing stress and moods by normalizing levels of norepinephrine, serotonin and dopamine).

Initially, in the first 10 days, she experienced a worsening of fatigue and foggy-headedness along with the onset of headaches, which was not a surprise, based on her caffeine withdrawal and the radical change in eating habits. By the third week, Tamiko's energy levels had stabilized and her cognition had improved dramatically. Her sleep and moods normalized in response, and her bloating had completely subsided by the second month. Compliance was good overall.

As a result of these improvements, we started to reintroduce foods to her diet. The eczema settled down, her skin became more supple and it had cleared entirely by the 6-month mark without the use of prescription creams. By this point, Tamiko's tolerance to aggravating foods had improved so that she could indulge occasionally without any repercussions.

How to Use the Meal Plans

The following meal plans (and the accompanying recipes in Part 5) are provided as templates for meals and snacks that will help reduce inflammation in your body, stabilize digestion and resolve hyperpermeability. You can try following the plans to the letter, but they are not set in stone. Don't worry too much if you slip up and eat a food that is not LGS-friendly. Just resolve to eat more gut-friendly foods for your next meal.

The meal plans and recipes provide a variety of foods to help you meet your nutritional requirements. Because the focus is not on weight management (whether loss, maintenance or gain), there are no specific portion sizes provided for the main meals, though all are roughly based on one serving of each recipe unless otherwise indicated. Portion sizes have been provided for the snacks and beverages, but only as a guide; we recommend that you continue eat the same amount of food you normally do. If you are concerned about your weight and feel you need guidance with portion sizes, ask your dietitian for help creating a weight management plan that will work within the parameters of the Leaky Gut Syndrome Diet Plan.

We have provided a 2-week meal plan for Phase 1 and a 4-week meal plan for Phase 2, to help you get the idea of how to put gut-healthy meals together before you set out to create your own meal plans with the help of the 150 recipes. Soon enough, the Leaky Gut Syndrome Diet Plan will become second nature. By the time you're in Phase 3, when your diet will be more individualized and much less restrictive, you'll be a pro at planning meals!

If you are concerned about your weight and feel you need guidance with portion sizes, ask your dietitian for help creating a weight management plan that will work within the parameters of the Leaky Gut Syndrome Diet Plan.

Starting Out

First you'll need to determine which diet phase you should be starting with, based on the severity of your current symptoms. Phase 1 is designed for people with severe inflammation, while Phase 2 is designed for those with mild to moderate inflammation.

If you're starting with Phase 1, try our 2-week meal plan, then repeat it as many times as necessary until you are ready to move on to Phase 2, or adapt our meal plan to suit your personal tastes or create your own meal plans within the parameters of the Phase 1 diet.

Similarly, if you are starting with Phase 2 (or once you progress to Phase 2 from Phase 1), follow our 4-week meal plan, then adapt it at will (within the parameters of the Phase 2 diet) until you are ready to move on to Phase 3.

Phase 3 is designed to help you maintain your renewed health. At this point, you will be creating your own meal plans as you gradually reintroduce foods, one at a time, into your diet, experimenting to see what works for you and what doesn't.

Adapt our meal plan to suit your personal tastes or create your own meal plans within the parameters of the diet.

Using the Recipes in This Book

The recipes in this book have some key features that will help make meal planning easier for you. First off, in the top left corner of each recipe, you'll see a tag identifying which phases the recipe is suitable for. If the tag says "Suitable for Phases 1, 2 & 3," feel free to enjoy it in any of the three phases (although you may need to make some adjustments to it, as noted below). If it states "Suitable for Phases 2 & 3," you should give it a pass while you're in Phase 1, as it contains some of the restricted ingredients. If the tag says "Suitable for Phase 3," you should wait to enjoy it until you are in Phase 3.

Some recipes also include an "Adjustment" box, which outlines what changes you will need to make to the recipe to make it suitable for a certain phase. For example, Fresh Basil Pesto (page 300) is suitable for Phase 1 if you adjust it by omitting the garlic, Parmesan cheese and pepper. Once you're in Phase 2, you can add the garlic and pepper back in, but you still need to leave out the cheese. In Phase 3, you can enjoy the recipe as written.

In addition to or in place of phase-specific adjustments, many recipes offer "Advice for a Healthy Gut": tips that will help you make the best choices for the health of your gut, regardless of what phase of the LGS Diet Plan you are in.

The final feature to look for in each recipe is the nutrient analysis, located in the bottom left corner. This table tells you the amount of calories, fat, carbohydrate, fiber, protein, vitamin A, iron and zinc provided by that recipe. Understanding the breakdown of calories, fat, carbohydrates and protein can help you customize your meal plan to ensure that you are getting balanced nutrition and are working within your parameters to manage your weight. Insoluble fiber can irritate an inflamed gut lining, so it's a good idea to keep an eye on your daily intake of fiber and adjust it according to guidelines established with your dietitian. Food-derived vitamin A and zinc support the health of the gut mucosa and the immune system; therefore, they are key nutrients to monitor and emphasize in your diet. As for iron, decreased serum levels of iron can occur in inflammatory bowel disease, potentially leading to anemia, so it's important to track your iron intake and ensure that you are consuming an adequate amount.

Insoluble fiber can irritate an inflamed gut lining, so it's a good idea to keep an eye on your daily intake of fiber and adjust it according to guidelines established with your dietitian.

LGS Diet Plan Timeline

One of the main questions people have when they embark on the LGS Diet Plan is how long they will have to spend in each phase. Of course, the answer depends largely on each individual's symptoms and recovery. But here are some general guidelines to help you know what to expect.

Phase 1: Calming Diet

If you are starting with Phase 1, eat within these parameters until your severe symptoms start to settle down to a mild to moderate level. Wait until the reduced symptoms have settled for 2 consecutive weeks before moving on to Phase 2. As a general guideline, expect to stay in Phase 1 for at least 1 month. If symptoms are improving but not fully settled by the end of 1 month, continue Phase 1 until symptoms are more tolerable. If they have settled by the end of 1 month, proceed to Phase 2.

The time needed to normalize inflammation is often determined by how long you have been unwell.

Phase 2: Restoring Diet

Expect to stay in Phase 2 for longer than Phase 1. The time needed to normalize inflammation is often determined by how long you have been unwell. As a general rule, you should expect to stay in Phase 2 for 6 to 8 weeks. Phase 2 ends when your symptoms have stayed under control for at least 2 consecutive weeks, and when you feel confident that you are ready to reintroduce foods and expand your diet.

Phase 3: Maintenance Diet

Phase 3 is the most variable phase of the diet plan. This is a reintroduction phase that occurs after inflammation has settled and symptoms have resolved. It is designed to slowly test and reintroduce foods to ensure that they do not aggravate your health. Introduce each new food individually and cautiously while monitoring for any potential negative effects on your health. The length of this phase is dependent on how many foods you decide to test and introduce back into your diet. You can introduce one new food item every 3 days, or you can be more cautious and introduce a new food item once a week.

Introduce each new food individually and cautiously while monitoring for any potential negative effects on your health.

Phase 3 is also intended to ensure that you have as much variety as possible in your diet in the long term, by slowly expanding the repertoire of foods that you are able to safely consume. Be patient in Phase 3. This is a maintenance phase, where you establish a safe and enduring diet plan for yourself. Don't rush the reintroduction of foods, as you don't want to rock the boat. You want a clear picture of which foods are safe and which are aggravating.

Phase 1 Meal Plan: Calming Diet

The recipes featured in these meal plans can be found in Part 5 of this book. Look up each recipe, record the ingredients, make a shopping list for the week and enjoy good food — and good health.

Week 1

Meal	Sunday	Monday	Tuesday	
Breakfast	Breakfast Rice* 1 tbsp (15 mL) virgin coconut oil, stirred into cereal Honey or maple syrup to taste (optional)	Agave Flax Muffin* 1–2 tbsp (15–30 mL) nut or seed butter Honey to taste (optional)	Cranberry Quinoa Porridge* 1 tbsp (15 mL) virgin coconut oil, stirred into cereal Honey or maple syrup to taste (optional)	
Snack	6–8 rice crackers	½ cup (125 mL) Apple-Cranberry Compote*	4–8 spears steamed asparagus and ¼ sliced avocado with lime juice and sea salt	
Lunch	Grilled Chicken Breast with Pesto* Italian-Style Green Rice* Roasted Vegetables*	Leftover turkey, beets and pilaf from Sunday dinner	Leftover turkey, beets and pilaf from Sunday dinner	
Snack	¼ cup (60 mL) cashews	¼ cup (60 mL) green pumpkin seeds (pepitas)	¾ cup (175 mL) coconut yogurt	
Dinner	Slow-Roasted Turkey* Cumin Beets* Quinoa Pilaf*	Whole Baked Fish* Old English Celery Bake* Fragrant Coconut Rice*	Butternut Squash Soup* Maple Ginger Salmon* Herbed Potatoes*	
Beverage	Warm water with manuka honey to taste	Marshmallow root tea	Mullein tea	

* The recipe is in the book; unless otherwise indicated, the amount is 1 serving.

Wednesday	Thursday	Friday	Saturday
Breakfast Rice* 1 tbsp (15 mL) virgin coconut oil, stirred into cereal Honey or maple syrup to taste (optional)	2–3 Home-Style Pancakes* 1 tbsp (15 mL) virgin coconut oil, spread on pancakes 1–2 tbsp (15–30 mL) maple syrup	Hot Millet Amaranth Cereal* 1 tbsp (15 mL) virgin coconut oil, stirred into cereal Honey to taste (optional)	Pumpkin Spice Muffin* 1–2 tbsp (15–30 mL) nut or seed butter Honey to taste (optional)
½–1 peeled medium cucumber with lime juice and sea salt	¾ cup (175 mL) coconut yogurt	½–1 oz (15–30 g) roasted seaweed snack	¼ cup (60 mL) blanched almonds
Leftover fish, celery bake and rice from Monday dinner	Leftover soup, salmon and potatoes from Tuesday dinner	Leftover lamb, vegetables and carrot-turnip purée from Wednesday dinner	Leftover chicken, green beans and fennel from Thursday dinner Quinoa Pilaf*
¼ cup (60 mL) sunflower seeds	¼ cup (60 mL) macadamia nuts with cinnamon	½–¾ cup (125–175 mL) Apple Butter*	6 spears steamed asparagus with lime juice and sea salt
Grilled Lamb and Vegetables with Roasted Garlic* Gingered Carrot-Turnip Purée*	Chicken Kabobs with Ginger Lemon Marinade* Braised Green Beans and Fennel* Sweet Potato Fries*	Foil-Roasted Halibut and Asparagus* Old English Celery Bake* Mashed Sweet Potatoes with Rosemary*	Leftover halibut, celery bake and sweet potatoes from Friday dinner
8 oz (250 mL) warm almond milk	8 oz (250 mL) room-temperature coconut water	Slippery elm tea	Nettle tea with manuka honey to taste

Week 2

Meal	Sunday	Monday	Tuesday	
Breakfast	Hot Millet Amaranth Cereal* 1 tbsp (15 mL) virgin coconut oil, stirred into cereal Honey or maple syrup to taste (optional)	Applesauce Raisin Muffin* 1–2 tbsp (15–30 mL) nut or seed butter Honey to taste (optional)	Multigrain Quinoa Muffin* 1–2 tbsp (15–30 mL) nut or seed butter Honey to taste (optional)	
Snack	6–8 rice crackers	½ cup (125 mL) Apple-Cranberry Compote*	½–¾ cup (125–175 mL) Apple Butter*	
Lunch	Grilled Lamb and Vegetables with Roasted Garlic* Old English Celery Bake* Fragrant Coconut Rice*	Whole Baked Fish* Braised Green Beans and Fennel* Cilantro-Ginger Quinoa*	Leftover turkey, mushroom and rice from Sunday dinner	
Snack	¼ cup (60 mL) cashews	¾ cup (175 mL) coconut yogurt	¼ cup (60 mL) green pumpkin seeds (pepitas)	
Dinner	Slow-Roasted Turkey* Baked Portobello Mushroom* Vegetable Rice*	Chicken with Root Vegetables*	Leftover lamb, celery bake and rice from Sunday lunch	
Beverage	Warm water with manuka honey to taste	Marshmallow root tea	Mullein tea	

* The recipe is in the book; unless otherwise indicated, the amount is 1 serving.

Wednesday	Thursday	Friday	Saturday
Hot Millet Amaranth Cereal* 1 tbsp (15 mL) virgin coconut oil, stirred into cereal Honey or maple syrup to taste (optional)	Breakfast Rice* 1 tbsp (15 mL) virgin coconut oil, stirred into cereal Honey or maple syrup to taste (optional)	Agave Flax Muffin* 1–2 tbsp (15–30 mL) nut or seed butter Honey to taste (optional)	2 to 3 Home-Style Pancakes* 1 tbsp (15 mL) virgin coconut oil, spread on pancakes 1–2 tbsp (15–30 mL) maple syrup
¼ cup (60 mL) sunflower seeds	6–8 rice crackers	¾ cup (175 mL) coconut yogurt	½–¾ cup (125–175 mL) stewed peeled pear and berries
Leftover fish, green beans, fennel and quinoa from Monday lunch	Leftover chicken and root vegetables from Monday dinner	Traditional Small Roast Chicken* Summer Zucchini* Baked Parsnip Fries*	Leftover lamb, vegetables and pilaf from Thursday dinner
½–1 peeled medium cucumber with lime juice and sea salt	¼ cup (60 mL) macadamia nuts with cinnamon	½–1 oz (15–30 g) roasted seaweed snack	¼ cup (60 mL) blanched almonds
Leftover turkey, mushroom and rice from Sunday dinner	Grilled Lamb and Vegetables with Roasted Garlic* Quinoa Pilaf*	Maple Ginger Salmon* Old English Celery Bake* Fragrant Coconut Rice*	Leftover salmon, celery bake and rice from Friday dinner
8 oz (250 mL) warm almond milk	8 oz (250 mL) room-temperature coconut water	Slippery elm tea	Nettle tea with manuka honey to taste

Phase 2 Meal Plan: Restoring Diet

The recipes featured in these meal plans can be found in Part 5 of this book. Look up each recipe, record the ingredients, make a shopping list for the week and enjoy good food — and good health.

Week 1

Meal	Sunday	Monday	Tuesday	
Breakfast	Quinoa Flake Granola* 1 tbsp (15 mL) virgin coconut oil, drizzled on cereal Honey or maple syrup to taste (optional)	Spiced Fruit and Grain Cereal* Honey to taste (optional)	Basic Nut Milk Smoothie*	
Snack	6–8 rice crackers	Apple Beet Pear Smoothie*	1 piece of fruit	
Lunch	Grilled Cilantro Shrimp Skewers* Simple Stir-Fried Kale* Roasted Cauliflower Quinoa*	Leftover turkey, green beans, fennel and wild rice casserole from Sunday dinner	Seared Salmon with Pineapple Mint Quinoa* Sautéed Spinach with Pine Nuts* Sweet Potato, Apple and Raisin Casserole*	
Snack	1 piece of fruit	¼ cup (60 mL) green pumpkin seeds (pepitas)	¾ cup (175 mL) coconut yogurt	
Dinner	Slow-Roasted Turkey* Braised Green Beans and Fennel* Wild Rice, Snow Pea and Almond Casserole*	Leftover shrimp, kale and quinoa from Sunday lunch	Traditional Small Roast Chicken* Cumin Beets* Mediterranean Vegetable Casserole*	
Beverage	Warm water with manuka honey to taste	Marshmallow root tea	Mullein tea	

* The recipe is in the book; unless otherwise indicated, the amount is 1 serving.

Wednesday	Thursday	Friday	Saturday
Agave Flax Muffin* 1 tbsp (15 mL) virgin coconut oil Honey or maple syrup to taste (optional)	1–2 Home-Style Pancakes* 1 tbsp (15 mL) virgin coconut oil, spread on pancakes 1–2 tbsp (15–30 mL) maple syrup	Baked Pumpkin Quinoa* 1 tbsp (15 mL) virgin coconut oil, stirred into cereal Honey or maple syrup to taste (optional)	Big-Batch Seed and Nut Granola* Honey or maple syrup to taste (optional)
Cucumber Fizz*	Orange Zinger*	1/2–1 oz (15–30 g) roasted seaweed snack	1/4 cup (60 mL) blanched almonds
Leftover turkey, green beans, fennel and wild rice casserole from Sunday dinner	Leftover chicken, beets and vegetable casserole from Tuesday dinner	Leftover lamb and potatoes from Wednesday dinner	Grilled Cilantro Shrimp Skewers* Simple Stir-Fried Kale* Gingered Carrot Turnip Puree*
Raw vegetables 1/3 cup (75 mL) Melizzano Despina (Eggplant Dip)*	1/4 cup (60 mL) macadamia nuts with cinnamon	1/2–3/4 cup (125–175 mL) Apple Butter*	Fennel Fantasy*
Moroccan-Style Lamb with Raisins and Apricots* Herbed Potatoes*	Leftover salmon, spinach and sweet potato casserole from Tuesday lunch	Grilled Chicken Breast with Pesto* Braised Green Beans and Fennel* Cauliflower Rice*	Leftover chicken, green beans, fennel and cauliflower rice from Friday dinner
8 oz (250 mL) warm almond milk	8 oz (250 mL) room-temperature coconut water	Slippery elm tea	Nettle tea with manuka honey to taste

Week 2

Meal	Sunday	Monday	Tuesday	
Breakfast	1–2 Toasted Sesame Quinoa Bars*	Pumpkin Spice Muffin* 1–2 tbsp (15–30 mL) nut or seed butter Honey to taste (optional)	Basic Berry Smoothie*	
Snack	Green Tea and Blueberries*	¾ cup (175 mL) coconut yogurt	Avocado Orange Smoothie*	
Lunch	Cedar-Baked Salmon* Sautéed Vegetables* Italian Broiled Tomatoes*	Leftover turkey, cabbage and wild rice casserole from Sunday dinner	Leftover turkey, cabbage and wild rice casserole from Sunday dinner	
Snack	¼ cup (60 mL) cashews	1 piece of fruit	¼ cup (60 mL) green pumpkin seeds (pepitas)	
Dinner	Slow-Roasted Turkey* Braised Red Cabbage* Wild Rice, Snow Pea and Almond Casserole*	Rosemary-Smoked Halibut with Balsamic Vinaigrette* Sautéed Spinach with Pine Nuts* Vegetable Rice*	Leftover halibut, spinach and rice from Monday dinner	
Beverage	Warm water with manuka honey to taste	Marshmallow root tea	Mullein tea	

* The recipe is in the book; unless otherwise indicated, the amount is 1 serving.

Wednesday	Thursday	Friday	Saturday
Mixed Fruit, Chia and Flaxseed Porridge* Honey or maple syrup to taste (optional)	1–2 Home-Style Pancakes* 1 tbsp (15 mL) virgin coconut oil, spread on pancakes 1–2 tbsp (15–30 mL) maple syrup	Breakfast Rice* 1 tbsp (15 mL) virgin coconut oil, stirred into cereal Honey or maple syrup to taste (optional)	1–2 Chewy Coconut Quinoa Bars*
¼ cup (60 mL) sunflower seeds	Raw vegetables ⅓ cup (75 mL) Melizzano Despina (Eggplant Dip)*	1 piece of fruit	½–¾ cup (125–175 mL) Apple-Cranberry Compote*
Leftover salmon, vegetables and tomatoes from Sunday lunch	Leftover lamb, Brussels sprouts, sweet potatoes and sweet pepper strips from Wednesday dinner	Leftover chicken, spinach and rice from Thursday dinner	Traditional Small Roast Chicken* Simple Stir-Fried Kale* Roasted Cauliflower Quinoa*
½–1 peeled medium cucumber with lime juice and sea salt	Autumn Refresher*	½–1 oz (15–30 g) roasted seaweed snack	Nip of Goodness*
Roasted Lamb with Marrakech Rub* Brussels Sprouts with Pecans and Sweet Potatoes* Roasted Garlic Sweet Pepper Strips*	Grilled Garlic-Ginger Chicken Breast* Sautéed Spinach with Pine Nuts* Fragrant Coconut Rice*	Seared Salmon with Pineapple Mint Quinoa* Sweet Potato, Apple and Raisin Casserole*	Leftover salmon and sweet potato casserole from Friday lunch
8 oz (250 mL) warm almond milk	8 oz (250 mL) room-temperature coconut water	Slippery elm tea	Nettle tea with manuka honey to taste

Week 3

Meal	Sunday	Monday	Tuesday	
Breakfast	Hot Millet Amaranth Cereal* 1 tbsp (15 mL) virgin coconut oil, stirred into cereal Honey or maple syrup to taste (optional)	Mixed Fruit, Chia, and Flaxseed Porridge*	1–2 Sugar-Free Quinoa Granola Bars*	
Snack	6–8 rice crackers	1 piece of fruit	½–¾ cup (125–175 mL) Apple Butter*	
Lunch	Foil-Roasted Halibut and Asparagus* Brussels Sprouts with Pecans and Sweet Potatoes*	Leftover turkey, celery bake and beets from Sunday dinner	Leftover halibut, asparagus, Brussels sprouts and sweet potatoes from Sunday lunch	
Snack	Chocolate Pecan Smoothie*	¼ cup (60 mL) green pumpkin seeds (pepitas)	Deep Orange Heart*	
Dinner	Slow-Roasted Turkey* Old English Celery Bake* Cumin Beets*	Salmon with Cranberry and Caper Vinaigrette* Roasted Garlic Sweet Pepper Strips* Roasted Cauliflower Quinoa*	Moroccan-Style Lamb with Raisins and Apricots* Wild Rice, Snow Pea and Almond Casserole*	
Beverage	Warm water with manuka honey to taste	Marshmallow root tea	Mullein tea	

* The recipe is in the book; unless otherwise indicated, the amount is 1 serving.

Wednesday	Thursday	Friday	Saturday
Mixed Fruit, Chia, and Flaxseed Porridge*	Cranberry Quinoa Porridge* 1 tbsp (15 mL) virgin coconut oil, stirred into cereal Honey or maple syrup to taste (optional)	Basic Berry Smoothie*	Big-Batch Seed and Nut Granola*
¼ cup (60 mL) sunflower seeds	¼ cup (60 mL) macadamia nuts with cinnamon	¾ cup (175 mL) coconut yogurt	1 piece of fruit
Leftover turkey, celery bake and beets from Sunday dinner	Leftover lamb and wild rice casserole from Tuesday dinner	Leftover chicken, kale and rice from Thursday dinner	Grilled Lamb and Vegetables with Roasted Garlic* Balsamic Asparagus with Walnuts* Sweet Potato, Apple and Raisin Casserole*
½–1 peeled medium cucumber with lime juice and sea salt	Creamy Fennel Smoothie*	½–1 oz (15–30 g) roasted seaweed snack	Raw vegetables ⅓ cup (75 mL) Melizzano Despina (Eggplant Dip)*
Leftover salmon, sweet pepper strips and quinoa from Monday dinner	Traditional Small Roast Chicken* Simple Stir-Fried Kale* Vegetable Rice*	Chicken Kabobs with Ginger-Lemon Marinade* Italian-Style Green Rice* Roasted Vegetables*	Leftover chicken, rice and vegetables from Friday dinner
8 oz (250 mL) warm almond milk	8 oz (250 mL) room-temperature coconut water	Slippery elm tea	Nettle tea with manuka honey to taste

Week 4

Meal	Sunday	Monday	Tuesday	
Breakfast	Pumpkin Spice Muffin* 1–2 tbsp (15–30 mL) nut or seed butter Honey to taste (optional)	Quinoa Flake Granola* Honey or maple syrup to taste (optional)	1–2 Toasted Sesame Quinoa Bars*	
Snack	Avocado Orange Smoothie*	¾ cup (175 mL) Apple-Cranberry Compote*	Spin Doctor*	
Lunch	Grilled Lamb and Vegetables with Roasted Garlic* Delicata Squash with Quinoa Stuffing*	Grilled Cilantro Shrimp Skewers* Wild Rice, Snow Pea and Almond Casserole* Sautéed Vegetables*	Leftover salmon, hearts of palm and artichoke and potatoes from Sunday dinner	
Snack	¼ cup (60 mL) cashews	¾ cup (175 mL) coconut yogurt	¼ cup (60 mL) green pumpkin seeds (pepitas)	
Dinner	Salmon with Cranberry and Caper Vinaigrette* Hearts of Palm and Artichoke* Herbed Potatoes*	Chicken Kabobs with Ginger-Lemon Marinade* Italian Broiled Tomatoes* Mashed Sweet Potatoes*	Leftover lamb, vegetables and stuffed squash from Sunday lunch	
Beverage	Warm water with manuka honey to taste	Marshmallow root tea	Mullein tea	

* The recipe is in the book; unless otherwise indicated, the amount is 1 serving.

Wednesday	Thursday	Friday	Saturday
Basic Nut Milk Smoothie*	Mixed Fruit, Chia and Flaxseed Porridge*	1–2 Chewy Coconut Quinoa Bars*	Breakfast Rice* 1 tbsp (15 mL) virgin coconut oil, stirred into cereal Honey or maple syrup to taste (optional)
¼ cup (60 mL) sunflower seeds	Orange Sunrise*	¾ cup (175 mL) coconut yogurt	½–¾ cup (125–175 mL) Apple Butter*
Leftover chicken, tomatoes and sweet potatoes from Monday dinner	Moroccan-Style Lamb with Raisins and Apricots* Wild Rice, Snow Pea and Almond Casserole*	Leftover halibut, asparagus, Brussels sprouts and sweet potatoes from Thursday dinner	Leftover lamb and wild rice casserole from Thursday lunch
½–1 peeled medium cucumber with lime juice and sea salt	¼ cup (60 mL) macadamia nuts with cinnamon	½–1 oz (15–30 g) roasted seaweed snack	Orange Zinger*
Grilled Cilantro Shrimp Skewers* Wild Rice, Snow Pea and Almond Casserole* Sautéed Vegetables*	Foil-Roasted Halibut and Asparagus* Brussels Sprouts with Pecans and Sweet Potatoes*	Slow-Roasted Turkey* Balsamic Asparagus with Walnuts* Herbed Potatoes*	Leftover turkey, asparagus and potatoes from Friday dinner
8 oz (250 mL) room-temperature coconut water	8 oz (250 mL) room-temperature coconut water	Slippery elm tea	Nettle tea with manuka honey to taste

Tips for Eating Out While on the LGS Diet

The advantage of making your own meals is that you can cook in bulk, freeze portions and take leftovers to work. But let's face it, life is busy. There isn't always time to make home-cooked meals, and there's nothing wrong with that. When a busy schedule gets in the way, you can still work on healing your gut while on the go.

Bring a copy of the basic guidelines for each phase with you, to help you navigate restaurant menus, and keep the following tips in mind:

- Stick with meat, fish, vegetables and plain rice. Try to get meat, fish and vegetables that are cooked as plainly as possible, without sauces or flavorings. Cooked grains that are appropriate for the LGS diet will likely be hard to find, with the exception of plain steamed rice and perhaps plain cooked quinoa.
- Choose grilled or poached foods. Grilling and poaching are the best cooking methods for the LGS Diet Plan, but sautéed foods are acceptable if necessary, so long as the restaurant uses vegetable oil for sautéing (ask your server). Avoid fried foods and dishes with sauces or flavorings made with unknown ingredients.

PART 5

Recipes for the LGS Diet Plan

About the Nutrient Analysis

The nutrient analysis done on the recipes in this book was derived from the Food Processor SQL Nutrition Analysis software, version 10.9, ESHA Research (2011). Where necessary, data was supplemented using the USDA National Nutrient Database for Standard Reference, release #27 (2014) (retrieved October 2014 from the USDA Agricultural Research Service website: www.nal. usda.gov/fnic/foodcomp/search/).

Recipes were evaluated as follows:

- The larger number of servings was used where there is a range.
- Where alternatives are given, the first ingredient and amount listed were used.
- Optional ingredients and ingredients that are not quantified were not included.
- Calculations were based on imperial measures and weights.
- The smaller quantity of an ingredient was used where a range is provided.
- Low-fat (1%) milk or fortified milk alternative beverages were used when the percentage of fat is not specified.
- Calculations involving meat and poultry used lean portions.
- Recipes were analyzed prior to cooking.

It is important to note that the cooking method used to prepare the recipe may alter the nutrient content per serving, as may ingredient substitutions and differences among brand-name products.

Breakfasts

Big-Batch Seed and Nut Granola

Suitable for Phases 2 & 3

Nuts and seeds are a great way to get vitamin E, an antioxidant with anti-inflammatory properties that helps to heal an inflamed gut. This granola can be eaten on its own or served simply with a milk alternative such as unsweetened, carrageenan-free rice, almond, hemp or coconut milk.

Tip

Layer dairy-free yogurt (such as coconut yogurt), fresh berries and granola in a tall glass or small Mason jar. Assemble in the evening, cover and place on a tray in the fridge. In the morning, open the fridge and enjoy!

- Preheat oven to 275°F (140°C)
- 2 baking sheets

1/2 cup	pure maple syrup	125 mL
2 tbsp	vegetable oil	30 mL
2 tbsp	liquid honey	30 mL
1 tsp	vanilla extract (gluten-free, if needed)	5 mL
2¾ cups	quick-cooking rolled oats (certified gluten-free, if needed)	675 mL
1/2 cup	sunflower seeds	125 mL
1/2 cup	pumpkin seeds	125 mL
1/2 cup	sliced almonds	125 mL
1/4 cup	sesame seeds	60 mL
2 tbsp	ground flax seeds (flaxseed meal)	30 mL
3/4 cup	dried fruit (raisins, blueberries, cranberries or cherries)	175 mL
3/4 cup	unsweetened flaked coconut	175 mL

1. In a large bowl, combine maple syrup, oil, honey and vanilla. Add oats, sunflower seeds, pumpkin seeds, almonds, sesame seeds and flax seeds. Mix well. Spread mixture evenly on baking sheets.

2. Bake in preheated oven for 15 minutes. Add dried fruit and coconut; mix well. Bake for 15 minutes or until lightly browned. Let cool on a clean baking sheet before storing in an airtight container for up to 1 month.

This recipe courtesy of Eileen Campbell.

Advice for a Healthy Gut

▶ "Vegetable oil" is a catchall term for any edible oil from a plant source, whether it be a vegetable, fruit, nut or seed. While you are following the LGS Diet Plan, the best choices for this recipe are grapeseed oil, macadamia nut oil and melted virgin coconut oil.

▶ Choose unsweetened dried fruit.

▶ Chew the granola well to ensure better digestion.

Nutrients per serving

Calories	191
Fat	10 g
Carbohydrate	23 g
Fiber	3 g
Protein	5 g
Vitamin A	1 IU
Iron	1.7 mg
Zinc	0.8 mg

Quinoa Flake Granola

Makes about 3½ cups (875 mL)

Suitable for Phases 2 & 3

Prepare yourself for the one of the crispiest, crunchiest and most delicious granolas you've ever had. It's all about the quinoa flakes, which are lighter in texture than oats and readily form the kinds of clusters you're looking for when making granola. The possibilities for variation are endless, so have fun with spices, sweeteners, nuts, seeds, flaked coconut and dried fruit.

- Preheat oven to 325°F (160°C)
- Large rimmed baking sheet, lined with parchment paper

2 cups	quinoa flakes	500 mL
½ cup	chopped pecans	125 mL
¼ cup	ground flax seeds (flaxseed meal)	60 mL
2 tsp	ground cinnamon	10 mL
½ cup	pure maple syrup or liquid honey	125 mL
2 tbsp	vegetable oil or unsalted butter, melted	30 mL
2 tsp	vanilla extract (gluten-free, if needed)	10 mL
½ cup	dried blueberries, cranberries or chopped cherries	125 mL

1. In a large bowl, combine quinoa flakes, pecans, flax seeds and cinnamon.

2. In a medium bowl, whisk together maple syrup, oil and vanilla until well blended.

3. Add the maple mixture to the quinoa mixture and stir until well coated. Spread mixture in a single layer on prepared baking sheet.

4. Bake in preheated oven for 22 to 27 minutes or until quinoa flakes are golden brown. Let cool completely on pan.

5. Transfer granola to an airtight container and stir in blueberries. Store at room temperature for up to 2 weeks.

Adjustment for Phase 2

▸ Use grapeseed oil, macadamia nut oil or melted virgin coconut oil for the vegetable oil. Do not use butter.

Advice for a Healthy Gut

▸ Once you're in Phase 3, you may choose to use organic butter.

▸ Choose unsweetened dried fruit.

▸ Chew the granola well to ensure better digestion.

Nutrients per ½ cup (125 mL)

Calories	381
Fat	14 g
Carbohydrate	57 g
Fiber	6 g
Protein	8 g
Vitamin A	13 IU
Iron	2.8 mg
Zinc	2.4 mg

Spiced Fruit and Grain Cereal

Suitable for Phases 2 & 3

A serving of this über-healthy cereal will let you sail through to lunchtime without feeling hungry. The pleasing mix of flavors and textures will make this your new favorite breakfast.

1/2 cup	quinoa, rinsed	125 mL
1/8 tsp	fine sea salt	0.5 mL
1 cup	water	250 mL
3/4 cup	milk or plain non-dairy milk (such as almond, rice or hemp)	175 mL
1/2 cup	large-flake (old-fashioned) rolled oats (certified gluten-free, if needed)	125 mL
3 tbsp	chopped dried figs or dried apricots	45 mL
2 tbsp	ground flax seeds (flaxseed meal)	30 mL
1/4 tsp	ground ginger	1 mL
1/4 tsp	ground cloves	1 mL
2 tbsp	chopped toasted walnuts	30 mL
2 tbsp	liquid honey	30 mL

1. In a medium saucepan, combine quinoa, salt, water and milk. Bring to a boil over medium–high heat. Reduce heat to low, cover and simmer for 10 minutes.

2. Stir in oats, figs, flax seeds, ginger and cloves. Cover and simmer for 5 to 8 minutes or until most of the liquid is absorbed and quinoa and oats are cooked through. Stir in walnuts and drizzle with honey.

Advice for a Healthy Gut

▸ While you are following the LGS Diet Plan, avoid dairy milk and soy milk. Use unsweetened, carrageenan-free rice, almond, hemp or coconut milk instead.

▸ Choose unsweetened dried fruit.

Nutrients per serving	
Calories	475
Fat	13 g
Carbohydrate	77 g
Fiber	9 g
Protein	16 g
Vitamin A	190 IU
Iron	4.4 mg
Zinc	2.4 mg

Hot Millet Amaranth Cereal

**Suitable for
Phases 1, 2 & 3**

*Here's a great way to start
your day and add variety
to your diet. Both millet
and amaranth are gluten-
free and relatively quick
and easy to cook — so
long as you keep the
temperature low, they
don't need to be stirred.
Use a sweetener of your
choice and add dried fruit
and nuts as you please.*

Tip

For best results, toast
the millet and amaranth
before cooking. Stir the
grains in a dry skillet
over medium heat until
they crackle and release
their aroma, about
5 minutes.

2½ cups	water	625 mL
½ cup	millet, toasted (see tip, at left)	125 mL
½ cup	amaranth, toasted	125 mL
	Liquid honey, pure maple syrup or raw cane sugar	
	Milk or non-dairy alternative	
	Dried cranberries, cherries or raisins (optional)	
	Toasted chopped nuts (optional)	

1. In a saucepan over medium heat, bring water to a boil. Add millet and amaranth in a steady stream, stirring constantly. Return to a boil. Reduce heat to low (see tip, page 164). Cover and simmer until grains are tender and liquid is absorbed, about 25 minutes. Serve hot, sweetened to taste and with milk or non-dairy alternative. Sprinkle with dried fruit and nuts, if desired.

Adjustments for Phase 1

▶ Do not add the optional dried fruit.

▶ Use only skin-free nuts.

Advice for a Healthy Gut

▶ While you are following the LGS Diet Plan, choose honey or maple syrup as the sweetener for this recipe.

▶ Avoid dairy milk and soy milk. Use unsweetened, carrageenan-free rice, almond, hemp or coconut milk instead.

▶ In Phases 2 and 3, if you decide to add dried fruit, choose unsweetened dried fruit.

▶ Once you're in Phases 2 and 3, you may use nuts with skins, if desired.

Nutrients per serving	
Calories	123
Fat	2 g
Carbohydrate	23 g
Fiber	3 g
Protein	4 g
Vitamin A	0 IU
Iron	1.7 mg
Zinc	0.8 mg

Baked Pumpkin Quinoa

Makes 4 servings

Suitable for Phases 2 & 3

Pumpkin provides beta-carotene, which the body converts to vitamin A, a nutrient essential for rebuilding and strengthening the digestive tract. Serve this cereal straight up or with any of the suggested accompaniments for a super-energizing breakfast.

Tip

It is important to give quinoa a quick rinse before use, to remove any saponin residue that may remain after processing. Place the quinoa in a fine-mesh strainer and rinse thoroughly under cold water for 30 to 60 seconds.

Nutrients per serving	
Calories	296
Fat	7 g
Carbohydrate	48 g
Fiber	4 g
Protein	11 g
Vitamin A	2630 IU
Iron	3.2 mg
Zinc	1.9 mg

- Preheat oven to 375°F (190°C)
- 8- or 9-inch (20 or 23 cm) square glass baking dish, sprayed with nonstick cooking spray

1 tbsp	unsalted butter or coconut oil	15 mL
1 cup	quinoa, rinsed	250 mL
1/4 cup	natural cane sugar or packed dark brown sugar	60 mL
1 tsp	ground cinnamon	5 mL
3/4 tsp	ground ginger	3 mL
1/2 tsp	salt	2 mL
1/4 tsp	ground cloves	1 mL
2 cups	milk or plain non-dairy milk (such as soy, almond, rice or hemp)	500 mL
3/4 cup	pumpkin purée (not pie filling)	175 mL
1/2 cup	water	125 mL
1 tsp	vanilla extract (gluten-free, if needed)	5 mL

Suggested Accompaniments

Pure maple syrup

Milk or plain non-dairy milk

Blueberries

Dried cranberries or dried cherries

1. In a medium saucepan, melt butter over medium heat. Add quinoa and cook, stirring, for 2 to 3 minutes or until fragrant and golden. Whisk in sugar, cinnamon, ginger, salt, cloves, milk, pumpkin, water and vanilla. Pour into prepared baking dish and cover tightly with foil.

2. Bake in preheated oven for 35 minutes. Transfer to a wire rack and carefully remove foil (steam will be released). Stir and let stand for 5 minutes.

3. Spoon into bowls and serve with any of the suggested accompaniments, as desired.

Tip

Let leftover cereal cool completely, cover and refrigerate for up to 2 days. Warm in the microwave.

Adjustments for Phase 2

▶ Use virgin coconut oil instead of butter.

▶ Replace the cane or brown sugar with an equal amount of pure maple syrup or liquid honey.

Advice for a Healthy Gut

▶ Once you're in Phase 3, you may choose to use organic butter instead of coconut oil.

▶ Continue to use maple syrup or honey as the sweetener for this recipe while you are following the LGS Diet Plan.

▶ Avoid dairy milk and soy milk. Use unsweetened, carrageenan-free rice, almond, hemp or coconut milk instead.

▶ Choose unsweetened dried fruit.

Breakfast Rice

**Suitable for
Phases 1, 2 & 3**

*Rice is a versatile
all-purpose grain that is
gluten-free and has very
low allergenic properties,
making it perfect to
include in any leaky
gut diet plan.*

Tip

Unless you have a stove
with a true simmer,
after reducing the
heat to low, place a heat
diffuser under the pot
to prevent the mixture
from boiling. This
also helps ensure even
cooking and prevents
hot spots, which might
cause scorching. Heat
diffusers are available
at kitchen supply and
hardware stores and are
made to work on gas or
electric stoves.

4 cups	vanilla-flavored enriched rice milk	1 L
1 cup	long- or short-grain brown rice, rinsed and drained	250 mL
½ cup	dried cherries, cranberries or blueberries	125 mL
	Raw cane sugar, liquid honey or pure maple syrup (optional)	
	Chopped toasted nuts (optional)	

1. In a large saucepan over medium heat, bring rice milk to a boil. Gradually stir in rice and cherries. Return to a boil. Reduce heat to low (see tip, at left). Cover and simmer until rice is tender, about 50 minutes. Stir well and serve with your favorite sweetener, if desired.

Variation

Slow Cooker Method: Use a small (3½-quart) lightly greased slow cooker. Combine ingredients in stoneware, adding ½ cup (125 mL) water or additional rice milk to mixture. (With the quantity of liquid recommended above, it will be a bit crunchy around the edges.) Place a clean tea towel, folded in half (so you will have two layers), over top of the stoneware to absorb moisture. Cover and cook on Low for up to 8 hours or overnight, or on High for 4 hours.

Adjustment for Phase 1

▶ Use only skin-free nuts.

Advice for a Healthy Gut

▶ While you are following the LGS Diet Plan, choose honey or maple syrup as the sweetener for this recipe.

▶ Choose an unsweetened, carrageenan-free rice milk.

▶ Choose unsweetened dried fruit.

▶ Once you're in Phases 2 and 3, you may use nuts with skins, if desired.

Nutrients per serving	
Calories	232
Fat	2 g
Carbohydrate	51 g
Fiber	2 g
Protein	3 g
Vitamin A	333 IU
Iron	0.5 mg
Zinc	0.6 mg

Cranberry Quinoa Porridge

Makes 6 servings

**Suitable for
Phases 1, 2 & 3**

*Here's a hot cereal you
can enjoy in less than
half an hour, start to
finish, and that doesn't
require any attention
while it's cooking. Quinoa
is a great gluten-free
source of magnesium,
iron, potassium, zinc
and protein.*

Tip

Unless you have a stove
with a true simmer,
after reducing the
heat to low, place a heat
diffuser under the pot
to prevent the mixture
from boiling. This
also helps ensure even
cooking and prevents
hot spots, which might
cause scorching. Heat
diffusers are available
at kitchen supply and
hardware stores and are
made to work on gas or
electric stoves.

3 cups	water	750 mL
1 cup	quinoa, rinsed and drained	250 mL
½ cup	dried cranberries	125 mL
	Pure maple syrup or liquid honey	
	Milk or non-dairy alternative (optional)	

1. In a saucepan over medium heat, bring water to a boil. Stir in quinoa and cranberries and return to a boil. Reduce heat to low. Cover and simmer until quinoa is cooked (look for a white line around the seeds), about 15 minutes. Remove from heat and let stand, covered, about 5 minutes. Serve with maple syrup and milk, if desired.

Variations

Substitute dried cherries or blueberries or raisins for the cranberries.

Use red quinoa for a change.

Advice for a Healthy Gut

▶ Choose unsweetened dried fruit.

▶ While you are following the LGS Diet Plan, avoid dairy milk and soy milk. Use unsweetened, carrageenan-free rice, almond, hemp or coconut milk instead.

Nutrients per serving	
Calories	136
Fat	2 g
Carbohydrate	27 g
Fiber	3 g
Protein	4 g
Vitamin A	4 IU
Iron	1.4 mg
Zinc	0.9 mg

Mixed Fruit, Chia and Flaxseed Porridge

Makes 2 to 3 servings

Suitable for Phases 2 & 3

This simple mixture is extremely nutritious. It is quick to prepare and will leave you feeling well satisfied throughout the morning. Soaking the flax seeds helps you digest them more easily — a good thing for a healing gut.

Tip

Flax seeds must be soaked or ground so your body can absorb the nutrients. In this recipe, soaked whole flax seeds add body to the porridge. Submerge the flax seeds in 6 tbsp (90 mL) water. Set aside for 30 minutes. Drain and rinse under cold running water.

¼ cup	chopped apple	60 mL
¼ cup	chopped banana	60 mL
¼ cup	chopped orange, skin and membrane removed	60 mL
¼ cup	chopped hulled strawberries	60 mL
¼ cup	blueberries	60 mL
3 tbsp	whole flax seeds, soaked (see tip, at left)	45 mL
3 tbsp	chia seeds	45 mL
½ cup	Coconut Milk (page 326)	125 mL
½ tsp	vanilla extract (gluten-free, if needed)	2 mL

1. In a bowl, combine apple, banana, orange, strawberries, blueberries, soaked flax seeds, chia seeds, coconut milk and vanilla. Set aside for 5 minutes so the chia seeds can swell and absorb some of the liquid.

Variation

Use ⅓ cup (75 mL) chia seeds and 1 tbsp (15 mL) flax seeds soaked in 2 tbsp (30 mL) water. The result will have a very similar texture and flavor but a higher content of omega–3 fatty acids, because the chia seeds contain more omega–3 fats than the flax seeds.

Nutrients per serving

Calories	237
Fat	17 g
Carbohydrate	19 g
Fiber	9 g
Protein	5 g
Vitamin A	56 IU
Iron	1.4 mg
Zinc	1.2 mg

Sugar-Free Quinoa Granola Bars

**Suitable for
Phases 2 & 3**

*When you've had your
fill of overly sweet granola
bars from the grocery
store, turn to this recipe.
Naturally sweetened
with dates and super-ripe
bananas, and bolstered
with protein-rich quinoa
flakes, these bars will
satisfy and energize you
in the most delicious way.*

Tip

Mash the bananas very
thoroughly so that no
large chunks remain.

- Preheat oven to 350°F (180°C)
- 8-inch (20 cm) square metal baking dish, lined with foil (see tip, page 168) and sprayed with nonstick cooking spray

1/2 tsp	fine sea salt	2 mL
1/4 tsp	ground cardamom or cinnamon	1 mL
1 cup	mashed very ripe bananas	250 mL
2 tbsp	coconut oil, warmed, or vegetable oil	30 mL
2 tsp	vanilla extract (gluten-free, if needed)	10 mL
2 cups	quinoa flakes	500 mL
1/2 cup	chopped pitted Medjool dates	125 mL
1/2 cup	chopped toasted nuts (such as walnuts, hazelnuts or pecans)	125 mL

1. In a large bowl, combine salt, cardamom, bananas, oil and vanilla. Stir in quinoa flakes, dates and nuts. Using your hands, a spatula or a large piece of waxed paper, press mixture firmly into prepared pan.

2. Bake in preheated oven for 25 to 30 minutes or until golden and edges appear crisp. Let cool completely in pan on a wire rack. Using foil liner, lift mixture from pan and invert onto a cutting board. Peel off foil and cut into 8 bars.

Advice for a Healthy Gut

▸ While you are following the LGS Diet Plan, use virgin coconut oil, or use grapeseed oil or macadamia nut oil for the vegetable oil.

▸ Choose unsweetened dates.

Nutrients per bar

Calories	292
Fat	11 g
Carbohydrate	43 g
Fiber	5 g
Protein	8 g
Vitamin A	27 IU
Iron	2.4 mg
Zinc	1.6 mg

Toasted Sesame Quinoa Bars

**Suitable for
Phases 2 & 3**

*Quinoa and rolled oats
provide protein, which is
needed to heal and repair
the digestive tract.*

Tip

Lining a pan with foil is
easy. Begin by turning
the pan upside down.
Tear off a piece of foil
longer than the pan,
then mold the foil over
the pan. Remove the
foil and set it aside. Flip
the pan over and gently
fit the shaped foil into
the pan, allowing the
foil to hang over the
sides (the overhang ends
will work as "handles"
when the contents of the
pan are removed).

- 9-inch (23 cm) square metal baking pan, lined with foil (see tip, at left)

¾ cup	quinoa, rinsed	175 mL
¼ cup	sesame seeds	60 mL
4 cups	large-flake (old-fashioned) rolled oats (certified gluten-free, if needed)	1 L
¾ cup	pitted dates, chopped	175 mL
¾ cup	chopped dried apricots	175 mL
¼ tsp	fine sea salt	1 mL
1 cup	tahini	250 mL
½ cup	liquid honey or brown rice syrup	125 mL
2 tsp	vanilla extract (gluten-free, if needed)	10 mL

1. In a large skillet, over medium heat, toast quinoa and sesame seeds, stirring, for 4 to 5 minutes or until seeds are golden and beginning to pop. Transfer to a large bowl and let cool completely.

2. To the quinoa mixture, add oats, dates, apricots and salt. Stir in tahini, honey and vanilla until blended.

3. Press mixture into prepared pan and refrigerate for at least 30 minutes, until firm. Using foil liner, lift mixture from pan and invert onto a cutting board; peel off foil and cut into 16 bars.

Advice for a Healthy Gut

▶ Choose unsweetened dates and dried apricots.

▶ Chew these bars well to ensure better digestion.

Nutrients per bar

Calories	294
Fat	11 g
Carbohydrate	43 g
Fiber	5 g
Protein	8 g
Vitamin A	232 IU
Iron	2.9 mg
Zinc	1.2 mg

Chewy Coconut Quinoa Bars

Suitable for Phases 2 & 3

How could something that tastes so good also be good for you? Eating is believing.

Tips

Any other variety of natural nut or seed butter, such as sunflower seed or cashew butter, may be used in place of the almond butter.

If the bars crumble while you're cutting them, refrigerate for 15 to 30 minutes, until they are more firm.

Store cooled bars in an airtight container at room temperature for up to 5 days. Or wrap them in plastic wrap, then foil, completely enclosing them, and freeze for up to 6 months. Let thaw at room temperature for 1 hour before serving.

- Preheat oven to 350°F (180°C)
- 8-inch (20 cm) square metal baking pan, lined with foil (see tip, page 168) and sprayed with nonstick cooking spray

2 cups	quinoa flakes	500 mL
2 cups	unsweetened flaked coconut	500 mL
1 tsp	ground ginger	5 mL
½ tsp	fine sea salt	2 mL
¾ cup	liquid honey or brown rice syrup	175 mL
6 tbsp	coconut oil, warmed, or vegetable oil	90 mL
⅓ cup	unsweetened natural almond butter	75 mL

1. In a large bowl, combine quinoa flakes, coconut, ginger and salt.

2. In a medium bowl, whisk together honey, oil and almond butter until blended.

3. Add the honey mixture to the quinoa mixture and stir until evenly coated. Using your hands, a spatula or a large piece of waxed paper, press mixture firmly into prepared pan.

4. Bake in preheated oven for 30 to 40 minutes or until browned at the edges but still slightly soft at the center. Let cool completely in pan on a wire rack. Using foil liner, lift mixture from pan and invert onto a cutting board. Peel off foil and cut into 15 bars.

Advice for a Healthy Gut

▸ Use virgin coconut oil, or use grapeseed oil or macadamia nut oil for the vegetable oil.

Nutrients per bar

Calories	268
Fat	13 g
Carbohydrate	35 g
Fiber	3 g
Protein	5 g
Vitamin A	3 IU
Iron	1.5 mg
Zinc	1.0 mg

Home-Style Pancakes

Suitable for Phases 1, 2 & 3

These fantastic pancakes are a great gluten-free option. Serve topped with fruit and drizzle with maple syrup.

Tips

Combine the dry ingredients and store in an airtight container for up to 2 weeks.

Cook the pancakes the night before and store them in the refrigerator. Toast them in the morning.

Cooled cooked pancakes can also be placed in an airtight container, with parchment paper between each one for easier separation, and stored in the freezer for up to 4 weeks. Toast to serve.

½ cup	sorghum flour	125 mL
½ cup	brown rice flour	125 mL
2 tbsp	psyllium husks	30 mL
1 tsp	gluten-free baking powder	5 mL
¼ tsp	baking soda	1 mL
¼ tsp	salt	1 mL
1	egg	1
1 cup	fortified gluten-free non-dairy milk or lactose-free 1% milk	250 mL
1 tbsp	liquid honey, pure maple syrup or agave nectar	15 mL
2 tsp	grapeseed oil	10 mL
1 tsp	vanilla extract (gluten-free, if needed)	5 mL
	Butter or grapeseed oil	

1. In a large bowl, combine sorghum flour, brown rice flour, psyllium, baking powder, baking soda and salt.

2. In another bowl, beat egg, milk, honey, oil and vanilla. Pour into flour mixture and whisk for about 1 minute or until smooth.

3. On a griddle or in a nonstick skillet, melt 1 tsp (5 mL) butter over medium heat. For each pancake, pour in ¼ cup (60 mL) batter. Cook for 1 to 2 minutes or until bubbles start to form and edges are firm. Flip over and cook other side for 1 to 2 minutes or until bottom is golden. Transfer to a plate and keep warm. Repeat with the remaining batter, greasing griddle and adjusting heat between batches as needed.

Nutrients per pancake

Calories	133
Fat	3 g
Carbohydrate	23 g
Fiber	3 g
Protein	4 g
Vitamin A	213 IU
Iron	1.0 mg
Zinc	0.5 mg

Tip

Psyllium husks are the outer part of psyllium seeds, which are from the plantain plant, *Plantago ovato*. Numerous large-scale studies have shown that daily consumption of small amounts of psyllium fiber (3 to 12 grams a day) can help reduce LDL cholesterol ("bad" cholesterol). Other research indicates that when psyllium is incorporated into food, it is more effective at reducing the blood glucose response than a soluble fiber supplement that is taken separately from food.

Adjustments for Phases 1 & 2

▶ Make an egg substitute by combining 1 tbsp (15 mL) ground flax seeds (flaxseed meal) with 3 tbsp (45 mL) water; let stand for 5 minutes. Use in place of the egg.

▶ Use grapeseed oil (or macadamia nut oil or virgin coconut oil) to cook the pancakes. Do not use butter.

Advice for a Healthy Gut

▶ In Phase 3, eggs can be gradually reintroduced (see page 130) and, if desired, you may choose to use organic butter instead of grapeseed oil.

▶ While you are following the LGS Diet Plan, avoid dairy milk and soy milk. Use unsweetened, carrageenan-free rice, almond, hemp or coconut milk instead.

Applesauce Raisin Muffins

Makes 12 muffins

Suitable for Phases 1, 2 & 3

Following a therapeutic diet can be challenging, especially when eating on the go. Muffins make it easier, as they are portable and can be eaten almost anywhere. Paired with phase-appropriate nuts and/or seeds, these muffins make the perfect breakfast or snack.

- Preheat oven to 400°F (200°C)
- 12-cup muffin pan, greased

2 cups	Brown Rice Flour Blend (see recipe, opposite)	500 mL
2 tsp	gluten-free baking powder	10 mL
1 tsp	ground cinnamon	5 mL
½ tsp	ground allspice	2 mL
½ tsp	baking soda	2 mL
½ tsp	salt	2 mL
1½ cups	unsweetened applesauce	375 mL
½ cup	liquid honey or agave nectar	125 mL
⅓ cup	vegetable oil	75 mL
1 tsp	gluten-free vanilla extract	5 mL
½ cup	unsulfured raisins	125 mL

1. In a large bowl, whisk together flour blend, baking powder, cinnamon, allspice, baking soda and salt.

2. In a medium bowl, whisk together applesauce, honey, oil and vanilla until blended.

3. Add the applesauce mixture to the flour mixture and stir until just blended. Gently fold in raisins.

4. Divide batter equally among prepared muffin cups.

5. Bake in preheated oven for 25 to 28 minutes or until tops are golden brown and a toothpick inserted in the center comes out clean. Let cool in pan on a wire rack for 5 minutes, then transfer to the rack to cool.

Advice for a Healthy Gut

▶ Use grapeseed oil, macadamia nut oil or melted virgin coconut oil for the vegetable oil.

▶ Choose unsweetened raisins.

Nutrients per muffin	
Calories	226
Fat	7 g
Carbohydrate	42 g
Fiber	2 g
Protein	2 g
Vitamin A	10 IU
Iron	0.7 mg
Zinc	0.5 mg

**Suitable for
Phases 1, 2 & 3**

*Brown rice flour, potato
starch and tapioca starch
are staple gluten-free
substitutes for wheat-based
flours. Avoiding gluten is
key when you're following
the LGS Diet Plan, as
gluten is both a common
trigger for and an irritant
to an inflamed gut. This
flour blend enables you
to include some favorite
baked goods in your diet
while allowing your gut to
heal at the same time.*

Tips

You can also make
the blend in smaller
amounts by using the
basic proportions:
2 parts finely ground
brown rice flour, ⅔ part
potato starch and ⅓ part
tapioca starch.

You can double, triple
or quadruple the recipe
to have it on hand.
Store the blend in an
airtight container in
the refrigerator for
up to 4 months, or
in the freezer for up
to 1 year. Let warm to
room temperature
before using.

Brown Rice Flour Blend

2 cups	finely ground brown rice flour	500 mL
⅔ cup	potato starch	150 mL
⅓ cup	tapioca starch	75 mL

1. In a bowl, whisk together brown rice flour, potato starch and tapioca starch. Use as directed in recipes.

Agave Flax Muffins

Suitable for Phases 1, 2 & 3

Another muffin option for a breakfast or snack on the go, this one has the added benefits of flax seeds. One muffin provides women with 52% of the recommended minimum daily intake of the plant-based omega-3 fat alpha-linoleic acid, and provides men with 37%.

- Preheat oven to 350°F (180°C)
- 12-cup muffin pan, lined with paper liners

1 cup	sorghum flour	250 mL
1 cup	Brown Rice Flour Blend (page 173)	250 mL
1/4 cup	ground flax seeds (flaxseed meal)	60 mL
1 tbsp	gluten-free baking powder	15 mL
1/2 tsp	ground cinnamon	2 mL
1/2 tsp	salt	2 mL
1/2 tsp	xanthan gum	2 mL
1/4 tsp	ground cloves	1 mL
1/4 cup	unsweetened applesauce	60 mL
1/4 cup	vegetable oil	60 mL
1/4 cup	agave nectar	60 mL
1 1/4 cups	hemp or rice milk	300 mL

1. In a large bowl, whisk together sorghum flour, flour blend, flax seeds, baking powder, cinnamon, salt, xanthan gum and cloves.

2. In a medium bowl, whisk together applesauce, oil and agave nectar until well blended. Whisk in hemp milk until blended.

3. Add the applesauce mixture to the flour mixture and stir until just blended.

4. Divide batter equally among prepared muffin cups.

5. Bake in preheated oven for 18 to 22 minutes or until a toothpick inserted in the center comes out clean. Let cool in pan on a wire rack for 5 minutes, then transfer to the rack to cool.

Advice for a Healthy Gut

▸ Use grapeseed oil, macadamia nut oil or melted virgin coconut oil for the vegetable oil.

▸ Choose an unsweetened, carrageenan-free hemp or rice milk.

Nutrients per muffin

Calories	179
Fat	7 g
Carbohydrate	29 g
Fiber	2 g
Protein	3 g
Vitamin A	96 IU
Iron	1.2 mg
Zinc	0.5 mg

Multigrain Quinoa Muffins

Suitable for Phases 1, 2 & 3

Cooked quinoa may be an unusual ingredient for muffins, but it and the rolled oats up the nutritional value by being good sources of phosphorus, magnesium, potassium, fiber and protein. And the delectable taste of these muffins may surprise you!

Tip

Consider pairing one of these muffins with ¾ cup (175 mL) non-dairy yogurt, such as coconut yogurt.

Nutrients per muffin	
Calories	171
Fat	4 g
Carbohydrate	32 g
Fiber	2 g
Protein	2 g
Vitamin A	7 IU
Iron	0.8 mg
Zinc	0.5 mg

- Blender
- Two 12-cup muffin pans, 18 cups greased

½ cup	quinoa, rinsed	125 mL
⅔ cup	boiling water	150 mL
2 cups	Brown Rice Flour Blend (page 173)	500 mL
½ cup	certified gluten-free large-flake (old-fashioned) rolled oats	125 mL
2 tsp	baking powder (gluten-free, if needed)	10 mL
1 tsp	baking soda	5 mL
1 tsp	ground cinnamon	5 mL
½ tsp	salt	2 mL
2 tbsp	ground flax seeds (flaxseed meal)	30 mL
1½ cups	unsweetened applesauce	375 mL
½ cup	agave nectar or liquid honey	125 mL
¼ cup	vegetable oil	60 mL
½ cup	unsulfured dried blueberries or raisins	125 mL

1. In a small bowl, combine quinoa and boiling water. Let stand for 20 minutes.

2. Preheat oven to 375°F (190°C).

3. In a large bowl, whisk together flour blend, oats, baking powder, baking soda, cinnamon and salt until blended.

4. In blender, process flax seeds, applesauce, agave nectar and oil for 1 minute or until just blended.

5. Add the applesauce mixture to the flour mixture and stir until just blended. Gently fold in quinoa and blueberries.

6. Divide batter equally among prepared muffin cups.

7. Bake for 18 to 23 minutes or until tops are golden and a toothpick inserted in the center comes out clean. Let cool in pans on a wire rack for 5 minutes, then transfer to the rack to cool.

Advice for a Healthy Gut

▶ Use grapeseed oil, macadamia nut oil or melted virgin coconut oil for the vegetable oil.

▶ Choose unsweetened dried fruit.

Pumpkin Spice Muffins

Suitable for Phases 1, 2 & 3

Pumpkin provides beta-carotene, which the body converts to vitamin A, a nutrient essential for rebuilding and strengthening the digestive tract.

- Preheat oven to 400°F (200°C)
- 12-cup muffin pan, greased

1½ cups	Brown Rice Flour Blend (page 173)	375 mL
¼ cup	ground flax seeds (flaxseed meal)	60 mL
1 tbsp	gluten-free baking powder	15 mL
2½ tsp	pumpkin pie spice	12 mL
¾ tsp	salt	3 mL
1 cup	pumpkin purée (not pie filling)	250 mL
⅔ cup	agave nectar or liquid honey	150 mL
½ cup	mashed ripe banana	125 mL
½ cup	vegetable oil	125 mL
⅓ cup	hemp or rice milk	75 mL
1½ tsp	gluten-free vanilla extract	7 mL

1. In a large bowl, whisk together flour blend, flax seeds, baking powder, pumpkin pie spice and salt.

2. In a medium bowl, whisk together pumpkin, agave nectar, banana, oil, hemp milk and vanilla until well blended.

3. Add the pumpkin mixture to the flour mixture and stir until just blended.

4. Divide batter equally among prepared muffin cups.

5. Bake in preheated oven for 18 to 22 minutes or until a toothpick inserted in the center comes out clean. Let cool in pan on a wire rack for 3 minutes, then transfer to the rack to cool.

Advice for a Healthy Gut

▶ Use grapeseed oil, macadamia nut oil or melted virgin coconut oil for the vegetable oil.

▶ Choose an unsweetened, carrageenan-free hemp or rice milk.

Nutrients per muffin

Calories	239
Fat	11 g
Carbohydrate	36 g
Fiber	2 g
Protein	2 g
Vitamin A	1051 IU
Iron	0.8 mg
Zinc	0.5 mg

Soups

Mushroom Broth

Suitable for Phase 3

This mushroom soup is nothing like the canned version. It is brown and brothy, full of the earthy mushroom essence. Mushrooms support immunity, which, in turn, supports gut healing.

- **Food processor or blender**

8 oz	shiitake mushrooms	250 g
1	leek, white and light green parts, sliced	1
1 cup	chopped onion	250 mL
1	clove garlic, finely chopped	1
2 tbsp	olive oil	30 mL
3 cups	ready-to-use vegetable broth (gluten-free, if needed), divided	750 mL
1 tbsp	pure maple syrup	15 mL
1 tsp	salt	5 mL
1 cup	coconut, rice or soy milk (optional)	250 mL

1. Trim and discard mushroom stems. Slice caps and set aside.

2. In a large saucepan, combine leek, onion, garlic and oil. Sauté over medium heat for about 10 minutes or until very soft. Add mushrooms and ½ cup (125 mL) broth. Bring to a gentle boil. Cover, reduce heat and simmer for 15 minutes.

3. Add the remaining broth, maple syrup and salt. Bring to a boil. Cover, reduce heat and simmer for 45 minutes.

4. Using a slotted spoon, lift out half the vegetables and transfer to food processor. Process for 30 seconds or until smooth. Pour into a bowl. Repeat with remaining vegetables. Keep remaining cooking liquids hot in the saucepan over low heat.

5. Return purée to the saucepan and stir well. Taste and add more salt, if required. Add milk (if using). Heat through and serve immediately.

Advice for a Healthy Gut

▶ While you are following the LGS Diet Plan, use unsweetened, carrageenan-free coconut or rice milk. Avoid soy milk.

▶ Choose extra virgin olive oil.

Nutrients per serving

Calories	131
Fat	7 g
Carbohydrate	17 g
Fiber	3 g
Protein	2 g
Vitamin A	747 IU
Iron	0.8 mg
Zinc	0.8 mg

Asparagus and Leek Soup

Suitable for Phase 3

*Asparagus is rich in folate,
a B vitamin that supports
cellular and tissue repair
and healing. It is an
essential nutrient for
healing the gut.*

Tips

Choose the greenest
asparagus with straight,
firm stalks. The tips
should be tightly closed
and firm.

This soup can be served
warm or cold.

The soup can be made
and refrigerated up to
1 day before. Reheat
gently before serving,
adding more broth if
too thick.

- Food processor

12 oz	asparagus	375 g
1½ tsp	vegetable oil	7 mL
1 tsp	crushed garlic	5 mL
1 cup	chopped onion	250 mL
2	leeks, sliced	2
3½ cups	ready-to-use chicken broth (gluten-free, if needed)	875 mL
1 cup	diced peeled potato	250 mL
	Salt and freshly ground black pepper	
2 tbsp	freshly grated Parmesan cheese	30 mL

1. Trim asparagus; cut stalks into pieces and set tips aside.

2. In large nonstick saucepan, heat oil; sauté garlic, onion, leeks and asparagus stalks just until softened, approximately 10 minutes.

3. Add broth and potato; reduce heat, cover and simmer for 20 to 25 minutes or until vegetables are tender. Purée in food processor until smooth. Taste and adjust seasoning with salt and pepper. Return to saucepan.

4. Steam or microwave reserved asparagus tips just until tender; add to soup. Serve sprinkled with Parmesan cheese.

Advice for a Healthy Gut

▶ "Vegetable oil" is a catchall term for any edible oil from a plant source, whether it be a vegetable, fruit, nut or seed. While you are following the LGS Diet Plan, the best choices for this recipe are extra virgin olive oil, macadamia nut oil, avocado oil and grapeseed oil.

Nutrients per serving
(1 of 6)

Calories	100
Fat	3 g
Carbohydrate	15 g
Fiber	3 g
Protein	6 g
Vitamin A	940 IU
Iron	2.3 mg
Zinc	0.7 mg

Borscht

Suitable for Phase 3

This soup has a dual personality. If made following the method below, it is thick and chunky, but if the cooked vegetables are strained and blended in a food processor and returned to the pot with the cooking liquid, a smooth and creamy sophisticated texture is achieved.

Tip

For a vegan version, omit the butter and use 2 tbsp (30 mL) olive oil in total instead.

1 lb	beets, peeled and finely chopped	500 g
1	onion, finely chopped	1
1	stalk celery, finely chopped	1
1	apple, finely chopped	1
1	carrot, shredded	1
1	parsnip, shredded	1
5 cups	ready-to-use vegetable broth (gluten-free, if needed), divided	1.25 L
1 tbsp	olive oil	15 mL
1 tbsp	butter	15 mL
2 tbsp	freshly squeezed lemon juice	30 mL
1 tbsp	fresh thyme leaves	15 mL
1 tsp	salt	5 mL
½ cup	Basic Almond Spread (page 309; optional)	125 mL

1. In a large saucepan, combine beets, onion, celery, apple, carrot, parsnip, ½ cup (125 mL) broth, oil and butter. Bring to a gentle boil over medium–high heat. Cover, reduce heat to medium and gently simmer for 15 minutes.

2. Stir in the remaining broth, lemon juice, thyme and salt. Bring to a boil. Cover, reduce heat and gently simmer for 30 minutes or until the vegetables are soft. Garnish with a dollop of Almond Spread, if desired. Serve immediately.

Advice for a Healthy Gut

▶ Choose extra virgin olive oil or avocado oil.

Nutrients per serving

Calories	128
Fat	5 g
Carbohydrate	22 g
Fiber	5 g
Protein	2 g
Vitamin A	2266 IU
Iron	1.0 mg
Zinc	0.4 mg

Cream of Broccoli Soup

Suitable for Phase 3

Every time you make this soup you will ask yourself why you don't do it more often. It is so easy to prepare and delicious served hot or cold — truly a year-round winner.

Advice for a Healthy Gut

▶ Choose extra virgin olive oil or avocado oil.

Nutrients per serving

Calories	206
Fat	12 g
Carbohydrate	21 g
Fiber	4 g
Protein	7 g
Vitamin A	2689 IU
Iron	2.4 mg
Zinc	1.7 mg

• **Food processor**

1 cup	raw cashews	250 mL
1 lb	broccoli	500 g
2 tsp	olive oil	10 mL
1/2	onion, chopped	1/2
5 cups	ready-to-use vegetable broth (gluten-free, if needed)	1.25 L
1	russet (Idaho) potato, peeled and cut into 1-inch (2.5 cm) cubes	1
1/4 tsp	freshly ground black pepper	1 mL
1/2 tsp	salt	2 mL

1. Place cashews in a bowl and add water to cover by 3 inches (7.5 cm). Cover bowl and let soak for at least 2 hours.

2. Cut broccoli into 2-inch (5 cm) florets. Peel stalk and cut in half lengthwise and then crosswise into 1-inch (2.5 cm) pieces. You should have about 8 cups (2 L) total. Set aside.

3. Place cashews and 2 tbsp (30 mL) soaking water into food processor and process to a semi-smooth paste. Leave in processor and set aside.

4. Place a large saucepan over medium heat and let pan get hot. Add oil and tip pan to coat. Add onion and cook, stirring occasionally, until softened, 3 to 4 minutes. Add broth and potato, increase heat to high and bring to a boil. Reduce heat and simmer until slightly softened, 5 to 6 minutes. Add broccoli and black pepper, increase heat to high and bring to a boil. Reduce heat and simmer until potatoes and broccoli are tender, 6 to 8 minutes.

5. Let cool slightly. Working in batches, ladle soup into food processor with cashews and blend until smooth. Return to pan. Stir in salt. Taste and adjust seasonings and heat over low heat, stirring often, until soup is heated through. Serve hot.

Variations

Add 1/8 tsp (0.5 mL) ground nutmeg or allspice or more to taste.

Refrigerate and serve soup chilled.

Roasted Corn Chowder

**Suitable for
Phase 3**

*Rich and velvety, this
soup uses every bit
of the delicious corn.
Even the cobs are roasted
and simmered with
the vegetable broth for
added flavor.*

Tip

To make this soup
year-round, use frozen
corn on the cob. Thaw
before cutting.

Nutrients per serving

Calories	180
Fat	7 g
Carbohydrate	29 g
Fiber	3 g
Protein	4 g
Vitamin A	2407 IU
Iron	1.2 mg
Zinc	0.5 mg

- Preheat oven to 400°F (200°C)
- Baking sheet, lined with parchment paper
- Blender

4	ears corn, husked	4
8 tsp	olive oil, divided	40 mL
6 cups	ready-to-use vegetable broth (gluten-free, if needed)	1.5 L
1	onion, chopped	1
2	stalks celery with leaves, chopped	2
1	carrot, peeled and chopped	1
½	green bell pepper, chopped	½
2	russet (Idaho) potatoes, peeled and cut into 1-inch (2.5 cm) cubes	2
1 tbsp	chopped fresh thyme	15 mL
1	bay leaf	1
¾ tsp	salt	3 mL
¾ tsp	freshly ground black pepper	3 mL
6	chives, chopped	6

1. Cut corn from cobs and spread kernels on prepared baking sheet. Toss kernels with 2 tsp (10 mL) oil. Add cobs to baking sheet. Roast in preheated oven until kernels are golden brown, 8 to 10 minutes. Set aside.

2. Pour broth into a stockpot. Add roasted corn cobs and place over medium heat. Bring just to a boil, reduce heat and simmer, 20 to 25 minutes. Remove corn cobs and discard. Set broth aside.

3. Place a large heavy-bottomed saucepan or Dutch oven over medium heat and let pan get hot. Add 2 tbsp (30 mL) oil and tip pan to coat. Add onion, celery, carrot and bell pepper. Reduce heat to low and sweat, stirring occasionally, until softened, 8 to 10 minutes. Add reserved broth, potatoes, roasted corn kernels, reserving ¼ cup (60 mL) kernels, thyme, bay leaf, salt and black pepper and simmer until potatoes are tender, about 15 minutes.

If you are using store-bought broth, check the label to make sure it doesn't contain gluten.

4. Let cool slightly. Remove bay leaf and transfer two-thirds of soup to blender and process until just smooth. Return soup to saucepan, stirring to thoroughly combine. Taste and adjust seasonings. Turn heat to low and simmer until soup is heated through. Serve topped with a sprinkle of roasted corn kernels and chives.

Variations

Add roasted poblano or green chiles; red bell pepper with chopped cilantro; or chopped parsley, lemon juice and lemon zest.

Advice for a Healthy Gut

▶ Choose extra virgin olive oil or avocado oil.

▶ If you decide to try the variation with poblano or green chiles, reintroduce them gradually (see page 130) and monitor your tolerance as your gut continues to heal.

Mushroom-Almond Bisque

Suitable for Phase 3

Mushrooms are an excellent source of potassium, magnesium, phosphorus and unique antioxidants that help to reduce inflammation — perfect for healing the gut.

Tip

This soup is meant to be served chilled, as a variation of vichyssoise, but may be reheated in step 5, if desired.

• **Food processor or blender**

20	shiitake mushrooms	20
1	leek, white and light green parts, sliced	1
2 tbsp	olive oil	30 mL
2 cups	ready-to-use vegetable broth (gluten-free, if needed), divided	500 mL
1	potato, peeled and cut into large chunks	1
2 tbsp	tahini paste	30 mL
2 tbsp	miso	30 mL
2 cups	rice or soy milk, divided	500 mL
1/4 cup	Basic Almond Spread (page 309) or ground almonds	60 mL
2	green onions, thinly sliced on the diagonal (optional)	2

1. Remove and discard stems from mushrooms. Slice caps thinly and set aside.

2. In a large saucepan, combine leek and oil. Sauté over medium heat for 5 minutes or until soft. Add mushrooms and 1/4 cup (60 mL) broth. Simmer for 5 minutes.

3. Stir in the remaining broth. Increase heat to high and bring to a boil. Add potato. Cover, reduce heat to low and simmer gently for 15 minutes or until tender. Let cool.

4. Using a slotted spoon, transfer solids to food processor. Add tahini, miso and 1 cup (250 mL) milk. Process for 1 minute or until smooth.

5. In a large bowl, combine purée, soup liquids from the saucepan, the remaining milk and Almond Spread. Stir to blend. Let cool and refrigerate for at least 2 hours, until chilled, or for up to 24 hours.

6. Ladle chilled soup into bowls. Garnish each with about 1 tbsp (15 mL) green onions, if desired.

Nutrients per serving

Calories	301
Fat	16 g
Carbohydrate	36 g
Fiber	6 g
Protein	7 g
Vitamin A	913 IU
Iron	2.2 mg
Zinc	2.1 mg

Advice for a Healthy Gut

▶ Choose extra virgin olive oil or avocado oil.

▶ Use unsweetened, carrageenan-free rice milk. Avoid soy milk.

Butternut Squash Soup

Makes 4 servings

Suitable for Phases 1, 2 & 3

Squash is an excellent source of beta-carotene, which the body can convert to vitamin A. It is also a source of vitamin C (an important antioxidant with anti-inflammatory properties), as well as potassium and magnesium.

- **Food processor or blender**

2 tbsp	garlic-infused olive oil	30 mL
1	butternut squash, peeled, seeded and cut into 1-inch (2.5 cm) cubes	1
5 cups	ready-to-use gluten-free vegetarian chicken-flavored broth	1.25 L
	Salt and freshly ground black pepper	
	Chopped fresh thyme	
	Chopped fresh basil	

1. In a large saucepan, heat oil over medium heat. Stir in squash until just coated and cook for 10 minutes or until softened.

2. Add broth and bring to a boil. Reduce heat to low, cover and simmer for about 20 minutes or until squash is very tender.

3. Transfer half of the squash mixture to food processor, purée until smooth and return to pot. Season to taste with salt and pepper. Ladle into individual warmed serving bowls. Garnish with thyme and basil.

Adjustments for Phase 1

▶ Use plain extra virgin olive oil or avocado oil.

▶ Omit the pepper, thyme and basil.

Advice for a Healthy Gut

▶ In Phases 2 and 3, you can introduce garlic-infused olive oil, but continue to choose extra virgin olive oil while you are following the LGS Diet Plan.

Nutrients per serving

Calories	98
Fat	7 g
Carbohydrate	10 g
Fiber	1 g
Protein	1 g
Vitamin A	6206 IU
Iron	0.4 mg
Zinc	0.1 mg

Spinach and Sea Vegetable Soup

Suitable for Phase 3

A thick purée is the perfect foil for the slightly crisp, nutty-tasting strands of wakame in this soup. Seaweeds have compounds that protect the mucous layer of the digestive tract.

Tip

If you are using store-bought broth, check the label to make sure it doesn't contain gluten.

- **Food processor or blender**

1 cup	chopped onion	250 mL
2 tbsp	olive oil	30 mL
2	cloves garlic, finely chopped	2
1	carrot, chopped	1
1	leek, white and light green parts, chopped	1
1	turnip, chopped	1
6 cups	ready-to-use vegetable broth (approx.), divided	1.5 L
8 oz	spinach, trimmed	250 g
½ cup	wakame or arame	125 mL
2 tbsp	fresh thyme leaves	30 mL

1. In a large saucepan, sauté onion in oil over medium heat for 7 minutes or until soft. Stir in garlic, carrot, leek, turnip and ½ cup (125 mL) broth. Bring to a boil. Cover, reduce heat and simmer, stirring occasionally, for 10 minutes.

2. Stir in 4 cups (1 L) broth. Bring to a boil. Cover, reduce heat and simmer for 10 minutes or until vegetables are tender. Stir in spinach. Cook for 2 minutes or until wilted. Let cool slightly.

3. Using a slotted spoon, lift out half the vegetables and transfer to food processor. Process for 30 seconds or until smooth. Pour into a bowl. Repeat with remaining vegetables. Keep remaining cooking liquids hot in the saucepan over low heat.

4. Return purée to the saucepan. Add wakame and thyme. Stir in the remaining broth, a small amount at a time, until desired consistency is achieved. Cover and simmer over medium heat for 10 minutes or until wakame is tender. Serve immediately.

Advice for a Healthy Gut

▶ Choose extra virgin olive oil or avocado oil.

Nutrients per serving

Calories	95
Fat	5 g
Carbohydrate	12 g
Fiber	2 g
Protein	2 g
Vitamin A	6053 IU
Iron	1.8 mg
Zinc	0.4 mg

Roasted Tomato and Red Pepper Soup

Suitable for Phase 3

Using the flavorful tomatoes of summer and fresh red peppers, this robust soup is perfect for the beginning of a light lunch or dinner. It's rich in potassium, as well as vitamin C and lycopene, both heavy-hitter antioxidants that reduce inflammation.

- Preheat oven to 375°F (190°C)
- Rimmed baking sheet, lightly oiled
- Blender or food processor

5	small tomatoes	5
2	red bell peppers, cut in half	2
1	onion, quartered	1
12	cloves garlic	12
2 tbsp	olive oil	30 mL
1 tbsp	chopped fresh rosemary or basil	15 mL
3 cups	ready-to-use vegetable broth (gluten-free, if needed) or water, divided	750 mL
1 tbsp	pure maple syrup (optional)	15 mL
	Sea salt and freshly ground black pepper	

1. On prepared baking sheet, combine tomatoes, red peppers, onion and garlic in one layer. Drizzle with oil and bake in preheated oven for 40 minutes. Remove onion and garlic, if tender, and continue roasting tomatoes and peppers for another 10 minutes or until skin on peppers is bubbly and black in places and tomatoes are soft and runny. Let cool.

2. In blender, combine half of the roasted tomatoes, red peppers, onion and garlic with 1½ cups (375 mL) broth. Blend until smooth. Pour into a saucepan. Repeat with the remaining vegetables and broth.

3. Add maple syrup (if using), and salt and pepper to taste. Soup may be transferred to a jar or bowl, tightly covered and refrigerated for up to 2 days before using. To serve, in a saucepan, bring to a boil over high heat. Reduce heat and simmer, stirring constantly, for 1 minute.

Nutrients per serving

Calories	88
Fat	5 g
Carbohydrate	11 g
Fiber	2 g
Protein	2 g
Vitamin A	2135 IU
Iron	0.6 mg
Zinc	0.3 mg

Advice for a Healthy Gut

▸ You may want to try using half the amount of garlic at first, monitoring your tolerance as your gut continues to heal.

▸ Choose extra virgin olive oil or avocado oil.

Cold Mango Soup

Suitable for Phase 3

This soup has a wonderful combination of fruity sweetness and savory flavors. Mango is loaded with potassium and the antioxidant beta-carotene, some of which is converted to vitamin A, which aids in healing.

Tips

Try to ensure that each mango is ripe. They can be stored in the refrigerator for up to 3 days. How can you tell if a mango is ripe? It should have a strong fragrance and feel slightly soft if you apply gentle pressure.

This soup can also be served at room temperature.

- Food processor

2 tsp	vegetable oil	10 mL
½ cup	chopped onions	125 mL
2 tsp	minced garlic	10 mL
2 cups	ready-to-use vegetable broth (gluten-free, if needed)	500 mL
2½ cups	chopped ripe mango (about 2 large)	625 mL

Garnish (optional)

2% plain yogurt

Fresh cilantro leaves

1. In a nonstick saucepan, heat oil over medium heat. Add onions and garlic; cook, stirring, 4 minutes or until browned.

2. Add broth. Bring to a boil; reduce heat to medium-low and cook 5 minutes or until onions are soft.

3. Transfer mixture to food processor. Add 2 cups (500 mL) mango. Purée until smooth. Stir in the remaining mango.

4. Cover and refrigerate for at least 2 hours, until chilled, or for up to 2 days.

5. If desired, serve with a dollop of yogurt and garnished with coriander.

Advice for a Healthy Gut

▶ While you are following the LGS Diet Plan, use a light-tasting oil, such as grapeseed oil, in this recipe, and use coconut yogurt instead of a dairy-based yogurt for the optional garnish.

Nutrients per serving

Calories	105
Fat	3 g
Carbohydrate	19 g
Fiber	3 g
Protein	1 g
Vitamin A	1116 IU
Iron	0.4 mg
Zinc	0.1 mg

Salads

Mexican Jicama Slaw

**Makes
1 main-course or
2 side salads**

Suitable for
Phase 3

*Jicama is a refreshing
vegetable that tastes
like a blend of apple,
celery and potato. In
this salad it is mixed
with cumin and chili
powder for an authentic
Mexican experience.*

Tip

To peel the jicama, use
a sharp chef's knife to
cut a small slice from
each end, exposing the
flesh. Starting from the
top, in a downward
motion, cut away the
dark brown skin around
the flesh and discard.

- **Food processor**

¼ cup	cold-pressed (extra virgin) olive oil	60 mL
3 tbsp	freshly squeezed lime juice	45 mL
1 tsp	chili powder	5 mL
½ tsp	ground cumin	2 mL
¼ tsp	fine sea salt	1 mL
2 cups	finely sliced peeled jicama (see tip, at left)	500 mL

1. In food processor, process oil, lime juice, chili powder, cumin and salt. Transfer to a bowl.

2. Add jicama to dressing and toss until well coated. Cover and set aside for 10 minutes, until softened. Serve immediately or cover and refrigerate for up to 2 days.

Advice for a Healthy Gut

▶ Consider using half the amount of the spices called for, monitoring your tolerance as your gut continues to heal.

Nutrients per side salad

Calories	296
Fat	27 g
Carbohydrate	13 g
Fiber	7 g
Protein	1 g
Vitamin A	443 IU
Iron	1.5 mg
Zinc	0.3 mg

Hearts of Palm and Artichoke

Suitable for Phases 2 & 3

Tip

The edible inner portion of the stem of the cabbage palm tree, hearts of palm are native to Florida and other tropical locales. They come in cans, packed in water, and can be found in the specialty canned vegetable section of your grocery store (usually beside canned artichokes). They resemble white asparagus, without the tips. The delicate flavor is a bit like an artichoke. Once opened, they should be transferred to an airtight nonmetal container. Refrigerate in their own liquid and use within 1 week in salads or main dishes. If hearts of palm are difficult to find in your area, add extra artichoke hearts.

2 cups	salad greens	500 mL
2	canned hearts of palm, cut into rounds	2
2	canned artichoke hearts, quartered	2
1 tbsp	sesame seeds	15 mL
1 tbsp	olive oil	15 mL
1 tsp	balsamic vinegar	5 mL
	Juice of 1 lemon or lime	
	Salt and freshly ground black pepper	
1	avocado, peeled and diced	1

1. In a large salad bowl, combine greens, hearts of palm and artichokes. Sprinkle with sesame seeds.

2. In a small bowl, combine oil, vinegar, lemon juice, and salt and pepper to taste.

3. Add avocado to the salad, then dressing; toss gently to combine.

This recipe courtesy of Valérie Murray.

Advice for a Healthy Gut

▶ Choose extra virgin olive oil or avocado oil.

Nutrients per serving

Calories	139
Fat	12 g
Carbohydrate	8 g
Fiber	5 g
Protein	3 g
Vitamin A	1090 IU
Iron	1.6 mg
Zinc	0.7 mg

Avocado Salad

Makes 2 servings

**Suitable for
Phase 3**

*Avocado is loaded with
potassium, fiber and
monounsaturated fats.
It is also a great source
of lutein, an antioxidant
and anti-inflammatory
carotenoid.*

1 tbsp	freshly squeezed lime juice	15 mL
1	ripe avocado	1
¼ cup	slivered red bell pepper	60 mL
¼ cup	slivered red onion	60 mL
2 tbsp	vegetable oil	30 mL
	Salt and freshly ground black pepper	
	Few sprigs fresh coriander, chopped	
	Salsa Cynthia (page 301)	
	Corn chips	

1. Put lime juice in a small bowl. Peel avocado and cut into slices (or scoop out with a small spoon) and add to the lime juice. Toss gently until well coated. Add red pepper and onion; drizzle with oil. Toss gently until all ingredients are thoroughly combined. Season to taste with salt and pepper.

2. Transfer salad to a serving plate and spread out attractively. Garnish with chopped coriander and serve within 1 hour, accompanied by salsa and corn chips.

Advice for a Healthy Gut

▶ "Vegetable oil" is a catchall term for any edible oil from a plant source, whether it be a vegetable, fruit, nut or seed. While you are following the LGS Diet Plan, the best choices for this recipe are extra virgin olive oil, avocado oil, macadamia nut oil and grapeseed oil.

Nutrients per serving	
Calories	298
Fat	29 g
Carbohydrate	12 g
Fiber	7 g
Protein	2 g
Vitamin A	734 IU
Iron	0.7 mg
Zinc	0.7 mg

Chunky Cucumber Corn Salad

**Makes
1 main-course or
2 side salads**

Suitable for Phase 3

Cucumbers give this salad a refreshing crunch.

Tip

To remove kernels from a cob of corn, cut pieces from the top and bottom of the cob to create flat surfaces. Stand up the cob on a flat end. Using a chef's knife in a downward motion, gently strip away the kernels, making sure not to remove too much of the starchy white body of the cob.

2 cups	roughly chopped peeled, seeded cucumber	500 mL
1 cup	fresh corn kernels (see tip, at left)	250 mL
1/4 cup	chopped red bell pepper	60 mL
3 tbsp	cold-pressed (extra virgin) olive oil	45 mL
2 tbsp	freshly squeezed lemon juice	30 mL
1/4 tsp	fine sea salt	1 mL

1. In a bowl, combine cucumber, corn, red pepper, oil, lemon juice and salt. Toss until well combined. Serve immediately or cover and refrigerate for up to 2 days.

Nutrients per side salad

Calories	271
Fat	21 g
Carbohydrate	20 g
Fiber	3 g
Protein	3 g
Vitamin A	717 IU
Iron	1.1 mg
Zinc	0.6 mg

Sautéed Eggplant Salad

Suitable for Phase 3

Eggplant is a huge favorite in southern Europe. This adaptation uses ratatouille as a base and touches on the various stewed and sautéed eggplant salads of the Middle East.

4 cups	eggplant, cut into ½-inch (1 cm) cubes	1 L
	Salted water	
3 tbsp	vegetable oil	45 mL
3 tbsp	olive oil	45 mL
½ tsp	salt	2 mL
¼ tsp	freshly ground black pepper	1 mL
¼ tsp	hot pepper flakes	1 mL
1	onion, cut into ¼-inch (0.5 cm) slices	1
½	green bell pepper, cut into ½-inch (1 cm) squares	½
½	red bell pepper, cut into ½-inch (1 cm) squares	½
4	cloves garlic, thinly sliced	4
4	sun-dried tomatoes, thinly sliced	4
1	tomato, cut into ½-inch (1 cm) wedges	1
1 tsp	red wine vinegar	5 mL
½ tsp	dried basil	2 mL
½ tsp	dried oregano	2 mL
¼ cup	water	60 mL
	Few sprigs chopped fresh basil and/or parsley	

1. Immerse cubed eggplant in cold salted water as soon as possible after cutting it (eggplant turns brown soon after it is cut); let soak 5 to 10 minutes.

2. In a large nonstick frying pan, heat vegetable oil over medium–high heat for 1 minute. Drain eggplant and add to the pan (watch for splutters). It will absorb all the oil almost immediately. Cook, stirring actively, for 6 to 7 minutes or until the eggplant is soft and browned all over. Transfer the cooked eggplant to a dish; set aside.

Nutrients per serving

Calories	241
Fat	21 g
Carbohydrate	13 g
Fiber	5 g
Protein	2 g
Vitamin A	880 IU
Iron	1.0 mg
Zinc	0.4 mg

If you like things less spicy, just omit the hot pepper flakes.

3. Using the same frying pan, heat olive oil over medium-high heat for 30 seconds. Add salt, black pepper and hot pepper flakes; stir-fry for 30 seconds. Add onion and green and red pepper; stir-fry 2 to 3 minutes or until wilted and beginning to char. Add garlic and sun-dried tomatoes; stir-fry 1 minute. Add tomato, vinegar, basil and oregano; stir-fry 2 minutes or until tomato has broken down and a sauce is forming. Add water and immediately reduce heat to medium. Stir in eggplant. Gently mix and fold all ingredients together; cook 2 minutes or until heated through.

4. Transfer to a flat dish and let rest for about 10 minutes. Garnish with fresh herbs. Serve lukewarm.

Advice for a Healthy Gut

▶ Use extra virgin olive oil, avocado oil, macadamia nut oil or grapeseed oil for the vegetable oil.

▶ While you are following the LGS Diet Plan, use natural balsamic vinegar (without color or sulfites) instead of red wine vinegar in this recipe.

Marinated Mushrooms

Makes 4 to 6 servings

Suitable for Phase 3

This is a refreshing appetizer or side vegetable that requires next to no cooking. It can sit nicely in the fridge for up to 2 days while waiting to be needed, improving its flavor all the while.

5 cups	mushrooms, washed and trimmed	1.25 L
1/4 cup	slivered red onion	60 mL
3	cloves garlic, minced	3
1/4 cup	walnut pieces	60 mL
1 tsp	olive oil	5 mL
6 tbsp	extra virgin olive oil	90 mL
2 tbsp	white wine vinegar	30 mL
1 tbsp	soy sauce (gluten-free, if needed)	15 mL
Pinch	cayenne pepper (optional)	Pinch
	Salt and freshly ground black pepper	
	Few sprigs fresh parsley and/or basil, chopped	

1. In a bowl, toss mushrooms, red onion and garlic until well mixed.

2. In a small frying pan over medium heat, stir-fry walnut pieces in 1 tsp (5 mL) olive oil for 1 to 2 minutes, being careful not to let them burn. Add to mushroom mixture.

3. In a small bowl, whisk together 6 tbsp (90 mL) olive oil, vinegar, soy sauce and cayenne (if using) until emulsified. Add dressing to salad and fold gently until the vegetables are well coated. Season to taste with salt and black pepper. Leave uncovered for at least 1 hour, gently folding every 15 minutes or so. Transfer to a serving bowl, and garnish liberally with the herb(s). Serve immediately or keep for up to 1 hour more, covered and unrefrigerated.

Advice for a Healthy Gut

▶ Choose extra virgin olive oil or avocado oil.

▶ While you are following the LGS Diet Plan, use rice vinegar instead of white wine vinegar in this recipe.

▶ Use gluten-free soy sauce or tamari.

Nutrients per serving (1 of 6)

Calories	176
Fat	18 g
Carbohydrate	4 g
Fiber	1 g
Protein	3 g
Vitamin A	1 IU
Iron	0.6 mg
Zinc	0.5 mg

Red Pepper, Snap Pea and Ginger Cashew Salad

**Suitable for
Phase 3**

Add some healthy fat, potassium and the anti-inflammatory carotenoid lutein to your diet with this salad, which combines the sweet, juicy pop of cherry tomatoes with smooth, creamy avocado.

Tip

To remove the stem and string from a snap pea, pinch its bottom tip to get a grip on the stem. Twist the stem to loosen the string along the spine, pull the string up the straight side of the pea pod and then pinch it off and discard.

Nutrients per side salad	
Calories	519
Fat	45 g
Carbohydrate	26 g
Fiber	4 g
Protein	9 g
Vitamin A	2466 IU
Iron	3.7 mg
Zinc	3.1 mg

- **Food processor**

1 cup	finely sliced red bell pepper (about 2 medium)	250 mL
½ cup	snap peas, strings removed (about 10 to 15)	125 mL
¾ cup	whole raw cashews	175 mL
3 tbsp	chopped gingerroot	45 mL
3 tbsp	cold-pressed sesame oil (untoasted)	45 mL
¼ tsp	fine sea salt	1 mL

1. In a serving bowl, toss together red pepper, snap peas and cashews until well combined. Set aside.

2. In food processor, process ginger, sesame oil and salt until smooth.

3. Add ginger-sesame dressing to the vegetable mixture and toss until well coated. Serve immediately or cover and refrigerate for up to 2 days.

Variation

Green Pepper, Spinach and Ginger Cashew Salad: Substitute green bell pepper for the red pepper and 2 cups (500 mL) baby spinach for the snap peas. After tossing the vegetables with dressing in step 3, set aside for 5 minutes to soften before serving.

Creamy Cherry Tomato Salad

**Suitable for
Phases 2 & 3**

Tips

To ripen avocados, place them in a brown paper bag with a tomato or an apple. If your avocado is ripe and won't be consumed within a day or two, place it in the coolest part of the refrigerator to lengthen its life by 3 to 4 days. Once you take an avocado out of the fridge, do not put it back in — it will turn black.

You can substitute $\frac{1}{4}$ cup (60 mL) fresh basil leaves for the dried basil.

- **Food processor**

2	avocados, divided	2
$\frac{1}{4}$ cup	freshly squeezed lemon juice	60 mL
2 tbsp	cold-pressed (extra virgin) olive oil	30 mL
$\frac{1}{4}$ cup	filtered water	60 mL
1 tbsp	dried basil	15 mL
$\frac{1}{2}$ tsp	fine sea salt	2 mL
2 cups	halved cherry tomatoes	500 mL

1. In food processor, combine 1 avocado, lemon juice, oil, water, basil and salt. Process until smooth.

2. Cut the remaining avocado into 1-inch (2.5 cm) cubes and place in a bowl. Add tomatoes and avocado purée. Toss well to coat. Serve immediately or cover and refrigerate for up to 1 day.

Nutrients per side salad

Calories	239
Fat	22 g
Carbohydrate	13 g
Fiber	8 g
Protein	3 g
Vitamin A	772 IU
Iron	1.3 mg
Zinc	0.8 mg

Tomato, Parsley and Onion Salad

Suitable for Phase 3

Italian cuisine marries bold flavors by using fresh produce. This salad is simple, fresh and delicious.

Tip

If you can, use heirloom tomatoes for this salad. Heirloom tomatoes have a meatier texture and are more flavorful than most commercial tomatoes. Look for varieties such as Green Zebra, Oaxacan Jewel, Brandywine and Purple Russian. Check out your local farmers' market to see what is available.

1 cup	chopped tomatoes	250 mL
1/2 cup	roughly chopped flat-leaf (Italian) parsley	125 mL
1/4 cup	finely sliced red onion	60 mL
3 tbsp	cold-pressed (extra virgin) olive oil	45 mL
2 tbsp	raw (unpasteurized) apple cider vinegar	30 mL
1/4 tsp	fine sea salt	1 mL

1. In a bowl, combine tomatoes, parsley and onion. Add oil, vinegar and salt. Toss until well combined. Serve immediately or cover and refrigerate for up to 1 day.

Nutrients per side salad

Calories	294
Fat	30 g
Carbohydrate	7 g
Fiber	2 g
Protein	1 g
Vitamin A	2030 IU
Iron	1.4 mg
Zinc	0.3 mg

Sesame Ginger Sea Veggies

Makes
1 main-course or
2 side salads

Suitable for
Phase 3

Packed with iodine, sea vegetables are not only nutritious and easy to use but also versatile and quick to absorb flavor. In addition, they help to heal and protect the lining of the gut.

Tip

Arame is a nutritious sea vegetable. Most sea vegetables are sold in a dry state. To rehydrate them, simply cover in twice their volume of warm water and set aside for 15 minutes or until softened.

¼ cup	dried arame (see tip, at left)	60 mL
1 cup	warm filtered water	250 mL
2	sheets nori, sliced thinly	2
¼ cup	finely sliced ginger	60 mL
3 tbsp	cold-pressed sesame oil (untoasted)	45 mL
2 tbsp	wheat-free tamari	30 mL

1. In a small bowl, combine arame and water. Cover and set aside for 15 minutes, until softened. Drain, discarding soaking liquid.

2. In a bowl, combine arame, nori, ginger, sesame oil and tamari. Toss until well combined. Serve immediately or cover and refrigerate for up to 3 days.

Variation

Substitute an equal amount of wakame for the arame.

Nutrients per side salad

Calories	208
Fat	21 g
Carbohydrate	4 g
Fiber	1 g
Protein	3 g
Vitamin A	242 IU
Iron	0.9 mg
Zinc	0.2 mg

Yam and Pecan Salad

Suitable for Phase 3

This is a spectacular salad that will gain new fans for the sweet smoothness of the neglected but nutritious yam — it's loaded with potassium and is high in fiber.

Advice for a Healthy Gut

▸ While you are following the LGS Diet Plan, the best choices for this recipe are extra virgin olive oil, macadamia nut oil, grapeseed oil and avocado oil.

Nutrients per serving (1 of 6)

Calories	203
Fat	14 g
Carbohydrate	18 g
Fiber	3 g
Protein	2 g
Vitamin A	11043 IU
Iron	0.7 mg
Zinc	0.5 mg

- Preheat oven to 450°F (230°C)
- Baking dish, greased with 1 tbsp (15 mL) vegetable oil

1 lb	yams, unpeeled but well scrubbed	500 g
½	red bell pepper, cut into thick strips	½
¼ cup	vegetable oil	60 mL
1 tsp	mustard seeds	5 mL
Pinch	cayenne pepper	Pinch
Pinch	ground cinnamon	Pinch
Pinch	ground cumin	Pinch
⅓ cup	pecan halves	75 mL
3 tbsp	freshly squeezed lime juice	45 mL
1 tsp	sesame oil	5 mL
½ tsp	salt	2 mL
½ cup	thinly slivered red onion	125 mL
	Few sprigs fresh coriander, chopped	

1. In a large saucepan, cover yams with plenty of water and bring to a boil. Cook for 10 minutes, then drain. Cut yams into rounds ½ inch (1 cm) thick.

2. In prepared baking dish, arrange the sliced yams and red pepper strips in a single layer. Bake in preheated oven for 12 to 15 minutes, until the yams are easily pierced with a fork.

3. Meanwhile, in a frying pan, heat oil over medium heat for 1 minute. Add mustard seeds, cayenne, cinnamon and cumin, and stir-fry for 2 minutes or until spices begin to pop. Add the pecans; stir-fry for 2 minutes until the nuts have browned a little on both sides (don't burn them). Remove from heat and reserve in pan.

4. Remove yams and red peppers from the oven. Using a spatula, carefully transfer them onto a serving plate, making a single layer.

5. Drizzle lime juice and sesame oil over the yams and sprinkle with salt. Scatter slivers of red onion on top. Using a spoon and a rubber spatula, scrape contents of the frying pan (pecans, oil and spices) evenly over the yams. Let salad rest for 10 to 15 minutes, then garnish with the chopped coriander and serve.

Quinoa Salad with Grapefruit and Avocado

Suitable for Phase 3

Quinoa, pronounced "KEEN-wah," is actually a seed that is a rich source of protein. Quinoa has roughly twice the protein of barley, corn and rice and is rich in iron, magnesium, zinc, potassium and vitamin E.

Advice for a Healthy Gut

▶ While you are following the LGS diet plan, replace the cane sugar with an equal amount of liquid honey.

2 cups	water	500 mL
1 tsp	salt	5 mL
1 cup	quinoa, rinsed	250 mL
2 tbsp	chopped fresh mint	30 mL
2 tbsp	freshly squeezed lime juice	30 mL
2 tsp	granulated natural cane sugar or other dry sweetener	10 mL
1/2 tsp	salt	2 mL
Pinch	freshly ground black pepper	Pinch
1/3 cup	vegetable oil	75 mL
1	red grapefruit, peeled, sectioned and each section cut into thirds	1
1	avocado, peeled, pitted and cut into 3/4-inch (2 cm) cubes	1
1/3 cup	Pickled Pink Onion Relish (page 307)	75 mL

1. In a pot, bring water and salt to a boil over high heat. Add quinoa, stirring to prevent lumps from forming, and return to a boil. Cover, reduce heat to low and simmer for 15 minutes or until tender and liquid is absorbed. Remove from heat and let stand, uncovered, for 5 minutes or until it reaches room temperature. Transfer to a serving bowl.

2. Meanwhile, in a small bowl, whisk together mint, lime juice, sugar, salt and pepper. Whisk in oil. Add grapefruit pieces, avocado and onion relish and toss lightly to coat. Spoon over quinoa, letting dressing drizzle down through the salad. Serve immediately.

Variations

Garnish this salad with a sprinkling of salted roasted pumpkin seeds. Substitute fresh cilantro for the mint.

Substitute 2 oranges or 2 blood oranges for the grapefruit.

Advice for a Healthy Gut

▶ Use extra virgin olive oil, macadamia nut oil, grapeseed oil or avocado oil for the vegetable oil.

Nutrients per serving (1 of 6)

Calories	296
Fat	19 g
Carbohydrate	28 g
Fiber	5 g
Protein	5 g
Vitamin A	519 IU
Iron	1.6 mg
Zinc	1.2 mg

Health Salad

Suitable for Phase 3

This salad makes a colorful and flavorful accompaniment to many meals. It also keeps very well; in fact, it improves after a day or two in the refrigerator.

Advice for a Healthy Gut

▶ While you are following the LGS Diet Plan, replace the cane sugar with an equal amount of liquid honey or pure maple syrup.

▶ Choose extra virgin olive oil or avocado oil.

Nutrients per serving (1 of 10)

Calories	37
Fat	0 g
Carbohydrate	9 g
Fiber	3 g
Protein	1 g
Vitamin A	2493 IU
Iron	0.5 mg
Zinc	0.2 mg

1	large apple (unpeeled), coarsely grated	1
1	small bulb fennel, cored and thinly sliced	1
2 tbsp	freshly squeezed lemon juice	30 mL
6 cups	thinly sliced red or green cabbage (about ½ head)	1.5 L
2	carrots, peeled and grated	2
1	red bell pepper, cut into quarters and thinly sliced crosswise	1

Dressing

3	green onions (white and green parts), finely chopped	3
½ cup	cider vinegar	125 mL
3 tbsp	coarsely chopped fresh Italian parsley	45 mL
2 tbsp	olive oil	30 mL
1 tbsp	granulated natural cane sugar or other dry sweetener	15 mL
	Salt and freshly ground black pepper	

1. In a large bowl, combine apple, fennel and lemon juice. Toss to coat. Add cabbage, carrots and red pepper and toss to combine.

2. *Dressing:* In a small bowl, whisk together green onions, vinegar, parsley, olive oil and sugar. Add to cabbage mixture, season to taste with salt and pepper and toss to coat. Cover and refrigerate for at least 2 hours or until flavors are developed, or for up to 2 days.

Variations

For a spicier version, add ½ tsp (2 mL) hot pepper sauce or a pinch of hot pepper flakes to the dressing.

Add 1 tbsp (15 mL) chopped fresh herbs, such as basil, dill, oregano or thyme, to the cabbage mixture along with the dressing.

Advice for a Healthy Gut

▶ If you want to try the spicier variation, start out with a smaller amount of hot pepper sauce or just a few hot pepper flakes, monitoring your tolerance as your gut continues to heal.

Blueberry Vinaigrette

Suitable for Phases 2 & 3

Serve this stunning dressing over mixed greens, garnished with fresh blueberries. Research suggests that honey provides antibacterial support to help heal the gut.

Tips

If you prefer, you can prepare the vinaigrette in a blender. Simply add all the ingredients and purée until smooth.

Keeps in the refrigerator for up to 5 days.

½ cup	fresh or frozen blueberries, thawed	125 mL
⅓ cup	liquid honey	75 mL
¼ cup	balsamic vinegar	60 mL
2 tbsp	vegetable oil	30 mL
2 tbsp	water	30 mL

1. In a small bowl, mash blueberries with a fork. Whisk in honey, vinegar, oil and water.

This recipe courtesy of dietitian Selina Chan.

Advice for a Healthy Gut

▶ Use extra virgin olive oil, macadamia nut oil, grapeseed oil or avocado oil for the vegetable oil.

▶ Choose natural balsamic vinegar (without color or sulfites).

Nutrients per serving

Calories	69
Fat	3 g
Carbohydrate	11 g
Fiber	0 g
Protein	0 g
Vitamin A	4 IU
Iron	0.1 mg
Zinc	0.0 mg

Vegetarian Dishes

Eggplant Caponata
with Roasted Potatoes

Suitable for Phase 3

Caponata is a Sicilian dish of eggplant and other vegetables with pine nuts cooked in olive oil and served at room temperature. If serving with bread, make sure it's gluten-free.

Advice for a Healthy Gut

▶ Choose extra virgin olive oil or avocado oil.

▶ While you are following the LGS Diet Plan, use rice vinegar or natural balsamic vinegar (without color or sulfites) instead of white wine vinegar.

Nutrients per serving

Calories	333
Fat	25 g
Carbohydrate	28 g
Fiber	12 g
Protein	4 g
Vitamin A	238 IU
Iron	1.4 mg
Zinc	0.8 mg

- Preheat oven to 450°F (230°C)
- Baking sheet, lined with parchment paper

1	large eggplant, cut into ½-inch (1 cm) cubes	1
1½ tsp	salt, divided	7 mL
2	Yukon Gold potatoes, cut into ½-inch (1 cm) cubes	2
7 tbsp	olive oil, divided	105 mL
¼ tsp	freshly ground black pepper, divided	1 mL
3	stalks celery, cut into matchsticks, or thinly sliced lengthwise, then cut into 1-inch (2.5 cm) pieces	3
6 oz	canned green olives, drained	175 g
¾ cup	fresh or frozen corn kernels (thawed if frozen)	175 mL
½ cup	pine nuts	125 mL
3 tbsp	drained capers	45 mL
3 tbsp	white wine vinegar	45 mL

1. Place eggplant in a colander, toss with 1 tsp (5 mL) salt and set aside to drain for about 20 minutes. Rinse and pat dry.

2. In a bowl, toss potatoes with 1 tbsp (15 mL) oil, ¼ tsp (1 mL) salt and ⅛ tsp (0.5 mL) pepper. Spread potatoes on prepared baking sheet and bake in preheated oven until fork tender, about 15 minutes. Remove and set aside.

3. Place a large heavy-bottomed skillet over medium heat and let pan get hot. Add remaining 6 tbsp (90 mL) oil and tip pan to coat. Add eggplant and cook, stirring frequently, until tender, 8 to 10 minutes. Using a slotted spoon, transfer eggplant to a dish and set aside.

4. Return skillet to medium-high heat. Add roasted potatoes, celery, green olives, corn kernels, pine nuts and capers and cook, stirring frequently, until celery is tender, about 5 minutes. Add vinegar and cook, stirring frequently, until evaporated, 1 to 2 minutes. Add the remaining salt and pepper. Serve hot or at room temperature.

Turkish Stuffed Baked Eggplant

Makes 4 servings

Suitable for Phase 3

Eggplant has modest amounts of vitamins and minerals but is rich in phytonutrients, plant compounds that promote optimal health and wellness.

- Preheat oven to 375°F (190°C)
- Baking sheet, lightly oiled

2	eggplants	2
3 tbsp	olive oil	45 mL
1	onion, coarsely chopped	1
1 cup	thinly sliced fennel bulb or celery	250 mL
3	cloves garlic, minced	3
2	large tomatoes, seeded and diced	2
1 tsp	ground coriander seeds	5 mL
1/2 tsp	ground cinnamon	2 mL
1/2 tsp	ground cumin	2 mL
1/2 tsp	ground turmeric	2 mL
1/2 tsp	salt	2 mL

1. Trim ends from eggplants and discard. Fill a large saucepan to the halfway point with water and bring to a boil over high heat. Add eggplants and cook for 7 minutes. Remove and rinse under cold water to stop the cooking. When cool, cut each in half lengthwise. Scoop out the flesh, leaving a 1/4-inch (0.5 cm) thick shell. Place shells cut side up on prepared baking sheet. Coarsely chop and reserve flesh.

2. Meanwhile, in a large skillet, heat oil over medium heat. Add onion and sauté for 10 minutes or until soft. Stir in fennel and garlic and sauté for 5 minutes. Stir in tomatoes, coriander, cinnamon, cumin, turmeric, salt and reserved eggplant. Cook, stirring, for 3 minutes or until vegetables are tender.

3. Spoon stuffing equally into each eggplant shell. Cover with foil and bake in preheated oven 30 minutes. Serve immediately or let cool and serve at room temperature.

Advice for a Healthy Gut

▸ Choose extra virgin olive oil or avocado oil.

Nutrients per serving	
Calories	193
Fat	11 g
Carbohydrate	24 g
Fiber	12 g
Protein	4 g
Vitamin A	864 IU
Iron	1.5 mg
Zinc	0.7 mg

Baked Portobello Mushrooms

Suitable for Phases 1, 2 & 3

Baked portobello mushrooms have many uses in the kitchen. They can be sliced and added to salads and sauces or served whole on a bun for a satisfying sandwich. They are also a great source of anti-inflammatory compounds that help to heal the body.

Tip

When removing the mushroom stem, carefully cut it out with a paring knife to leave the mushroom cap intact.

- Preheat oven to 350°F (180°C)
- 13- by 9-inch (33 by 23 cm) baking dish, greased

| 4 | portobello mushrooms, cleaned and stems removed (see tip, at left) | 4 |

Marinade

¼ cup	olive oil	60 mL
2 tbsp	balsamic vinegar	30 mL
	Salt and freshly ground black pepper	

1. *Marinade:* In a small bowl, whisk together olive oil, balsamic vinegar, and salt and pepper to taste.

2. Place mushrooms in prepared baking dish, gill side up, and pour marinade over top, making sure each mushroom cap is completely covered. Cover dish and refrigerate for 1 to 2 hours to allow mushrooms to absorb some of the marinade.

3. Drain off excess marinade. Bake mushrooms in preheated oven for 35 minutes or until soft.

Variation

Portobello Mushroom Burgers: Serve whole baked mushrooms on a gluten-free bun or soft roll.

Adjustment for Phase 1

▶ Omit the pepper.

Advice for a Healthy Gut

▶ Choose extra virgin olive oil and natural balsamic vinegar (without color or sulfites).

Nutrients per serving

Calories	94
Fat	7 g
Carbohydrate	6 g
Fiber	1 g
Protein	2 g
Vitamin A	0 IU
Iron	0.6 mg
Zinc	0.5 mg

Baked Winter Greens

Winter greens — cabbage, beet tops, Swiss chard, kale, spinach — add important nutrients to a winter diet, and this easy dish is a tasty way to enjoy them.

- Preheat oven to 350°F (180°C)
- 8-inch (20 cm) baking dish, lightly oiled

2 cups	shredded green or Savoy cabbage	500 mL
2 cups	chopped kale leaves, thick ribs removed	500 mL
2 cups	chopped Swiss chard leaves	500 mL
2 cups	Garlic White Sauce (page 304)	500 mL

1. In a bowl, toss cabbage, kale and Swiss chard together. Pour about $\frac{1}{4}$ cup (60 mL) Garlic White Sauce into bottom of prepared baking dish. Pile greens on top and pour the remaining white sauce over. Cover and bake in preheated oven for 30 minutes or until sauce is bubbly and greens are soft.

Nutrients per serving
(1 of 6)

Calories	140
Fat	6 g
Carbohydrate	20 g
Fiber	4 g
Protein	3 g
Vitamin A	4504 IU
Iron	1.5 mg
Zinc	0.6 mg

Mediterranean Vegetable Casserole

Suitable for Phases 2 & 3

This delectable combination of vegetables seasoned with fresh oregano bakes into a mouthwatering lunch or dinner.

Tip

Salting and sweating eggplant leaches moisture and some of the bitterness from the eggplant as well as reducing the spongy texture that is likely to absorb grease while cooking. Rinse salt from eggplant and dry with a kitchen towel to eliminate as much moisture as possible before cooking.

- Preheat oven to 350°F (180°C)
- 13- by 9-inch (33 by 23 cm) baking pan, lightly oiled

1	large eggplant, peeled and cut into ½-inch (1 cm) slices	1
	Salt	
1	red onion, sliced	1
8 oz	cremini mushrooms, sliced	250 g
1	green bell pepper, sliced	1
2	tomatoes, sliced	2
¼ cup	olive oil, divided	60 mL
2 tbsp	chopped fresh Greek oregano, divided	30 mL
1 tsp	freshly ground black pepper, divided	5 mL

1. Arrange eggplant slices in colander, sprinkle with 2 tsp (10 mL) salt and set aside to drain for about 20 minutes. Rinse and pat dry.

2. In prepared baking pan, layer half each of eggplant, red onion, mushrooms, green pepper and tomatoes. Drizzle with 2 tbsp (30 mL) oil and sprinkle with 1 tbsp (15 mL) oregano and ½ tsp (2 mL) each salt and pepper. Repeat with remaining ingredients.

3. Bake casserole in preheated oven until vegetables are tender and top is slightly browned with crisp edges, 40 to 45 minutes. Let stand for 10 minutes before serving.

Variation

Fry eggplant slices in olive oil before layering in baking pan.

Advice for a Healthy Gut

▶ Choose extra virgin olive oil or avocado oil.

Nutrients per serving (1 of 6)

Calories	131
Fat	10 g
Carbohydrate	11 g
Fiber	5 g
Protein	3 g
Vitamin A	469 IU
Iron	0.7 mg
Zinc	0.5 mg

Big-Batch Oven-Roasted Ratatouille

Suitable for Phases 2 & 3

Ratatouille, a popular Mediterranean dish, combines eggplant, tomatoes, onions, peppers, zucchini, garlic and herbs, all usually simmered in olive oil. This version cooks in the oven with a little oil and takes on a toasty flavor. It's perfect in the summer months, when fresh produce is abundant, but it's delicious all year round.

- Preheat oven to 450°F (230°C)
- 16- by 12-inch (40 by 30 cm) shallow roasting pan

4	tomatoes, chopped	4
4	cloves garlic, chopped	4
3	small Italian eggplants, cut into ½-inch (1 cm) rounds	3
2	large zucchini, cut into ½-inch (1 cm) rounds	2
1	red bell pepper, cut into chunks	1
1	yellow bell pepper, cut into chunks	1
1	large red onion, cut into chunks	1
3 tbsp	olive oil	45 mL
	Salt and freshly ground black pepper	
1	small bunch fresh basil, roughly torn	1
½ cup	freshly grated Parmesan cheese	125 mL

1. In a large bowl, combine tomatoes, garlic, eggplants, zucchini, red pepper, yellow pepper and red onion. Add olive oil and toss to coat. Transfer to roasting pan and season to taste with salt and pepper.

2. Roast on the top rack of preheated oven for 15 minutes. Stir and roast for 15 minutes or until vegetables are just soft and tinged brown on the edges.

3. Transfer to a serving bowl and stir in basil. Sprinkle with cheese.

This recipe courtesy of Eileen Campbell.

Adjustment for Phase 2

▸ Omit the Parmesan cheese.

Advice for a Healthy Gut

▸ Choose extra virgin olive oil or avocado oil.

Nutrients per serving	
Calories	106
Fat	5 g
Carbohydrate	14 g
Fiber	6 g
Protein	4 g
Vitamin A	868 IU
Iron	0.8 mg
Zinc	0.7 mg

Roasted Squash and Parsnip Stew

Suitable for Phase 3

Roasting vegetables mellows their flavor and brings out their natural sugars. Cooking also makes carotenoids, such as beta-carotene, easier for the body to absorb.

Tip

You can prepare this stew the day before. Complete through to the point of adding squash, onions, parsnips, garlic and pan juices to the saucepan in step 3 but do not simmer. Let cool, cover and refrigerate for up to 24 hours. Bring to room temperature and simmer on medium-low heat for 12 minutes.

- Preheat oven to 375°F (190°C)
- 2 rimmed baking sheets, lightly oiled

1	butternut squash, cut in half lengthwise, seeds removed	1
3	large onions, quartered	3
2	parsnips, cut into chunks	2
10	cloves garlic	10
3 tbsp	olive oil, divided	45 mL
2 tbsp	balsamic vinegar	30 mL
2	leeks, white and light green parts, sliced	2
3 cups	tomato sauce	750 mL
	Sea salt and freshly ground black pepper	

1. Arrange squash, cut side down, on prepared baking sheet. Bake in preheated oven for 40 minutes or until tender when pierced with the tip of a knife. Let cool completely. Peel off skin and cut into 1-inch (2.5 cm) pieces. Set aside.

2. Meanwhile, on second prepared baking sheet, combine onions, parsnips and garlic. Drizzle with 2 tbsp (30 mL) oil and vinegar. Bake alongside squash for 30 minutes or until caramelized and tender when pierced with the tip of a knife.

3. In a large saucepan, heat remaining oil over high heat. Add leeks and reduce heat to medium. Cook, stirring occasionally, for 6 to 8 minutes or until soft. Add tomato sauce, squash, onions, parsnips, garlic and pan juices and simmer over low heat for 12 minutes to blend flavors and heat through. Season to taste with salt and pepper.

Advice for a Healthy Gut

▶ Choose extra virgin olive oil and natural balsamic vinegar (without color or sulfites).

Nutrients per serving

Calories	182
Fat	7 g
Carbohydrate	28 g
Fiber	5 g
Protein	4 g
Vitamin A	4747 IU
Iron	2.6 mg
Zinc	0.7 mg

Delicata Squash with Quinoa Stuffing

Suitable for Phases 2 & 3

Delicata squash at its seasonal best lends subtle sweetness and rich, mellow flavor to a protein-, vitamin- and antioxidant-rich stuffing of quinoa, peppery arugula and tart cranberries.

Advice for a Healthy Gut

▶ While you are following the LGS Diet Plan, lightly brush cut sides of squash with extra-virgin olive oil in step 1 instead of using cooking spray.

Nutrients per serving

Calories	348
Fat	9 g
Carbohydrate	61 g
Fiber	7 g
Protein	10 g
Vitamin A	9865 IU
Iron	3.7 mg
Zinc	1.6 mg

- Preheat oven to 350°F (180°C)
- Large rimmed baking sheet

2	delicata squash (each about 1 lb/500 g), halved lengthwise and seeded	2
	Nonstick cooking spray (preferably olive oil)	
1 tsp	fine sea salt, divided	5 mL
1 cup	black, red or white quinoa, rinsed	250 mL
2 cups	ready-to-use reduced-sodium vegetable broth (gluten-free, if needed)	500 mL
1/3 cup	dried cranberries, chopped	75 mL
1/4 tsp	freshly cracked black pepper	1 mL
1 tbsp	white wine vinegar	15 mL
2 tsp	liquid honey or agave nectar	10 mL
2 cups	packed arugula, roughly chopped	500 mL
1/2 cup	packed fresh mint leaves, chopped	125 mL
1/3 cup	chopped toasted hazelnuts or almonds	75 mL

1. Lightly spray cut sides of squash with cooking spray. Sprinkle with half the salt. Place cut side down on baking sheet. Bake in preheated oven for 40 to 45 minutes or until tender.

2. Meanwhile, in a medium saucepan, combine quinoa and broth. Bring to a boil over medium–high heat. Reduce heat to low, cover and simmer for 10 minutes. Stir in cranberries, cover and simmer for 2 to 5 minutes or until liquid is absorbed. Let stand, covered, for 5 minutes. Fluff with a fork.

3. In a large bowl, whisk together the remaining salt, pepper, vinegar and honey. Add quinoa mixture, arugula, mint and hazelnuts, gently tossing to combine.

4. Fill squash cavities with quinoa mixture.

Advice for a Healthy Gut

▶ Use unsweetened cranberries.

▶ While you are following the LGS Diet Plan, use rice vinegar instead of white wine vinegar in this recipe.

Mandarin Rice and Walnut–Stuffed Acorn Squash

Suitable for Phases 2 & 3

A delightfully unexpected combination of exotic aromas and fragrant flavors merge in this hearty and warm stuffed squash.

- Preheat oven to 375°F (190°C)
- 13- by 9-inch (33 by 23 cm) glass baking dish

1	acorn squash, halved lengthwise, seeds and pulp removed	1
2 tsp	olive oil	10 mL
2 tsp	pure maple syrup	10 mL

Stuffing

¼ cup	dried figs, diced	60 mL
1	can (11 oz or 284 mL) unsweetened mandarin oranges, with juice	1
1 tbsp	olive oil	15 mL
2	shallots, chopped	2
1 tsp	grated gingerroot	5 mL
2 tsp	garam masala	10 mL
¼ cup	toasted walnuts	60 mL
2 tbsp	golden raisins (sultanas)	30 mL
1 cup	cooked long-grain brown rice	250 mL
2 tbsp	chopped fresh cilantro	30 mL
	Salt and freshly ground black pepper	

1. Place squash in baking dish cut side up and drizzle inside of each half with 1 tsp (5 mL) oil and 1 tsp (5 mL) maple syrup. Add ½ inch (1 cm) water and bake in preheated oven for 45 minutes.

2. *Stuffing:* In a small bowl, combine figs and oranges with juice. Set aside.

3. Place a skillet over medium heat and let pan get hot. Add oil and tip pan to coat. Add shallots, ginger and garam masala and cook, stirring occasionally, until shallots are softened, 2 to 3 minutes. Stir in walnuts, raisins, rice and cilantro. Remove from heat and season to taste with salt and pepper. Mix in fig and orange mixture.

Nutrients per serving (1 of 8)

Calories	230
Fat	11 g
Carbohydrate	33 g
Fiber	3 g
Protein	3 g
Vitamin A	545 IU
Iron	1.0 mg
Zinc	0.8 mg

Tip

To remove the skin from gingerroot with the least amount of waste, use the edge of a teaspoon. With a brushing motion, scrape off the skin to reveal the yellow root.

4. Transfer par-cooked squash to a cutting board and, when cool enough to handle, stuff each half with rice mixture, mounding high without compacting. Return squash to baking dish, cover loosely with foil and bake until squash is tender and stuffing is slightly crunchy on top, 10 to 15 minutes. Let cool slightly before serving.

Advice for a Healthy Gut

▶ Choose extra virgin olive oil or avocado oil.

▶ Use unsweetened dried figs and raisins.

Vegetable Paella

Makes 6 to 8 servings

Suitable for Phase 3

This recipe is rich in fiber, potassium, phytonutrients and the anti-inflammatory antioxidant lycopene. As cooking with seasonal vegetables produces superior flavors, use green beans if asparagus is unavailable.

Advice for a Healthy Gut

▸ Choose extra virgin olive oil.

▸ Choose sun-dried tomatoes packed in olive oil.

Nutrients per serving (1 of 8)

Calories	325
Fat	7 g
Carbohydrate	51 g
Fiber	4 g
Protein	7 g
Vitamin A	586 IU
Iron	4.3 mg
Zinc	0.9 mg

- Preheat oven to 350°F (180°C)
- Paella pan or large ovenproof skillet

3 tbsp	olive oil	45 mL
1	onion, diced	1
1	large fennel bulb, trimmed and cut into bite-size pieces	1
4	cloves garlic, chopped	4
2 cups	short- or medium-grain white rice	500 mL
2 cups	warm water	500 mL
1½ cups	dry white wine	375 mL
½ tsp	paprika	2 mL
¾ tsp	saffron threads or ground turmeric	3 mL
1 tsp	salt	5 mL
1	can (14 oz/400 mL) artichoke hearts in water, drained	1
¾ cup	sliced drained oil-packed sun-dried tomatoes	175 mL
8 oz	thin asparagus or green beans, trimmed and halved	250 g
⅓ cup	green olives	75 mL
3 tbsp	chopped fresh Italian (flat-leaf) parsley	45 mL

1. Place paella pan over medium heat and let pan get hot. Add oil and tip pan to coat. Add onion and fennel and cook, stirring frequently, until vegetables begin to soften, 4 to 5 minutes. Add garlic and cook, stirring frequently, until onions and fennel are lightly browned, 3 to 5 minutes. Mix in rice, lightly coating all grains with oil. Stir in water, wine, paprika, saffron, salt, artichoke hearts and sun-dried tomatoes. Gently shake pan to distribute rice evenly. Reduce heat and simmer for 10 minutes.

2. Remove pan from heat and scatter asparagus and green olives over rice. Cover pan and bake in preheated oven until rice is tender with a slightly crusted bottom, about 30 minutes.

3. Scatter chopped parsley over top and serve hot.

Italian-Style Baked Tofu

Suitable for Phase 3

This recipe is versatile. Serve it as an appetizer, in salads, or crumbled and used as a cheese substitute in Italian dishes.

Tip

To drain tofu, place the cubes on a plate lined with a double layer of paper towels. Cover with another paper towel, then another plate. Place a weight on top of the plate to press the water out of the tofu. Let stand for 30 minutes. Drain off water.

- Preheat oven to 350°F (180°C)
- 8-inch (20 cm) square glass baking dish

1 lb	firm or extra-firm tofu, cut into 1-inch (2.5 cm) cubes and drained (see tip, at left)	500 g
2	cloves garlic, minced (about 2 tsp/10 mL)	2
1 tsp	dried oregano	5 mL
1 tsp	dried basil	5 mL
1/4 tsp	salt (or to taste)	1 mL
	Freshly ground black pepper	
1/4 cup	prepared Italian salad dressing	60 mL

1. In baking dish, combine tofu, garlic, oregano, basil, and salt and pepper to taste. Drizzle with dressing, then stir until tofu is evenly coated. Marinate for 1 hour at room temperature or in the refrigerator for at least 2 hours or for up to 8 hours.

2. Bake, uncovered, in preheated oven, for 35 to 40 minutes, stirring and turning pieces over after 20 minutes, until tofu is firm and liquid is absorbed.

Advice for a Healthy Gut

- Use only non-GMO, organic tofu.
- Choose an extra virgin olive oil–based Italian salad dressing that is free of preservatives, gluten and artificial colors and flavors.

Nutrients per serving (1 of 6)

Calories	140
Fat	9 g
Carbohydrate	5 g
Fiber	2 g
Protein	12 g
Vitamin A	133 IU
Iron	2.3 mg
Zinc	1.2 mg

Mushroom-Topped Polenta Tart with Mushroom Sauce

Suitable for Phase 3

Served piping hot, this savory polenta tart will warm you on a cold day. What could be better than guilt-free comfort food? Mushrooms are loaded with potassium and a unique form of carbohydrate that boosts the immune system.

Tip

This tart is delicious with any and all mushrooms. Try wild mushrooms such as chanterelles, porcini and morels or domesticated mushrooms such as cremini or button or a mixture of a few.

Nutrients per serving

Calories	262
Fat	11 g
Carbohydrate	33 g
Fiber	4 g
Protein	6 g
Vitamin A	686 IU
Iron	2.5 mg
Zinc	0.9 mg

- **2 baking sheets, lined with parchment paper**

6 cups	ready-to-use vegetable broth (gluten-free, if needed), divided	1.5 L
1 cup	cornmeal	250 mL
4 tbsp + 1 tsp	olive oil, divided	65 mL
1½ lbs	mixed wild and domestic mushrooms, divided	750 g
1	red bell pepper	1
½ cup	minced onion	125 mL
1 tsp	fresh thyme leaves	5 mL
1 tsp	minced fresh sage	5 mL
⅛ tsp	freshly ground black pepper	0.5 mL
½ cup	dry white wine	125 mL
2 tbsp	cornstarch	30 mL
3 tbsp	water	45 mL
	Salt	

1. In a saucepan, bring 4 cups (1 L) broth to a boil over high heat. Gradually whisk in cornmeal and cook, stirring, for 2 minutes. Cover, reduce heat to low and simmer for 25 minutes, uncovering and stirring vigorously 2 or 3 times during cooking. Remove from heat. Brush one parchment-lined baking sheet with 1 tsp (5 mL) oil and pour polenta on prepared baking sheet, spreading to ½ inch (1 cm) thickness. Refrigerate for 1 hour and brush top with 1 tbsp (15 mL) oil. You can cover polenta and refrigerate for up to 1 day.

2. Preheat oven to 450°F (230°C) with racks positioned in the middle and bottom of oven.

3. Slice half of the mushrooms and half of the red pepper into ¼-inch (0.5 cm) thick strips. Brush remaining baking sheet with 2 tbsp (30 mL) oil. Spread sliced mushrooms and pepper evenly over baking sheet. Place baking sheet with vegetables on bottom rack and baking sheet with polenta on middle rack of oven. Bake for 20 minutes, turning vegetables halfway through cooking.

Tip

No time for do-ahead tart? Serve the roasted mushrooms and sauce over soft polenta, skipping the step of spreading it on the baking sheet, chilling and baking.

4. Coarsely chop remaining mushrooms and red pepper. Place a large skillet over medium heat and let pan get hot. Add the remaining oil and tip pan to coat. Add mushrooms, red pepper, onion, thyme, sage and pepper and cook, stirring frequently, until softened, 4 to 6 minutes. Add wine and the remaining 2 cups (500 mL) broth and bring to a boil. Reduce heat and simmer until flavors are combined and mixture is slightly reduced, 10 to 15 minutes. Whisk cornstarch into water and gradually drizzle into pan, adding enough to thicken. Add more wine or water to thin if necessary. Adjust seasoning, adding salt to taste.

5. To serve, top polenta tart with roasted mushrooms and peppers. Slice into squares and serve with sauce on the side.

Advice for a Healthy Gut

▶ Choose extra virgin olive oil or avocado oil.

Nutty Tofu and Green Vegetable Stir-Fry

Suitable for Phase 3

This spicy, nutty tofu recipe has the flavor of an Asian satay dish and is guaranteed to please both vegetarians and non-vegetarians!

Tips

Freeze the tofu cubes prior to preparation; this enhances the texture of the tofu so it's more poultry-like.

This dish goes well with jasmine rice or gluten-free noodles.

1 tbsp	vegetable oil	15 mL
8 oz	firm tofu, cubed	250 g
1	green bell pepper, thinly sliced	1
1½ cups	green beans, trimmed	375 mL
½ tsp	salt	2 mL
4	cloves garlic, minced	4
1	onion, chopped	1
1	tomato, chopped	1
¼ cup	coarsely ground almonds	60 mL
½ cup	water (approx.), divided	125 mL
½ tsp	granulated sugar	2 mL
½ tsp	ground turmeric	2 mL
½ tsp	ground cumin	2 mL
½ tsp	ground coriander	2 mL

1. In a large skillet, heat oil over medium heat. Lightly brown tofu on all sides, then remove from pan and set aside.

2. Add green pepper, green beans and salt to skillet; stir-fry until tender-crisp, about 5 minutes. Add garlic, onion and tomato; stir-fry for 5 minutes. Stir in tofu pieces. Stir in almonds, ¼ cup (60 mL) water and sugar. Reduce heat to low and cook for 5 minutes. Stir in turmeric, cumin and coriander, then the remaining water (add more if the mixture becomes too dry and sticks to the pan).

This recipe courtesy of dietitian Colleen Joice.

Nutrients per serving

Calories	191
Fat	12 g
Carbohydrate	13 g
Fiber	5 g
Protein	12 g
Vitamin A	723 IU
Iron	2.7 mg
Zinc	1.4 mg

Advice for a Healthy Gut

▸ Use extra virgin olive oil, macadamia nut oil, grapeseed oil or avocado oil for the vegetable oil.

▸ Use only non-GMO, organic tofu.

▸ While you are following the LGS Diet Plan, replace the granulated sugar with an equal amount of liquid honey.

Orange Saffron Rice with Tofu

Suitable for Phase 3

The best preparation makes the best-tasting tofu. A soy-based protein, tofu can complete any meal.

Tip

Increase the protein by doubling the tofu in the recipe (for those with larger appetites).

Advice for a Healthy Gut

▸ Choose extra virgin olive oil or avocado oil.

▸ Use only non-GMO, organic tofu.

Nutrients per serving

Calories	215
Fat	13 g
Carbohydrate	16 g
Fiber	2 g
Protein	12 g
Vitamin A	98 IU
Iron	2.9 mg
Zinc	1.0 mg

- Preheat oven to 400°F (200°C)
- 9-inch (23 cm) baking dish, lightly oiled

Orange Saffron Rice

1 tbsp	hot water	15 mL
1/4 tsp	saffron threads	1 mL
2 cups	basmati rice	500 mL
3/4 tsp	salt, divided	3 mL
2 tsp	garlic-infused olive oil	10 mL
1 tsp	orange extract	5 mL
1/2 tsp	ground turmeric	2 mL
1/2 tsp	ground cardamom	2 mL

Baked Tofu

1	package (12 1/2 oz/350 g) firm tofu, cubed	1
1/4 cup	gluten-free soy sauce	60 mL
2 tbsp	garlic-infused olive oil	30 mL

1. *Orange Saffron Rice:* In a small bowl, combine hot water and saffron. Let soak for 1 hour.

2. Meanwhile, in a strainer, thoroughly rinse rice under cold running water. Drain. In a medium bowl, stir together rice, 5 cups (1.25 L) water and 1/2 tsp (2 mL) salt. Let soak for 30 minutes. Drain.

3. In a large saucepan, heat oil over medium-high heat. Stir in orange extract, turmeric, cardamom, remaining salt and saffron with soaking water, stirring for 30 seconds until combined. Stir in rice, stirring for 1 minute until rice is coated with oil mixture.

4. Stir in 2 1/4 cups (550 mL) water and bring to a boil. Reduce heat to lowest setting, cover and cook, stirring occasionally, for 20 minutes or until rice is tender.

5. *Baked Tofu:* In a large bowl, stir together tofu, soy sauce and oil. Arrange tofu in a single layer in prepared baking dish. Bake in preheated oven, gently stirring and turning once or twice, for 25 to 35 minutes or until browned.

6. Transfer rice to a serving platter. Spoon tofu over rice.

Tofu Vegetarian Pilaf

**Suitable for
Phase 3**

*Here's a simple and tasty
way to include tofu in
your diet. The cinnamon,
cardamom and turmeric
add wonderful flavor
and color.*

Tip

Increase the protein by
doubling the tofu in the
recipe (for those with
larger appetites).

3 to 4	cinnamon sticks (each about 3 inches/7.5 cm)	3 to 4
3 to 4	cardamom pods	3 to 4
2 tbsp	vegetable oil	30 mL
½ tsp	ground turmeric	2 mL
2	large potatoes, peeled and cubed	2
2	carrots, peeled and diced	2
2 tbsp	grated gingerroot	30 mL
	Salt	
3 cups	water	750 mL
1½ cups	basmati rice, well rinsed	375 mL
5 oz	firm tofu, diced	150 g

1. In a large saucepan over medium heat, combine cinnamon sticks, cardamom pods, oil and turmeric and cook, stirring, for about 2 minutes or until fragrant.

2. Stir in potatoes, carrots, ginger and salt to taste and cook, stirring, for 3 to 4 minutes or until vegetables start to brown.

3. Stir in water and rice until combined and bring to a boil. Reduce heat to low, cover and simmer, stirring occasionally to prevent rice from sticking to bottom of pan, for 10 minutes. If rice mixture begins to dry out during cooking, add small amounts of water to prevent sticking and burning.

4. Gently stir in tofu, cover and cook for 5 to 10 minutes or until water has been absorbed and rice and potatoes are tender. Remove and discard cinnamon sticks and cardamom pods. Serve immediately.

Advice for a Healthy Gut

▶ Use only non-GMO, organic tofu.

▶ Use extra virgin olive oil, macadamia nut oil, grapeseed oil or avocado oil for the vegetable oil.

Nutrients per serving	
Calories	256
Fat	5 g
Carbohydrate	46 g
Fiber	4 g
Protein	7 g
Vitamin A	2586 IU
Iron	1.7 mg
Zinc	0.6 mg

Fish and Seafood

Whole Baked Fish

Suitable for Phases 1, 2 & 3

Fish is a great source of omega-3 fats, which reduce inflammation and promote normalization of gut function. Fish is also a source of zinc, protein and selenium.

- Preheat oven to 375°F (190°C)
- Baking dish, greased

1	whole oily fish (about 3 lbs/1.5 kg)	1
1 tbsp	vegetable oil	15 mL
	Salt and freshly ground black pepper	
	Juice of 1 lemon	
	Mushroom Ragoût (see recipe, opposite)	

1. Cut 3 to 4 slits in each side of the fish and rub fish with oil, salt, pepper and lemon juice. Place fish in prepared baking dish.

2. Bake in preheated oven for 10 minutes per inch (2.5 cm) of thickness or until fish is opaque and flakes easily with a fork. Serve with Mushroom Ragoût.

Adjustment for Phase 1

▶ Omit the pepper.

Advice for a Healthy Gut

▶ Use extra virgin olive oil, macadamia nut oil, grapeseed oil or avocado oil for the vegetable oil.

Nutrients per serving (based on salmon, without ragoût)

Calories	151
Fat	10 g
Carbohydrate	1 g
Fiber	1 g
Protein	13 g
Vitamin A	500 IU
Iron	0.7 mg
Zinc	0.0 mg

**Suitable for
Phases 1, 2 & 3**

Mushroom Ragoût

¼ oz	dried wild mushrooms	7 g
¾ cup	warm water	175 mL
2 tbsp	butter	30 mL
4 oz	mushrooms, sliced	125 g
1	leek (white part only), thinly sliced	1
1	tomato, peeled, seeded and chopped	1
1 tbsp	chopped fresh Italian (flat-leaf) parsley	15 mL
Pinch	dried thyme	Pinch

1. Soak dried mushrooms in warm water for 15 minutes. Strain through cheesecloth or a coffee filter, reserving mushrooms and soaking liquid separately.

2. In a large skillet, melt butter over medium heat. Sauté soaked and fresh mushrooms and leek until tender. Add mushroom soaking liquid, tomato, parsley and thyme; bring to a boil. Reduce heat and simmer for 3 minutes.

Adjustments for Phase 1

▸ Use extra virgin olive oil, avocado oil, macadamia nut oil or grapeseed oil instead of butter.

▸ Omit the leek.

Advice for a Healthy Gut

▸ Once you're in Phase 3, you may choose to use organic butter.

Nutrients per ½ cup
(125 mL)

Calories	87
Fat	6 g
Carbohydrate	7 g
Fiber	2 g
Protein	2 g
Vitamin A	885 IU
Iron	1.3 mg
Zinc	0.3 mg

Foil-Roasted Halibut and Asparagus

Makes 4 servings

Suitable for Phases 1, 2 & 3

Halibut is a light-tasting and versatile white fish. It's loaded with phosphorus and selenium, a mineral the body uses to make an antioxidant. One serving also has more potassium than a medium banana.

Tips

Sea bass, cod or any other firm white fish fillets may be used in place of the halibut.

Four 12-inch (30 cm) squares of parchment paper may be used in place of the foil. To seal the packets, fold the parchment over the fish and asparagus, then fold and crimp the edges tightly to enclose the filling completely.

Nutrients per serving	
Calories	191
Fat	6 g
Carbohydrate	7 g
Fiber	3 g
Protein	29 g
Vitamin A	1007 IU
Iron	2.9 mg
Zinc	1.2 mg

- Preheat oven to 400°F (200°C)
- Four 12-inch (30 cm) squares foil
- Large rimmed baking sheet

	Nonstick cooking spray (preferably olive oil)	
4	skinless Pacific halibut fillets (each about 5 oz/150 g)	4
1 tbsp	minced fresh tarragon	15 mL
2 tsp	finely grated orange zest	10 mL
1/4 tsp	fine sea salt	1 mL
1/4 tsp	freshly cracked black pepper	1 mL
1 lb	thin asparagus spears, trimmed and cut into 1-inch (2.5 cm) pieces	500 g
1/4 cup	freshly squeezed orange juice	60 mL
1 tbsp	extra virgin olive oil	15 mL

1. Place foil squares on a work surface and spray with cooking spray. Top each square with a fish fillet and sprinkle with tarragon, orange zest, salt and pepper. Arrange asparagus around each fillet, then drizzle fish and asparagus with orange juice and oil. Fold foil over fish and asparagus, crimping edges tightly to seal. Place packets on baking sheet.

2. Bake in preheated oven for 13 to 15 minutes or until fish is opaque and flakes easily when tested with a fork. Slide packets onto plates.

Adjustments for Phase 1

▶ Omit the tarragon and pepper.

Advice for a Healthy Gut

▶ While you are following the LGS Diet Plan, brush the foil squares with extra-virgin olive oil in step 1 instead of using cooking spray.

Rosemary-Smoked Halibut with Balsamic Vinaigrette

Makes 6 servings

Suitable for Phases 2 & 3

It's hard to believe this impressive-sounding recipe is so easy to make. Just lighting the sprigs of rosemary gives the fish a tantalizing herb flavor and aroma.

- Preheat oven to 425°F (220°C)
- Baking dish

2 or 3	sprigs fresh rosemary	2 or 3
1½ lbs	halibut fillets	750 g

Balsamic Vinaigrette

¼ cup	olive oil	60 mL
2 tbsp	balsamic vinegar	30 mL
¼ tsp	coarsely crushed black pepper	1 mL
⅛ tsp	salt	0.5 mL
½ cup	diced seeded tomato	125 mL
1 tsp	finely chopped shallot	5 mL

1. In a baking dish, place rosemary beside halibut; light rosemary with match (rosemary may not remain lit). Cover tightly with foil. Bake in preheated oven for 8 to 12 minutes or until fish flakes easily when tested with fork.

2. *Balsamic Vinaigrette:* Meanwhile, in a small bowl, whisk together oil, balsamic vinegar, pepper and salt; stir in tomato and shallot. Serve with halibut.

This recipe courtesy of chef Pamela Good and dietitian Carrie Roach.

Advice for a Healthy Gut

▶ Choose extra virgin olive oil and natural balsamic vinegar (without color or sulfites).

Nutrients per serving

Calories	191
Fat	11 g
Carbohydrate	2 g
Fiber	0 g
Protein	21 g
Vitamin A	223 IU
Iron	0.4 mg
Zinc	0.5 mg

Grilled Salmon Steaks with Lemon and Olive Oil

Suitable for Phases 1, 2 & 3

Salmon is one of the best sources of anti-inflammatory omega-3 fats, which help maintain gut integrity by reducing gut permeability. Plus, salmon provides zinc, iron, potassium and selenium.

• **Preheat barbecue grill to high**

¼ cup	extra virgin olive oil	60 mL
	Juice of ½ lemon	
	Salt and freshly ground black pepper	
4	salmon steaks (1 inch/2.5 cm thick)	4

1. In a shallow dish, whisk together oil, lemon juice, salt and pepper. Add salmon and turn to coat. Cover and refrigerate for 1 hour, turning halfway through.

2. Remove salmon from marinade and discard marinade. Grill salmon, turning once, for 4 minutes per side or until fish is opaque and flakes easily with a fork.

Adjustment for Phase 1

▶ Omit the pepper.

Nutrients per serving

Calories	483
Fat	23 g
Carbohydrate	0 g
Fiber	0 g
Protein	65 g
Vitamin A	372 IU
Iron	1.3 mg
Zinc	1.2 mg

Cedar-Baked Salmon

Makes 6 servings

Suitable for Phases 2 & 3

Salmon is a great source of omega-3 fats, which reduce inflammation and promote normalization of gut function. Salmon is also a source of protein, zinc and selenium.

Tips

Cedar shingles and shims, available at lumberyards, impart a unique flavor to salmon when baking. For this recipe, you'll need to soak 2 untreated cedar shingles or 1 package cedar shims in water for at least 2 hours or preferably overnight. Soaking the wood ensures that it is damp enough to produce lots of aromatic smoke.

When soaking shingles or shims, weight them down. Otherwise they will float to the surface.

Nutrients per serving

Calories	178
Fat	5 g
Carbohydrate	7 g
Fiber	2 g
Protein	26 g
Vitamin A	5227 IU
Iron	2.9 mg
Zinc	1.0 mg

* Preheat oven to 425°F (220°C)
* Soaked cedar shingles or shims (see tips, at left)
* Steamer basket

1½ lbs	salmon fillets	750 g
	Grated zest and juice of 1 lime	
1½ cups	diagonally sliced asparagus	375 mL
¼ cup	julienned leek	60 mL
4	thin slices red onion	4
¼ cup	diagonally sliced celery	60 mL
½ cup	thickly sliced shiitake mushrooms	125 mL
2	tomatoes, seeded and cut into strips	2
8	fresh basil leaves, slivered	8
1	bag (10 oz/300 g) fresh spinach, trimmed	1
	Salt and freshly ground black pepper	

1. Place soaked shingles or shims on baking sheet; lightly brush with oil. Remove skin and any bones from salmon; cut into 6 serving-size pieces and place on cedar. Sprinkle with lime zest and juice. Bake in preheated oven for 10 to 15 minutes or until fish flakes easily when tested with fork.

2. Meanwhile, in steamer basket, combine asparagus, leek, onion and celery; steam until partially cooked. Add mushrooms, tomatoes, basil and spinach; steam just until tender-crisp and spinach has wilted. Place on 6 individual plates; season to taste with salt and pepper. Top each with salmon.

This recipe courtesy of chef Judson Simpson and dietitian Violaine Sauvé.

Broiled Cilantro Ginger Salmon

Makes 6 servings

Suitable for Phase 3

Broiling the fish on only one side keeps it moist, delicious and full of flavor. Salmon is a great source of omega-3 fats, which promote normalization of gut function.

Tips

This can also be cooked on a barbecue with two or more burners. Preheat one side to medium, place salmon on the other side and close the lid. This indirect cooking method is great for delicate proteins like fish. There will be enough heat to cook the salmon without burning it or drying it out.

Extra salmon is great served cold with a salad.

- **Rimmed baking sheet, greased**

3	cloves garlic, roughly chopped	3
2 tbsp	grated gingerroot	30 mL
1/2 tsp	salt	2 mL
1/2 cup	chopped fresh cilantro	125 mL
2 tbsp	olive oil	30 mL
1/2 tsp	freshly ground black pepper	2 mL
	Grated zest of 2 limes	
6	salmon fillets (about 2 1/4 lbs/1.125 kg total)	6

1. Using a mortar and pestle (or a food processor), crush garlic, ginger and salt to form a paste. Stir in cilantro, olive oil, pepper and lime zest.

2. Place salmon on a plate and coat top evenly with paste. Cover and refrigerate for at least 30 minutes or for up to 2 hours. Preheat broiler, with rack set 4 inches (10 cm) from the top.

3. Transfer salmon to prepared baking sheet and broil for 7 to 10 minutes or until salmon is opaque and flakes easily with a fork.

This recipe courtesy of Eileen Campbell.

Advice for a Healthy Gut

▶ Choose extra virgin olive oil.

Nutrients per serving	
Calories	260
Fat	12 g
Carbohydrate	1 g
Fiber	0 g
Protein	35 g
Vitamin A	209 IU
Iron	0.7 mg
Zinc	0.7 mg

Seared Salmon with Pineapple Mint Quinoa

Makes 4 servings

Suitable for Phases 2 & 3

Orange marmalade might seem like an odd addition here, but it's a handy ingredient that can perform amazing feats even when used in small amounts.

Tip

A pineapple is ripe enough to eat when a leaf is easily pulled from the top. To prepare it, cut off the leafy top and a small layer of the base, then slice off the tough skin and "eyes." Cut the flesh into slices, then remove the chewy central core from each slice. Cut each slice into chunks.

1 cup	diced fresh pineapple	250 mL
2 tbsp	chopped fresh mint	30 mL
2 tsp	minced gingerroot	10 mL
2 tbsp	orange marmalade	30 mL
1 tbsp	freshly squeezed lime juice	15 mL
1½ cups	cooked quinoa, cooled	375 mL
4	skinless wild salmon fillets (each about 5 oz/150 g)	4
2 tsp	vegetable oil	10 mL
¼ tsp	fine sea salt	1 mL
⅛ tsp	cayenne pepper	0.5 mL

1. In a medium bowl, combine pineapple, mint, ginger, orange marmalade and lime juice. Add quinoa, gently tossing to combine. Cover and refrigerate until ready to use.

2. Brush both sides of fish with oil and sprinkle with salt and cayenne. Heat a large skillet over medium-high heat. Add fish and cook, turning once, for 3 to 4 minutes per side or until fish is opaque and flakes easily when tested with a fork. Serve with pineapple quinoa.

Advice for a Healthy Gut

▸ Use only 100% no-sugar-added marmalade.

▸ "Vegetable oil" is a catchall term for any edible oil from a plant source, whether it be a vegetable, fruit, nut or seed. While you are following the LGS Diet Plan, the best choices for this recipe are extra virgin olive oil, macadamia nut oil, grapeseed oil and avocado oil.

Nutrients per serving

Calories	332
Fat	10 g
Carbohydrate	28 g
Fiber	3 g
Protein	32 g
Vitamin A	259 IU
Iron	1.8 mg
Zinc	1.4 mg

Salmon with Cranberry and Caper Vinaigrette

Suitable for Phases 2 & 3

Here is a stylish and unusual dish that couldn't be easier to make. Prepare the tangy vinaigrette the day before and then warm it up while the salmon fillets are grilling.

Tip

Use ½ tsp (2 mL) chopped fresh thyme instead of the dried thyme, if available.

• **Preheat barbecue or broiler**

½ cup	red wine vinegar	125 mL
¼ cup	vegetable oil	60 mL
¼ cup	water	60 mL
¼ cup	sliced cranberries	60 mL
2 tbsp	capers	30 mL
1 tbsp	finely chopped shallots	15 mL
1 tsp	minced fresh or dried chives	5 mL
1 tsp	minced garlic	5 mL
½ tsp	pink peppercorns	2 mL
½	small lemon, peeled and cut into 4 wedges	½
½	small lime, peeled and cut into 4 wedges	½
¼ to ½ tsp	cayenne pepper	1 to 2 mL
Pinch	dried thyme	Pinch
6	skin-on salmon fillets (each 4 oz/125 g)	6

1. In a jar, combine vinegar, oil, water, cranberries, capers, shallots, chives, garlic, pink peppercorns, lemon wedges, lime wedges, cayenne and thyme; shake well and let stand for 6 to 8 hours.

2. Broil or grill salmon fillets over medium-high heat for 3 to 4 minutes per side or until fish flakes easily when tested with fork.

3. Warm vinaigrette on stove or in microwave; remove lemon and lime wedges. Remove skin from salmon. Serve with vinaigrette spooned over fillets.

This recipe courtesy of chef Daryle Ryo Nagata and dietitian Jane Thornthwaite.

Nutrients per serving

Calories	190
Fat	13 g
Carbohydrate	2 g
Fiber	1 g
Protein	16 g
Vitamin A	156 IU
Iron	0.5 mg
Zinc	0.3 mg

Tips

Always preheat the broiler when broiling meats or fish. Lightly oil the broiling rack and position it 4 to 6 inches (10 to 15 cm) from the heat.

For best results, use salmon fillets that are about 1 inch (2.5 cm) thick.

Adjustments for Phase 2

▶ Omit the shallots, chives, garlic and cayenne pepper.

▶ Substitute rice vinegar or natural balsamic vinegar (without color or sulfites) for the red wine vinegar.

Advice for a Healthy Gut

▶ Continue to choose rice vinegar or natural balsamic vinegar over red wine vinegar while you are following the LGS Diet Plan.

▶ Use extra virgin olive oil, macadamia nut oil, grapeseed oil or avocado oil for the vegetable oil.

Maple Ginger Salmon

Makes 4 servings

Suitable for Phases 1, 2 & 3

This is a North American twist on an Asian classic. Fish provides zinc, iron and selenium, key nutrients for a healthy immune system, which aids in healing.

- Preheat oven to 350°F (180°C)
- Rimmed baking sheet, lined with foil

4	skinless salmon fillets	4
¼ cup	pure maple syrup	60 mL
2 tbsp	rice vinegar	30 mL
1 tsp	finely grated gingerroot	5 mL

1. Place salmon on prepared baking sheet.

2. In a small bowl, whisk together maple syrup, vinegar and ginger. Pour over fillets.

3. Bake in preheated oven for 10 to 15 minutes or until fish is opaque and flakes easily when tested with a fork.

Nutrients per serving

Calories	461
Fat	14 g
Carbohydrate	15 g
Fiber	0 g
Protein	65 g
Vitamin A	372 IU
Iron	1.2 mg
Zinc	1.5 mg

Salmon, Potato and Green Bean Salad

Suitable for Phases 2 & 3

This main-meal salad makes a great summer supper when fresh vegetables and herbs are in season.

Tips

For a change, replace the salmon with canned tuna packed in water.

If desired, make your own vinaigrette rather than using the bottled variety.

1 lb	small new white potatoes, halved or quartered	500 g
1 cup	green beans, cut into 2-inch (5 cm) pieces	250 mL
1	green onion, chopped	1
1 cup	halved cherry tomatoes or diced tomatoes	250 mL
2 tbsp	chopped fresh basil (or 1 tsp/5 mL dried)	30 mL
1/3 cup	bottled oil-and-vinegar-type dressing	75 mL
2	cans (each 7 1/2 oz/213 g) salmon, drained, bones and skin removed	2
	Salt and freshly ground black pepper	

1. In a medium saucepan, gently boil potatoes for 10 to 15 minutes or until tender but firm, adding beans during last 4 minutes of cooking time. Drain and transfer vegetables to a large bowl.

2. Add green onion, tomatoes and basil. Add dressing; toss gently to combine. Gently stir in salmon. Season to taste with salt and pepper. Chill until serving.

This recipe courtesy of Colette Villeneuve.

Adjustment for Phase 2

▶ Omit the green onion.

Advice for a Healthy Gut

▶ Choose an extra virgin olive oil–based salad dressing that is free of preservatives, gluten and artificial colors and flavors, and that is made with rice vinegar or natural balsamic vinegar.

Nutrients per serving	
Calories	283
Fat	10 g
Carbohydrate	23 g
Fiber	4 g
Protein	29 g
Vitamin A	581 IU
Iron	1.8 mg
Zinc	0.5 mg

Grilled Cilantro Shrimp Skewers

Suitable for Phase 3

Shrimp is a great source of protein and has the immune-supporting nutrients selenium and zinc. It is also an excellent source of phosphorus and niacin.

Tips

Barbecue Method: Preheat barbecue to 350°F (180°C) and cook for $2\frac{1}{2}$ minutes per side or until shrimp are pink and opaque.

Cook extra shrimp and serve over a green salad for a main course another day.

- Six 6-inch (15 cm) wooden skewers
- Baking sheet, greased

2	cloves garlic, minced	2
$\frac{1}{4}$ cup	chopped fresh cilantro	60 mL
2 tbsp	olive oil	30 mL
$\frac{1}{2}$ tsp	ground coriander	2 mL
	Grated zest and juice of 2 limes	
	Salt and freshly ground black pepper	
1 lb	extra-large shrimp, peeled and deveined	500 g

1. In a small bowl, combine garlic, cilantro, olive oil, coriander, lime zest, lime juice, and salt and pepper to taste.

2. Place shrimp in a shallow dish and pour in marinade. Cover and refrigerate for at least 30 minutes or for up to 2 hours. Meanwhile, soak skewers in hot water for 30 minutes and preheat broiler.

3. Thread shrimp evenly onto skewers and place on prepared baking sheet.

4. Broil, turning once, for $2\frac{1}{2}$ minutes per side or until shrimp are pink and opaque.

This recipe courtesy of Eileen Campbell.

Advice for a Healthy Gut

▸ Choose extra virgin olive oil.

Nutrients per serving

Calories	97
Fat	5 g
Carbohydrate	1 g
Fiber	0 g
Protein	10 g
Vitamin A	141 IU
Iron	0.2 mg
Zinc	0.8 mg

Turkey and Chicken

Slow-Roasted Turkey

Suitable for Phases 1, 2 & 3

Turkey is an excellent source of protein, potassium, magnesium and the immune-supporting and healing mineral zinc. It also boasts a lot of selenium, a mineral the body uses to create an important antioxidant that is needed to heal the gut.

Tip

In Phases 2 and 3, the turkey can be flavored with herbs and spices to enhance the versatility of this recipe.

- Preheat oven to 450°F (230°C)
- Roasting pan with rack

| 1 | turkey (about 15 lbs/7.5 kg), without giblets | 1 |
| | Salt and freshly ground black pepper | |

1. Season turkey inside and out with salt and pepper. Place on rack in roasting pan and roast in preheated oven for 1 hour.

2. Reduce oven temperature to 170°F (80°C) and roast for at least 14 hours (if your oven is well calibrated, the turkey will not overcook; the bird will be amazingly juicy and tender). Remove from oven and let rest for 20 minutes before carving.

Adjustment for Phase 1

▶ Omit the pepper.

Nutrients per serving (1 of 15)

Calories	365
Fat	9 g
Carbohydrate	1 g
Fiber	0 g
Protein	66 g
Vitamin A	0 IU
Iron	4.4 mg
Zinc	7.2 mg

Traditional Small Roast Chicken

Makes 8 servings

Suitable for Phases 1, 2 & 3

This simple roast chicken is perfect for all phases of the LGS Diet Plan. It's an excellent source of protein, iron and zinc.

Tip

In Phases 2 and 3, the chicken can be flavored with herbs and spices to enhance the versatility of this recipe.

- Preheat oven to 400°F (200°C)
- Roasting pan with rack, rack sprayed with vegetable cooking spray

1	whole chicken (about 4 lbs/2 kg)	1
2 tsp	salt	10 mL
1 tsp	freshly ground black pepper	5 mL
2 tbsp	olive oil, divided	30 mL

1. Rinse chicken inside and out and pat dry. Trim off visible fat. Combine salt and pepper, and rub into the walls of the interior cavity of the chicken.

2. Run your fingers under the skin of the breast and legs, separating it gently from the meat underneath. Rub half the oil over the meat under the skin and the rest over surface of the skin. Place chicken, breast side down, on prepared rack in roasting pan.

3. Roast in preheated oven for 30 minutes. Reduce oven temperature to 375°F (190°C) and turn chicken breast side up. Roast for 45 minutes, until skin is golden brown and a thermometer inserted into the thickest part of a thigh registers 170°F to 175°F (77°C to 80°C). Let rest for 10 minutes before carving.

Adjustment for Phase 1

▸ Omit the pepper.

Advice for a Healthy Gut

▸ Choose extra virgin olive oil.

Nutrients per serving	
Calories	300
Fat	10 g
Carbohydrate	0 g
Fiber	0 g
Protein	49 g
Vitamin A	120 IU
Iron	2.1 mg
Zinc	3.5 mg

Grilled Chicken Breasts with Pesto

Makes 4 servings

Suitable for Phases 1, 2 & 3

Grilling the pesto-stuffed chicken adds a new twist to this classic flavor combination. Even the modified versions for Phases 1 and 2 still have lots of flavor.

• Preheat barbecue grill to medium-high

4	bone-in chicken breasts	4
1/2 cup	pesto (store-bought or see recipe, page 300)	125 mL
2 tsp	olive oil	10 mL

1. Make a pocket in the center of each chicken breast. Place 2 tsp (10 mL) pesto inside each breast and rub with 1/2 tsp (2 mL) olive oil.

2. Grill, turning once, for 8 to 10 minutes per side or until no longer pink inside. Serve dolloped with the remaining pesto.

Adjustment for Phases 1 & 2

▶ Use the homemade pesto on page 300, following the phase-specific adjustment instructions. Avoid using store-bought pesto.

Advice for a Healthy Gut

▶ Choose extra virgin olive oil.

Nutrients per serving

Calories	309
Fat	20 g
Carbohydrate	2 g
Fiber	1 g
Protein	31 g
Vitamin A	325 IU
Iron	1.5 mg
Zinc	1.2 mg

Grilled Garlic-Ginger Chicken Breasts

Makes 4 servings

Suitable for Phases 2 & 3

This simple grilled chicken can be enhanced with one of the great salsas or dips in this book.

Tips

Broiler Method: After removing chicken from marinade, place in a lightly greased 9-inch (23 cm) square baking pan and pour in marinade. Broil, turning once, for 5 to 6 minutes per side or until chicken is no longer pink inside and has reached an internal temperature of 170°F (77°C).

Extra cooked chicken is always useful to add a quick protein boost to salads, stir-fries and soups.

2 tbsp	freshly squeezed lemon juice	30 mL
2 tsp	minced garlic	10 mL
2 tsp	minced gingerroot	10 mL
2 tsp	olive oil	10 mL
1 tsp	ground cumin	5 mL
4	boneless skinless chicken breasts (1 lb/500 g total)	4
	Freshly ground black pepper	

1. In a shallow dish, whisk together lemon juice, garlic, ginger, olive oil and cumin. Add chicken and turn to coat. Let stand at room temperature for 10 minutes, or cover and refrigerate for up to 4 hours. Preheat barbecue to medium.

2. Remove chicken from marinade and discard marinade. Place chicken on barbecue and cook, turning once, for 3 to 5 minutes per side or until chicken is no longer pink inside and has reached an internal temperature of 170°F (77°C). Season to taste with pepper.

This recipe courtesy of dietitian Judy Jenkins.

Advice for a Healthy Gut

▸ Choose extra virgin olive oil.

▸ You may want to try using a smaller amount of cumin at first, monitoring your tolerance as your gut continues to heal.

Nutrients per serving	
Calories	161
Fat	6 g
Carbohydrate	1 g
Fiber	0 g
Protein	24 g
Vitamin A	37 IU
Iron	0.6 mg
Zinc	0.7 mg

Lemon Garlic Chicken

Suitable for Phase 3

The herbs and spices in this tangy, light dish smell wonderful when you're cooking and taste wonderful when it's time to eat.

Tips

Chicken can be marinated at room temperature for up to 30 minutes if you are short on time. Any longer, make sure it is refrigerated. Throw out the plastic bag used for marinating.

Can't find the cover that fits your casserole? Cover it with foil, dull side out. Trace around the rim with your fingers to be sure foil forms a tight seal.

- 8-cup (2 L) covered casserole dish

1	clove garlic, minced	1
2 tbsp	freshly squeezed lemon juice	30 mL
1 tbsp	extra virgin olive oil	15 mL
1 tsp	dried thyme	5 mL
1/4 tsp	salt	1 mL
Pinch	ground nutmeg	Pinch
Pinch	paprika	Pinch
Pinch	freshly ground white pepper	Pinch
4	boneless skinless chicken breasts	4

1. In a sealable plastic freezer bag set in a bowl, combine garlic, lemon juice, olive oil, thyme, salt, nutmeg, paprika and white pepper. Add chicken breasts to marinade, seal bag and refrigerate for 1 hour.

2. Preheat oven to 375°F (190°C). Place chicken breasts with marinade in the casserole dish and cover tightly. Bake for 45 minutes or until chicken is no longer pink inside and a meat thermometer inserted in the thickest part of a breast registers 165°F (74°C).

Variations

Rather than baking the chicken, barbecue or grill it for 5 to 8 minutes per side.

Substitute an equal amount of oregano for the thyme. Or use 1 tbsp (15 mL) snipped fresh thyme or oregano.

Nutrients per serving	
Calories	170
Fat	7 g
Carbohydrate	1 g
Fiber	0 g
Protein	25 g
Vitamin A	81 IU
Iron	1.0 mg
Zinc	0.7 mg

Moroccan-Style Chicken with Prunes and Quinoa

Suitable for Phases 2 & 3

Traditionally, this dish is served with couscous, but quinoa is every bit as tasty, more nutritious and gluten-free.

Tips

You can halve this recipe, but be sure to use a small (1½- to 3½-quart) slow cooker.

If you are marinating the chicken overnight, refrigerate the prune mixture separately.

If you have difficulty digesting grains, you may want to soak your quinoa overnight in plenty of water, preferably with 1 tbsp (15 mL) apple cider vinegar. Drain and rinse thoroughly before using.

Nutrients per serving	
Calories	333
Fat	8 g
Carbohydrate	47 g
Fiber	3 g
Protein	20 g
Vitamin A	482 IU
Iron	3.3 mg
Zinc	2.6 mg

- Medium to large (3½- to 5-quart) slow cooker

1½ cups	chopped pitted prunes	375 mL
1½ cups	water	375 mL
1 tbsp	liquid honey	15 mL
1 tsp	grated lemon zest	5 mL
4	cloves garlic, minced	4
1 tbsp	dried oregano, crumbled	15 mL
1 tbsp	grated lemon zest	15 mL
½ tsp	sea salt	2 mL
½ tsp	cracked black peppercorns	2 mL
2 lbs	skinless bone-in chicken thighs (about 8 thighs)	1 kg
2 cups	ready-to-use chicken broth (gluten-free, if needed)	500 mL
¼ cup	freshly squeezed lemon juice	60 mL
3 cups	water	750 mL
1½ cups	quinoa, rinsed	375 mL

1. In a bowl, combine prunes, water, honey and lemon zest. Cover and set aside (see Tips, left).

2. In a bowl, combine garlic, oregano, lemon zest, salt and peppercorns. Add chicken and toss until evenly coated. Cover and refrigerate for at least 1 hour or overnight.

3. Transfer reserved chicken mixture to stoneware. Add broth and lemon juice and stir well. Cover and cook on Low for 5 hours or on High for 2½ hours, until juices run clear when chicken is pierced with a fork. Add prunes with liquid. Cover and cook on High for 30 minutes to meld flavors.

4. Meanwhile, in a pot over high heat, bring 3 cups (750 mL) water to a boil. Reduce heat to medium. Add quinoa in a steady stream, stirring to prevent lumps from forming, and return to a boil. Cover, reduce heat to low and simmer until tender and liquid is absorbed, about 15 minutes. Set aside.

5. To serve, spoon quinoa onto a plate and top with chicken mixture.

Chicken with Root Vegetables

Makes 6 servings

Suitable for Phases 1, 2 & 3

This hearty one-pot meal is full of antioxidant-packed garden-fresh vegetables. Chicken is a good source of zinc, potassium and phosphorus.

3 lbs	whole chicken, skin removed	1.5 kg
	Salt and freshly ground black pepper	
8	small russet potatoes, peeled and quartered	8
4	stalks celery, peeled and coarsely chopped	4
4	carrots, peeled and coarsely chopped	4
4	parsnips, peeled and coarsely chopped	4
8 cups	ready-to-use gluten-free chicken broth	2 L
8	sprigs parsley	8
4	bay leaves	4

1. Sprinkle chicken all over (including cavity) with salt and pepper to taste. Place in a large, heavy-bottomed pot or Dutch oven.

2. Arrange potatoes, celery, carrots and parsnips around chicken. Pour in broth, immersing chicken (add enough water to cover, if necessary). Sprinkle with parsley and bay leaves.

3. Over medium heat, simmer, uncovered and checking occasionally to ensure chicken is covered (add more water, if necessary), for 50 minutes or until drumsticks wiggle when touched, a meat thermometer inserted in the thickest part of a thigh registers 185°F (85°C) and vegetables are tender.

Adjustment for Phase 1

▶ Omit the pepper.

Nutrients per serving	
Calories	502
Fat	9 g
Carbohydrate	46 g
Fiber	6 g
Protein	59 g
Vitamin A	7157 IU
Iron	3.7 mg
Zinc	4.5 mg

Chicken Kabobs with Ginger Lemon Marinade

Makes 4 servings

Suitable for Phases 1, 2 & 3

Chicken is a versatile lean protein and provides immune-supporting nutrients, such as B vitamins and zinc. It's also an excellent source of potassium and phosphorus.

Advice for a Healthy Gut

▶ Use extra virgin olive oil, macadamia nut oil or avocado oil for the vegetable oil.

▶ Continue to use rice vinegar and honey in this recipe while you are following the LGS Diet Plan.

Nutrients per serving

Calories	166
Fat	8 g
Carbohydrate	12 g
Fiber	2 g
Protein	13 g
Vitamin A	706 IU
Iron	0.6 mg
Zinc	0.5 mg

Ginger Lemon Marinade

3 tbsp	freshly squeezed lemon juice	45 mL
2 tbsp	water	30 mL
1 tbsp	vegetable oil	15 mL
2 tsp	sesame oil	10 mL
1½ tsp	red wine vinegar	7 mL
4 tsp	packed brown sugar	20 mL
1 tsp	minced gingerroot (or ¼ tsp/1 mL ground ginger)	5 mL
½ tsp	ground coriander	2 mL
½ tsp	ground fennel seeds (optional)	2 mL

Chicken Kabobs

8 oz	boneless skinless chicken breasts, cut into 2-inch (5 cm) cubes	250 g
16	squares green bell pepper	16
16	pineapple chunks (fresh or canned)	16
16	cherry tomatoes	16

1. *Ginger Lemon Marinade:* In small bowl, combine lemon juice, water, vegetable oil, sesame oil, vinegar, brown sugar, ginger, coriander, and fennel seeds (if using); mix well. Add chicken and mix well; marinate for 20 minutes.

2. *Chicken Kabobs:* Alternately thread chicken cubes, green pepper, pineapple and tomatoes onto 4 long or 8 short barbecue skewers. Barbecue for 15 to 20 minutes or just until chicken is no longer pink inside, brushing often with marinade and rotating every 5 minutes.

Adjustments for Phase 1

▶ Substitute rice vinegar for the red wine vinegar.

▶ Replace the brown sugar with an equal amount of liquid honey.

▶ Omit the cherry tomatoes.

Cornish Game Hens with Cranberry and Wild Rice Stuffing

Suitable for Phase 3

This recipe is rich in both flavor and nutrition. The wild and brown rice stuffing adds crunch and texture, and it is healthier than a traditional stuffing made with bread crumbs.

Tip

When purchasing dried sage or thyme, use dried leaves and avoid the powdered variety.

* **Roasting pan**

4 cups	ready-to-use gluten-free chicken broth	1 L
¾ cup	brown rice	175 mL
½ cup	wild rice, rinsed	125 mL
1 tbsp	crumbled dried sage	15 mL
1 tbsp	crumbled dried thyme	15 mL
1 tbsp	butter	15 mL
1 tbsp	vegetable oil	15 mL
1	large onion, chopped	1
1 cup	sliced cremini mushroom caps (halved, then cut into ¼-inch/0.5 cm slices)	250 mL
1 cup	diced celery	250 mL
1 cup	diced carrots	250 mL
¼ tsp	salt	1 mL
¼ tsp	freshly ground black pepper	1 mL
1 cup	dried cranberries	250 mL
2 tbsp	balsamic vinegar	30 mL
4 to 6	Cornish game hens (each about 1 to 1¼ lbs/500 to 625 g)	4 to 6
	Plum Dipping Sauce (see recipe, page 303)	

1. In a large saucepan, over high heat, combine broth, brown rice, wild rice, sage and thyme and bring to a boil. Reduce heat, cover and simmer gently for 45 to 55 minutes or until rice is tender. Remove from heat and fluff with a fork. Set aside to cool completely.

2. In a skillet, heat butter and oil over medium–high heat. Add onion, mushrooms, celery, carrots, salt and pepper and cook, stirring constantly, until tender, about 8 to 10 minutes. Stir in dried cranberries and balsamic vinegar.

Nutrients per serving (1 of 6)	
Calories	571
Fat	14 g
Carbohydrate	53 g
Fiber	4 g
Protein	56 g
Vitamin A	3936 IU
Iron	3.3 mg
Zinc	4.8 mg

This recipe makes enough stuffing for 4 to 6 Cornish game hens or a 10-lb (4.5 kg) turkey.

3. Add vegetable mixture to rice mixture and stir gently to combine. Loosely stuff into the game hens and place them breast side up in roasting pan.

4. Preheat oven to 350°F (180°C). Roast hens, uncovered, for 45 to 60 minutes or until meat thermometer inserted in thigh registers 180°F (82°C). Remove the stuffing immediately.

5. Serve with Plum Dipping Sauce.

Advice for a Healthy Gut

▶ Use only organic butter.

▶ Use extra virgin olive oil, macadamia nut oil, grapeseed oil or avocado oil for the vegetable oil.

▶ Choose unsweetened dried cranberries.

▶ Choose natural balsamic vinegar (without color or sulfites).

Warm Chicken Salad with Fruit

Suitable for Phases 2 & 3

This salad is packed with phytonutrient-rich, anti-inflammatory berries. Use any fresh fruit in this delicious and eye-appealing salad.

Tip

For variety, replace one of the lettuces in this recipe with shredded spinach or red leaf lettuce. Vary the lettuce and the fruit to create a different salad every time you make this recipe.

- Food processor or blender

Dressing

1 cup	fresh or thawed frozen unsweetened raspberries	250 mL
½ tsp	grated orange zest	2 mL
¼ cup	freshly squeezed orange juice	60 mL
1 tsp	grated lemon zest	5 mL
1 tbsp	freshly squeezed lemon juice	15 mL
1 tbsp	chopped fresh mint	15 mL
1 tsp	liquid honey	5 mL
¼ tsp	salt	1 mL

Salad

4	boneless skinless chicken breasts (3 oz/90 g each)	4
½	head butter or Boston lettuce	½
½	head romaine lettuce	½
½	cantaloupe, peeled	½
2 cups	strawberries, hulled and halved	500 mL
1 cup	blueberries or blackberries	250 mL

1. *Dressing:* In food processor, purée raspberries; press through sieve to remove seeds and return to food processor. Add orange zest and juice, lemon zest and juice, mint, honey and salt; process until well blended. Pour into jar; refrigerate for up to 24 hours. Shake well before serving.

2. *Salad:* Broil or barbecue chicken until no longer pink inside. Cut into strips.

3. Meanwhile, tear butter lettuce and romaine into bite-size pieces; arrange on 4 large plates. Slice cantaloupe into 8 wedges; cut wedges in half crosswise. Arrange on greens along with strawberries and blueberries. Place chicken on top. Drizzle with dressing. Serve immediately.

This recipe courtesy of chef Dean Mitchell and dietitian Suzanne Journault-Hemstock.

Nutrients per serving

Calories	214
Fat	3 g
Carbohydrate	28 g
Fiber	7 g
Protein	21 g
Vitamin A	9939 IU
Iron	2.2 mg
Zinc	1.2 mg

Lamb, Beef and Pork

Roast Lamb with Marrakech Rub

Suitable for Phases 2 & 3

This simple roast with the flavors of Morocco is easy to prepare if you have a batch of Marrakech Rub on hand. It's great served hot but would also be good cold, with salad.

- Roasting pan with rack, lightly sprayed with vegetable cooking spray

3 lbs	boneless leg of lamb, trimmed	1.5 kg
2 tbsp	Marrakech Rub (see recipe, opposite)	30 mL
2 cups	ready-to-use reduced-sodium chicken broth (gluten-free, if needed)	500 mL
1 cup	sliced dried apricots	250 mL

1. Place lamb in a large container and rub with Marrakech Rub. Cover and refrigerate for at least 1 hour or overnight. Preheat oven to 375°F (190°C).

2. Place lamb on rack in roasting pan and roast for 25 minutes. Add 1 cup (250 mL) broth and the apricots to the drippings in the pan. Roast, adding more broth as the liquid evaporates, for 20 to 35 minutes or until lamb has reached an internal temperature of 150°F (65°C) for medium–rare, or until desired doneness. Remove to a plate and cover with foil. Let rest for 15 minutes before carving.

This recipe courtesy of Eileen Campbell.

Advice for a Healthy Gut

▶ You may want to try using a smaller amount of Marrakech Rub at first, monitoring your tolerance as your gut continues to heal.

Nutrients per serving

Calories	243
Fat	8 g
Carbohydrate	5 g
Fiber	2 g
Protein	37 g
Vitamin A	1191 IU
Iron	3.9 mg
Zinc	6.8 mg

**Suitable for
Phases 2 & 3**

*Mix up a batch of this
zesty rub and keep it
for days when you want
to make Roast Lamb
with Marrakech Rub
(opposite). It's also great
for seasoning vegetables for
roasting or chicken, pork
or lamb for grilling.*

Big-Batch Marrakech Rub

¼ cup	paprika	60 mL
2 tbsp	ground coriander	30 mL
2 tbsp	ground cumin	30 mL
2 tbsp	ground cinnamon	30 mL
1 tbsp	cayenne pepper	15 mL
1 tbsp	ground allspice	15 mL
1 tsp	ground ginger	5 mL
1 tsp	ground cloves	5 mL

1. Combine all ingredients and store in a covered
   container for up to 6 months.

Nutrients per 1 tbsp
(15 mL)

Calories	6
Fat	0 g
Carbohydrate	1 g
Fiber	1 g
Protein	0 g
Vitamin A	457 IU
Iron	0.4 mg
Zinc	0.1 mg

Moroccan-Style Lamb with Raisins and Apricots

Suitable for Phases 2 & 3

This classic Middle Eastern tagine-style recipe, in which lamb is braised in spices and honey, is an appetizing combination of savory and sweet. Serve it with quinoa for a New World twist.

Tip

You can halve this recipe, but be sure to use a small (1½- to 3½-quart) slow cooker.

Nutrients per serving

Calories	253
Fat	8 g
Carbohydrate	22 g
Fiber	2 g
Protein	24 g
Vitamin A	604 IU
Iron	3.3 mg
Zinc	4.9 mg

• **Medium to large (3½- to 5-quart) slow cooker**

1 to 2 tbsp	olive oil	15 to 30 mL
2 lbs	trimmed stewing lamb, cut into 1-inch (2.5 cm) cubes	1 kg
1	onion, finely chopped	1
1 tbsp	minced gingerroot	15 mL
1 tbsp	ground cumin (see tip, opposite)	15 mL
1 tsp	ground coriander	5 mL
1 tsp	grated lemon zest	5 mL
½ tsp	salt	2 mL
½ tsp	cracked black peppercorns (approx.)	2 mL
1	1-inch (2.5 cm) piece cinnamon stick	1
½ cup	ready-to-use chicken broth (gluten-free, if needed)	125 mL
1 tbsp	freshly squeezed lemon juice	15 mL
1 tbsp	liquid honey	15 mL
	Salt (optional)	
1 cup	dried apricots, chopped	250 mL
½ cup	raisins	125 mL
½ cup	finely chopped fresh cilantro	125 mL

1. In a skillet, heat 1 tbsp (15 mL) oil over medium-high heat. Add lamb, in batches, and cook, stirring, adding more oil if necessary, until browned, about 4 minutes per batch. Transfer to slow cooker stoneware.

2. Reduce heat to medium. Add onion to pan and cook, stirring, until softened. Add ginger, cumin, coriander, lemon zest, salt, peppercorns and cinnamon stick and cook, stirring, for 1 minute. Add broth and bring to a boil.

Tips

For best results, toast and grind the cumin and coriander seeds yourself. Place seeds in a dry skillet over medium heat and cook, stirring, until fragrant, about 3 minutes. Using a mortar and pestle or a spice grinder, pound or grind as finely as you can.

This recipe can be partially prepared ahead of time. Heat 1 tbsp (15 mL) oil and complete step 2. Cover and refrigerate overnight or for up to 2 days. When you're ready to cook, either brown the lamb as outlined in step 1 or add it to the stoneware without browning. Stir well and continue with step 3.

3. Transfer to slow cooker stoneware. Stir well. Cover and cook on Low for 6 to 8 hours or on High for 3 to 4 hours, until lamb is tender. Add lemon juice and honey and stir well. Season to taste with salt (if using). Stir in apricots and raisins. Cover and cook on High for 20 minutes, until fruit is warmed through. Garnish with cilantro. Discard cinnamon stick.

Advice for a Healthy Gut

▸ Choose extra virgin olive oil.

▸ You may want to try using a smaller amount of gingerroot and cumin at first, monitoring your tolerance as your gut continues to heal.

Grilled Lamb and Vegetables with Roasted Garlic

Suitable for Phases 1, 2 & 3

The subtle flavor of roasted garlic blends perfectly with the warm vegetables and thinly sliced lamb in this delicious recipe.

Tip

Roasted garlic has a milder taste than fresh garlic and is easier on the digestive system.

- Preheat oven to 400°F (200°C)

2	stalks celery, cut into 1-inch (2.5 cm) thick slices	2
1	red bell pepper, cut into strips	1
1	zucchini, sliced	1
1	eggplant, cut into 1/4-inch (5 mm) thick slices	1
1 tsp	crushed dried thyme	5 mL
2	heads garlic	2
1/4 cup	olive oil, divided	60 mL
2 tbsp	white wine vinegar	30 mL
1/4 tsp	salt	1 mL
1/4 tsp	freshly ground black pepper	1 mL
1	package (400 g) frozen boneless lamb loins, thawed	1
	Fresh thyme (optional)	

1. In a bowl, combine celery, red pepper, zucchini, eggplant and thyme; let stand for 1 hour.

2. Cut tops off garlic heads; place in a small baking dish or custard cups. Set aside 1 tbsp (15 mL) oil. Cover garlic with remaining oil. Bake in preheated oven for 30 to 35 minutes or until cloves come out of their skins. (Do not burn.) Remove garlic from skins and mash with fork. Stir in vinegar, salt and pepper. Keep warm (or reheat in microwave for 15 seconds).

3. Preheat broiler. Brush lamb and vegetables with reserved oil. Grill lamb loins and vegetables for 2 to 3 minutes per side. (Or heat reserved oil in large skillet; brown lamb for about 5 minutes. Remove; keep warm. Add vegetables to skillet and sauté for about 5 minutes or until tender.)

Nutrients per serving	
Calories	485
Fat	40 g
Carbohydrate	14 g
Fiber	6 g
Protein	19 g
Vitamin A	1128 IU
Iron	2.7 mg
Zinc	2.4 mg

Tips

Use 1 tbsp (15 mL) fresh thyme instead of dried, and fresh rather than frozen lamb, if available.

If desired, cook this dish on the barbecue, bearing in mind that because foods cooked at high temperatures may present a risk for cancer, they should be served less often.

4. To serve, pour 1 tbsp (15 mL) garlic sauce onto 1 side of each of 4 plates. Slice lamb and place on top. Place vegetables beside lamb. Garnish with fresh thyme, if desired.

This recipe courtesy of chef Philippe Guiet and dietitian Dawn Palin.

Adjustment for Phase 1

▸ Omit the roasted garlic sauce (made with the garlic, vinegar, salt and pepper).

Advice for a Healthy Gut

▸ Choose extra virgin olive oil.

▸ While you are following the LGS Diet Plan, use rice vinegar or natural balsamic vinegar (without color or sulfites) instead of white wine vinegar in this recipe.

Chile-Spiked Lamb Shanks

Makes 4 to 8 servings

Suitable for Phase 3

You'll love the flavors in this dish — a sweet-and-sour combination with a bit of heat.

Tips

You can halve this recipe, but be sure to use a small (2- to 3½-quart) slow cooker.

Whether you cook the lamb shanks whole or halved or have them cut into pieces is a matter of preference. However, if the shanks are left whole, you will be able to serve only four people — each will receive one large shank.

● **Large (approx. 5-quart) slow cooker**

2 tbsp	clarified butter, divided	30 mL
4	large lamb shanks (about 4 lbs/2 kg), patted dry (see tip, at left)	4
2	onions, finely chopped	2
2	carrots, peeled and diced	2
2	stalks celery, diced	2
6	cloves garlic, minced	6
1 tsp	dried thyme	5 mL
1 tsp	cracked black peppercorns	5 mL
½ tsp	sea salt	2 mL
1 cup	dry red wine	250 mL
2 tbsp	coconut sugar	30 mL
2 tbsp	red wine vinegar	30 mL
2 cups	ready-to-use chicken broth (gluten-free, if needed)	500 mL
2 to 4	jalapeño peppers, seeded and diced	2 to 4
	Finely chopped parsley (optional)	

1. In a large skillet, heat 1 tbsp (15 mL) butter over medium-high heat. Add lamb, in batches, and brown on all sides, about 8 minutes per batch. Transfer to slow cooker stoneware as completed. Drain off fat from pan.

2. Reduce heat to medium. Add the remaining butter to pan. Add onions, carrots and celery to pan and cook, stirring, until carrots are soft, about 7 minutes. Add garlic, thyme, peppercorns and sea salt and cook, stirring, for 1 minute. Add wine, bring to a boil and boil for 2 minutes, scraping up brown bits from bottom of pan. Add coconut sugar and vinegar and stir well.

Nutrients per serving (1 of 8)	
Calories	491
Fat	30 g
Carbohydrate	7 g
Fiber	1 g
Protein	45 g
Vitamin A	2712 IU
Iron	4.5 mg
Zinc	8.3 mg

Tips

For a more sophisticated version, after the dish has finished cooking, transfer the lamb to a deep platter and keep warm. Transfer the sauce to a saucepan and cook over medium heat until reduced by a third, about 10 minutes. Purée using an immersion blender. Pour over shanks and garnish liberally with parsley, if desired.

This recipe can be partially prepared ahead of time. Complete step 2. Cover and refrigerate for up to 2 days. When you're ready to cook, complete the recipe.

3. Transfer to slow cooker stoneware. Stir in broth. Cover and cook on Low for 8 to 10 hours or on High for 4 to 5 hours, until meat is falling off the bone. Stir in jalapeños to taste and cook on High for 15 minutes, until flavors meld. Garnish with parsley, if desired.

Advice for a Healthy Gut

▸ Use only organic clarified butter.

▸ While you are following the LGS Diet Plan, use rice vinegar instead of red wine vinegar in this recipe.

▸ You may want to start with a smaller amount of jalapeño peppers, monitoring your tolerance as your gut continues to heal.

Beef with Baby Bok Choy

Suitable for Phase 3

For a healthy and quick weekday meal, marinate the beef the night before. Beef is a great source of protein and zinc, which help the gut heal.

Tip

Serve over rice, gluten-free noodles or rice vermicelli.

2 tbsp	gluten-free soy sauce, divided	30 mL
2 tbsp	cornstarch	30 mL
1½ tsp	granulated sugar, divided	7 mL
⅓ cup	water, divided	75 mL
1 lb	beef flank steak, trimmed and thinly sliced	500 g
¾ cup	ready-to-use gluten-free beef broth, divided	175 mL
1 tsp	cornstarch	5 mL
1 lb	baby bok choy, trimmed and coarsely chopped	500 g
2 tsp	canola oil	10 mL
3 tbsp	coarsely chopped gingerroot	45 mL
2	hot red chile peppers, peeled, seeded and finely chopped (optional)	2

1. In a medium bowl, stir together 1 tbsp (15 mL) soy sauce, 2 tbsp (30 mL) cornstarch, 1 tsp (5 mL) sugar and ¼ cup (60 mL) water. Add beef, turning to coat. Cover, refrigerate and let marinate for at least 30 minutes or overnight.

2. In a small bowl, stir together ¼ cup (60 mL) broth, 1 tsp (5 mL) cornstarch and the remaining soy sauce and water. Set aside.

3. In a large skillet, heat the remaining broth over medium-high heat. Stir in the remaining sugar until dissolved. Add bok choy and cook, stirring, for 1 minute. Cover and cook for 5 minutes or until tender. Uncover and cook, stirring, for 3 to 5 minutes or until liquid has evaporated. Using tongs, transfer bok choy to a bowl, cover and keep warm.

Nutrients per serving	
Calories	115
Fat	4 g
Carbohydrate	5 g
Fiber	1 g
Protein	14 g
Vitamin A	2533 IU
Iron	1.5 mg
Zinc	2.3 mg

Tips

For larger appetites, double the serving size.

To remove the skin from gingerroot with the least amount of waste, use the edge of a teaspoon. With a brushing motion, scrape off the skin to reveal the yellow root.

4. In same skillet, heat canola oil over high heat. Add ginger and chiles (if using) and cook, stirring, for 1 minute. Reduce heat to medium-high. Using tongs, transfer beef to skillet and cook, stirring occasionally, for 7 to 8 minutes or until browned.

5. Stir in broth mixture from step 2 and bring to a boil. Cook, stirring, for about 1 minute or until sauce has thickened. Stir in bok choy and cook for 3 to 5 minutes or until heated through.

Advice for a Healthy Gut

▶ While you are following the LGS Diet Plan, replace the granulated sugar with an equal amount of honey, and use extra virgin olive oil, macadamia nut oil, grapeseed oil or avocado oil in place of the canola oil.

▶ If you decide to use the chile peppers, you may want to start with a smaller amount, monitoring your tolerance as your gut continues to heal.

Beef with Cumin and Lime

Lime adds extra flavor to this Mexican-inspired dish. Beef is an excellent source of zinc, which supports the immune system and helps with repair and healing.

1 tsp	ground cumin	5 mL
1/4 tsp	salt	1 mL
1/4 tsp	freshly ground black pepper	1 mL
1/8 tsp	cayenne pepper	0.5 mL
1 tsp	olive oil	5 mL
2 lbs	stewing beef, cubed	1 kg
2	whole cloves	2
1 cup	water	250 mL
1 tbsp	freshly squeezed lime juice	15 mL
1/4 cup	chopped fresh cilantro	60 mL

1. In a small bowl, stir together cumin, salt, black pepper and cayenne.

2. In a large nonstick skillet, heat oil over medium–high heat. Brown beef on all sides. Sprinkle cumin mixture over beef and stir in cloves, water and lime juice. Reduce heat to medium, cover and simmer, adding more water if mixture becomes dry, for 1 hour or until beef is tender.

3. Remove and discard cloves. Using a slotted spoon, transfer beef to a plate. Cover with foil and keep warm. Increase heat to high and boil cooking liquid for 5 to 10 minutes or until reduced to 1/4 cup (60 mL). Stir in cilantro. Divide beef evenly among 8 individual serving plates. Spoon sauce on top.

Advice for a Healthy Gut

▶ Choose extra virgin olive oil or avocado oil.

Nutrients per serving

Calories	183
Fat	9 g
Carbohydrate	0 g
Fiber	0 g
Protein	24 g
Vitamin A	18 IU
Iron	1.9 mg
Zinc	4.2 mg

Ginger Beef

Suitable for Phase 3

This is a classic Asian-inspired main course. Ginger has well-known anti-inflammatory and gut-calming properties.

Tip

To roast bell peppers, place an oven rack 4 inches (10 cm) below element and preheat oven to 450°F (230°C) or turn broiler on high. Line a baking sheet with foil. Cut each pepper in half, then core and seed it thoroughly to remove insoluble fiber. Place each half, skin side up, on prepared baking sheet. Bake or broil for 5 to 7 minutes or until skins have charred and bubbled. Remove from oven and let stand until cool enough to handle. Peel to remove remaining insoluble fiber.

Nutrients per serving	
Calories	265
Fat	4 g
Carbohydrate	35 g
Fiber	2 g
Protein	21 g
Vitamin A	779 IU
Iron	2.0 mg
Zinc	3.3 mg

2½ cups	water	625 mL
1 cup	basmati rice	250 mL
½ cup	ready-to-use gluten-free vegetarian beef-flavored broth	125 mL
¼ cup	dry white wine	60 mL
1 tbsp	gluten-free soy sauce	15 mL
2 tbsp	cornstarch	30 mL
2 tbsp	finely grated gingerroot	30 mL
2 tbsp	packed brown sugar	30 mL
1 lb	sirloin grilling steak, sliced	500 g
1 cup	sliced seeded peeled roasted red bell peppers (see tip, at left)	250 mL
1 cup	bean sprouts	250 mL

1. In a medium saucepan, combine water and rice and bring to a boil over high heat. Reduce heat to low, cover and simmer for 25 minutes or until rice is tender and water has been absorbed.

2. Meanwhile, in a large nonstick skillet over medium-high heat, stir together broth, wine, soy sauce, cornstarch, ginger and sugar and cook until warm. Add beef and cook, stirring occasionally, for 10 minutes or until beef is tender and browned.

3. Add roasted peppers and bean sprouts and cook, stirring, for 3 minutes or until vegetables are tender and sauce has thickened.

4. Spoon rice onto a serving platter or divide evenly among 6 bowls. Top with beef mixture.

Advice for a Healthy Gut

▶ While you are following the LGS Diet Plan, replace the brown sugar with an equal amount of honey.

Beef and Quinoa Power Burgers

Suitable for Phase 3

With these burgers, along with incredibly delicious flavor, you also get complete protein from the quinoa, vitamin C from the tomatoes and substantial B vitamins from the spinach.

- Food processor

⅔ cup	quinoa, rinsed	150 mL
1⅓ cups	water	325 mL
1 lb	extra-lean ground beef	500 g
½ cup	finely chopped green onions	125 mL
2 tsp	ground cumin	10 mL
1 tsp	fine sea salt	5 mL
1 tsp	extra virgin olive oil	5 mL
4	whole-grain hamburger buns, split and toasted	4
¼ cup	hummus	60 mL
4	large tomato slices	4
2 cups	packed baby spinach or tender watercress sprigs	500 mL

1. In a medium saucepan, combine quinoa and water. Bring to a boil over medium-high heat. Reduce heat to low, cover and simmer for 15 to 18 minutes or until water is absorbed. Remove from heat and let cool to room temperature. Transfer to a large bowl.

2. In food processor, combine cooled quinoa, beef, green onions, cumin and salt; pulse until blended. Form into four ¾-inch (2 cm) thick patties.

3. In a large skillet, heat oil over medium-high heat. Add patties and cook for 4 minutes. Turn and cook for 5 minutes or until no longer pink inside.

4. Spread top halves of buns with hummus. Transfer patties to bottom halves and top with tomato and spinach. Cover with top halves, pressing down gently.

Variation

Substitute lean ground turkey or extra-lean ground pork for the beef.

Advice for a Healthy Gut

▸ Make sure to choose gluten-free hamburger buns.

Nutrients per serving

Calories	441
Fat	12 g
Carbohydrate	49 g
Fiber	4 g
Protein	33 g
Vitamin A	108 IU
Iron	6.0 mg
Zinc	6.9 mg

Blackened Cajun Burgers

Suitable for Phase 3

Beef is packed with protein, zinc and glutamine, an amino acid that is needed for the repair of the digestive tract.

1½ lbs	ground beef	750 g
¼ cup	ice water	60 mL
2 tbsp	ground fennel seeds	30 mL
2 tbsp	garlic powder	30 mL
2 tbsp	salt	30 mL
2 tbsp	freshly ground white pepper	30 mL
2 tbsp	freshly ground black pepper	30 mL
2½ tsp	dry mustard	12 mL
2½ tsp	cayenne pepper	12 mL
4	hamburger buns, split	4
¼ cup	water	60 mL
3 tbsp	Worcestershire sauce	45 mL

1. Using your hands, combine beef and ice water. Form into 4 patties, 1 to 1½ inches (2.5 to 4 cm) thick (do not pack too tightly). Combine all spices and rub the surface of the patties with this mixture.

2. In a large, white-hot iron skillet, cook burgers, turning once, for 5 to 6 minutes per side or until no longer pink inside. Remove pan from heat and transfer burgers to buns.

3. Add water and Worcestershire sauce to pan and scrape up any brown bits from the bottom. Pour liquid over burgers.

Advice for a Healthy Gut

▶ Make sure to choose gluten-free hamburger buns and Worcestershire sauce.

▶ You may want to start with a smaller amount of the various spices, monitoring your tolerance as your gut continues to heal.

Nutrients per serving

Calories	422
Fat	12 g
Carbohydrate	34 g
Fiber	4 g
Protein	43 g
Vitamin A	503 IU
Iron	7.7 mg
Zinc	9.3 mg

Roasted Pork Tenderloin with Pear Slaw

Makes 4 servings

Suitable for Phase 3

Pork and pears make a very fine couple. Napa cabbage adds a fresh crunch, as well as fiber. Pork also provides protein and zinc and is rich in niacin.

- Preheat oven to 400°F (200°C)
- Large ovenproof skillet

½ tsp	fine sea salt, divided	2 mL
½ tsp	freshly ground black pepper, divided	2 mL
2 tbsp	cider vinegar	30 mL
4 tsp	extra virgin olive oil, divided	20 mL
1 tbsp	liquid honey	15 mL
1 tsp	Dijon mustard	5 mL
1	firm-ripe Bosc pear, cut into very thin wedges	1
4 cups	thinly sliced napa cabbage	1 L
½ cup	thinly sliced green onions	125 mL
1 lb	pork tenderloin, trimmed	500 g

1. In a large bowl, whisk together half the salt, half the pepper, vinegar, half the oil, honey and mustard. Add pear, cabbage and green onions, gently tossing to combine. Set aside.

2. Sprinkle pork with the remaining salt and pepper. In ovenproof skillet, heat the remaining oil over medium-high heat. Add pork and cook, turning several times, for 3 to 4 minutes or until browned all over.

3. Transfer skillet to preheated oven and roast for 12 to 14 minutes or until an instant-read thermometer inserted in the thickest part of the tenderloin registers 145°F (63°C) for medium-rare, or until desired doneness. Let rest for at least 5 minutes before slicing. Serve with slaw.

Nutrients per serving

Calories	240
Fat	9 g
Carbohydrate	16 g
Fiber	3 g
Protein	25 g
Vitamin A	1139 IU
Iron	1.5 mg
Zinc	2.2 mg

Herb-Crusted Roasted Pork Loin

Makes 6 to 8 servings

Suitable for Phase 3

Pork provides a handful of immune-supporting nutrients, including zinc, iron and selenium, which the body needs to make the antioxidant glutathione.

- Preheat oven to 375°F (190°C)
- Roasting pan with rack

2	cloves garlic, minced	2
1/4 cup	finely chopped fresh Italian (flat-leaf) parsley	60 mL
2 tbsp	dried rosemary, crumbled	30 mL
1 tsp	kosher salt	5 mL
1 tsp	freshly ground black pepper	5 mL
1	boneless center-cut pork loin roast (3 to 4 lbs/1.5 to 2 kg)	1
2 tbsp	extra virgin olive oil	30 mL
1 tbsp	freshly squeezed lemon juice	15 mL

1. Combine garlic, parsley, rosemary, salt and pepper. Rub pork with oil and the spice mixture. Place on rack in roasting pan.

2. Roast in preheated oven for about 1 hour or until a meat thermometer inserted in the center registers 150°F (65°C). Transfer to a carving board and let rest for 15 minutes before slicing.

3. Meanwhile, spoon fat from pan drippings and stir in lemon juice. Drizzle juice over pork slices before serving.

Nutrients per serving (1 of 8)

Calories	255
Fat	12 g
Carbohydrate	1 g
Fiber	0 g
Protein	34 g
Vitamin A	184 IU
Iron	1.2 mg
Zinc	3.9 mg

Sautéed Pork Chops with Balsamic Onions, Kale and Cherries

Makes 4 servings

Suitable for Phase 3

Pork chops and kale revel in a sweet-tart sauce. Kale is rich in carotenoids, which help rebuild and strengthen the lining of the gut.

Tip

Unlike other greens, kale stems are so tough they are virtually inedible. Hence, they, along with the tougher part of the center rib, must be removed before cooking. To do so, lay a leaf upside down on a cutting board and use a paring knife to cut a V shape along both sides of the rib, cutting it and the stem free from the leaf.

4	boneless pork loin chops (each about 6 oz/175 g)	4
½ tsp	fine sea salt, divided	2 mL
½ tsp	freshly cracked black pepper, divided	2 mL
4 tsp	extra virgin olive oil, divided	20 mL
1	small red onion, cut into ¼-inch (0.5 cm) thick rings	1
1	large bunch curly kale, stems and ribs removed, leaves very thinly sliced crosswise (about 5 cups/1.25 L)	1
¼ cup	dried cherries or cranberries, chopped	60 mL
¼ cup	balsamic vinegar	60 mL
2 tsp	liquid honey	10 mL

1. Sprinkle pork with half the salt and half the pepper. In a large skillet, heat half the oil over medium–high heat. Add pork and cook, turning once, for 5 to 6 minutes per side or until just a hint of pink remains inside. Transfer to a plate and tent with foil to keep warm.

2. In the same skillet, heat the remaining oil over medium–high heat. Add red onion and cook, stirring, for 3 minutes. Add kale, cherries, vinegar, honey and the remaining salt and pepper; cook, stirring, for 2 minutes. Reduce heat to low, cover and simmer, stirring occasionally, for 8 to 10 minutes or until kale is tender. Serve with pork.

Advice for a Healthy Gut

▸ Use unsweetened dried cherries or cranberries.

▸ Choose natural balsamic vinegar (without color or sulfites).

Nutrients *per serving*	
Calories	289
Fat	11 g
Carbohydrate	22 g
Fiber	4 g
Protein	26 g
Vitamin A	13,168 IU
Iron	2.5 mg
Zinc	3.0 mg

Pork Braised in Apple Cider

Suitable for Phase 3

This recipe makes eating well simple, with minimal preparation. Pork is a good source of protein, zinc, iron and selenium — nutrients that are needed for healing and repair of the gut.

12 oz	lean boneless center-cut pork loin, trimmed	375 g
	Salt and freshly ground black pepper	
	Vegetable cooking spray	
1	clove garlic, chopped	1
½ cup	chopped onion	125 mL
2 tsp	chopped fresh thyme	10 mL
1 cup	unsweetened apple cider	250 mL
½ cup	dry white wine	125 mL

1. Season pork with salt and pepper. Coat a nonstick skillet with cooking spray and place over medium–high heat. Cook pork until browned on all sides.

2. Reduce heat to medium and scatter garlic, onion and thyme around pork. Cover and cook for 3 to 4 minutes or until onion browns on the edges.

3. Add cider and wine; simmer, covered, for 35 minutes. Remove pork to a plate. Boil pan liquid until slightly thickened.

4. Slice pork against the grain and return to the pan; heat through.

Advice for a Healthy Gut

▶ While you are following the LGS Diet Plan, coat the skillet with extra virgin olive oil in Step 1 instead of using cooking spray.

Nutrients per serving

Calories	175
Fat	4 g
Carbohydrate	10 g
Fiber	0 g
Protein	17 g
Vitamin A	23 IU
Iron	0.6 mg
Zinc	2.0 mg

Savory Braised Pork

Makes 6 to 8 servings

Suitable for Phase 3

This pork is very easy to make but it's disproportionately delicious because marinating it overnight imbues the meat with deep flavor. It makes a terrific Sunday dinner.

Tips

To purée garlic, use a fine, sharp-toothed grater, such as those made by Microplane.

You can use a bone-in or boneless roast for this recipe, ranging in weight from about 3 to 4 lbs (1.5 to 2 kg).

Advice for a Healthy Gut

▸ Use only organic clarified butter.

Nutrients per serving (1 of 8)

Calories	292
Fat	14 g
Carbohydrate	6 g
Fiber	2 g
Protein	34 g
Vitamin A	2656 IU
Iron	2.8 mg
Zinc	5.0 mg

- **Medium (3- to 4-quart) slow cooker**

2 tsp	coriander seeds	10 mL
2 tsp	cumin seeds	10 mL
1 tsp	cracked black peppercorns	5 mL
6	cloves garlic, puréed (see tip, at left)	6
1 tsp	coarse sea salt	5 mL
1 tbsp	extra virgin olive oil	15 mL
3 lb	pork shoulder or blade (butt) roast	1.5 kg
1 tbsp	clarified butter or pure lard	15 mL
2	onions, finely chopped	2
2	stalks celery, diced	2
2	carrots, peeled and diced	2
2	bay leaves	2
½ cup	water or ready-to-use chicken broth (gluten-free, if needed)	125 mL

1. In a skillet over medium heat, toast coriander and cumin seeds until fragrant, about 3 minutes. Transfer to a mortar or a spice grinder. Add peppercorns and coarsely pound or grind. Transfer to a bowl and combine with garlic, sea salt and oil. Make slits all over meat and fill with spice paste. Rub remainder all over meat. Cover and refrigerate overnight or for up to 24 hours, turning several times, if possible.

2. In a skillet, heat clarified butter over medium-high heat. Add pork and brown on all sides, about 10 minutes. Transfer to slow cooker stoneware.

3. Reduce heat to medium. Add onions, celery and carrots and cook, stirring, until softened, about 7 minutes. Stir in bay leaves and water and bring to a boil, scraping up brown bits from bottom of pan.

4. Pour over pork. Cover and cook on Low for 8 hours or on High for 4 hours, until pork is very tender. Transfer meat to a deep platter and keep warm. Transfer sauce to a saucepan and skim off fat. Bring to a boil over medium-high heat and cook until reduced by one-quarter, about 7 minutes. Taste and adjust seasoning. Spoon over pork and serve.

Side Dishes

Balsamic Asparagus with Walnuts

Suitable for Phases 2 & 3

Fresh asparagus pairs well with a splash of tangy balsamic vinegar and the rich flavor of walnuts. Asparagus is rich in folate, a B vitamin that is needed during the healing process as new cells are formed.

2 tbsp	olive oil	30 mL
1	shallot, minced	1
2 lbs	asparagus (about 16 to 20 spears), trimmed and cut into 2-inch (5 cm) pieces	1 kg
½ cup	toasted walnut halves	125 mL
3 tbsp	balsamic vinegar	45 mL
¾ tsp	salt	3 mL
½ tsp	freshly ground black pepper	2 mL

1. Place a large nonstick skillet over medium-high heat and let pan get hot. Add oil and tip pan to coat. When hot, add shallot and cook, stirring frequently, until slightly softened and slightly browned, 3 to 5 minutes.

2. Add asparagus, tossing to coat, and cook, turning occasionally, for 5 to 6 minutes. Add walnuts and balsamic vinegar and cook until al dente and slightly browned, 3 to 4 minutes. Sprinkle with salt and pepper and serve immediately.

Advice for a Healthy Gut

▶ Choose extra virgin olive oil and natural balsamic vinegar (without color or sulfites).

Nutrients per serving (1 of 6)

Calories	132
Fat	10 g
Carbohydrate	9 g
Fiber	4 g
Protein	5 g
Vitamin A	1154 IU
Iron	3.6 mg
Zinc	1.1 mg

Cumin Beets

**Suitable for
Phases 1, 2 & 3**

*Beets have a long
history of being used
medicinally. They contain
phytonutrients that
support liver health.*

Tips

Peeling the beets before
they are cooked ensures
that all the delicious
cooking juices end up
on your plate.

This dish can be
assembled the night
before it is cooked.
Complete step 1, add
beets to mixture and
refrigerate overnight.
The next day, continue
cooking as directed in
step 2.

- Slow cooker

1 tbsp	vegetable oil	15 mL
1	onion, finely chopped	1
3	cloves garlic, minced	3
1 tsp	cumin seeds	5 mL
1 tsp	salt	5 mL
$\frac{1}{2}$ tsp	freshly ground black pepper	2 mL
2	tomatoes, peeled and coarsely chopped	2
1 cup	water	250 mL
1 lb	beets, peeled and used whole, if small, or sliced thinly (see tip, at left)	500 g

1. In a skillet, heat oil over medium-high heat. Add
   onion and cook, stirring, until softened. Stir in garlic,
   cumin, salt and pepper and cook for 1 minute. Add
   tomatoes and water and bring to a boil.

2. Place beets in slow cooker stoneware and pour tomato
   mixture over them. Cover and cook on Low for 8 to
   10 hours or on High for 4 to 5 hours, until beets
   are tender.

Adjustments for Phase 1

▶ Omit the onion, garlic and pepper, and remove the
   seeds from the tomatoes. In step 1, simply bring
   the tomatoes, cumin, salt and water to a boil over
   medium-high heat.

Advice for a Healthy Gut

▶ Use extra virgin olive oil, macadamia nut oil,
   grapeseed oil or avocado oil for the vegetable oil.

Nutrients per serving	
Calories	66
Fat	3 g
Carbohydrate	10 g
Fiber	3 g
Protein	2 g
Vitamin A	78 IU
Iron	0.9 mg
Zinc	0.4 mg

Brussels Sprouts with Pecans and Sweet Potatoes

Suitable for Phases 2 & 3

Brussels sprouts are loaded with potassium and beta-carotene, which the body converts to vitamin A, a nutrient needed for gut repair. The addition of sweet potatoes and pecans balances the flavor of these mighty vegetables.

Tip

Toast pecans in a 400°F (200°C) oven or in a skillet on the stovetop for 2 minutes or until brown.

1½ cups	cubed peeled sweet potatoes	375 mL
12 oz	Brussels sprouts, cut in half	375 g
1 tbsp	margarine	15 mL
½ cup	chopped onion	125 mL
1 tsp	crushed garlic	5 mL
¼ cup	ready-to-use chicken broth (gluten-free, if needed)	60 mL
4 tsp	packed brown sugar or liquid honey	20 mL
¼ tsp	ground cinnamon	1 mL
2 tbsp	chopped pecans, toasted (see tip, at left)	30 mL

1. In saucepan of boiling water, cook sweet potatoes until just tender; drain and reserve. Repeat with Brussels sprouts. Set aside.

2. In nonstick skillet, melt margarine; sauté onion and garlic just until tender. Add sweet potatoes, Brussels sprouts, broth, sugar, cinnamon and pecans; cook for 3 minutes or until vegetables are tender.

Adjustment for Phase 2

▸ Replace the margarine with extra virgin olive oil, macadamia nut oil, grapeseed oil or avocado oil.

Advice for a Healthy Gut

▸ Extra virgin olive oil, macadamia nut oil, grapeseed oil and avocado oil continue to be the best fat choices, but in Phase 3, you may use organic butter instead, if desired.

▸ While you are following the LGS Diet Plan, use honey as the sweetener for this recipe.

Nutrients per serving	
Calories	160
Fat	6 g
Carbohydrate	25 g
Fiber	6 g
Protein	5 g
Vitamin A	7845 IU
Iron	1.7 mg
Zinc	0.7 mg

Braised Red Cabbage

Suitable for Phases 2 & 3

Long, slow cooking develops the flavors in this fabulous fall or winter dish. It will reheat well and may be stored for 1 week in the refrigerator.

Adjustments for Phase 2

▶ Substitute rice vinegar for the red wine vinegar.

▶ Replace the granulated sugar with an equal amount of liquid honey.

▶ Omit the bacon and cook the onion and apples in 1 tbsp (15 mL) olive, macadamia nut, grapeseed or avocado oil.

Nutrients per serving

Calories	53
Fat	1 g
Carbohydrate	12 g
Fiber	2 g
Protein	1 g
Vitamin A	655 IU
Iron	0.6 mg
Zinc	0.2 mg

- Preheat oven to 325°F (160°C)
- 8-cup (2 L) baking dish

1	small red cabbage (about 1½ lbs/750 g)	1
⅓ cup	red wine vinegar	75 mL
1 tbsp	granulated sugar	15 mL
1 tsp	salt	5 mL
1	slice bacon, chopped	1
⅓ cup	chopped onion	75 mL
2	Granny Smith apples, peeled, cored and cut into eighths	2
1	whole clove	1
1	small onion	1
1	bay leaf	1
½ cup	boiling water	125 mL
2 tbsp	dry red wine (optional)	30 mL

1. Remove outer leaves of cabbage and discard. Cut cabbage into quarters; trim off excess white heart. Shred about ⅛ inch (3 mm) thick to make 6 cups (1.5 L). Place in bowl; toss with vinegar, sugar and salt.

2. In a large skillet, brown bacon; remove bacon, reserving drippings in pan. Set bacon aside. Add chopped onion; cook, stirring, for 2 minutes. Add apples; cook for 5 minutes.

3. Push clove into onion; add to skillet along with cabbage mixture, bay leaf, boiling water and bacon. Mix well. Pour into 8-cup (2 L) baking dish. Cover and bake in preheated oven for 2 hours, stirring occasionally. (If it becomes dry, add more water.) Remove onion and bay leaf. Stir in wine, if desired.

This recipe courtesy of chef Alastair Gray and dietitian Mary Margaret Laing.

Advice for a Healthy Gut

▶ Continue to use rice vinegar and honey in this recipe while you are following the LGS Diet Plan.

Gingered Carrot-Turnip Purée

Suitable for Phases 1, 2 & 3

Warm the plates and serve immediately, because if the purée hits a cold plate or sits too long before being served, some of the liquid may separate out.

- **Blender or food processor**

3	large carrots, cut into chunks	3
1/2	rutabaga, cut into chunks	1/2
1 tsp	finely grated orange zest (optional)	5 mL
	Juice of 1 orange	
1 tbsp	agave nectar or brown rice syrup	15 mL
1 tsp	finely grated fresh gingerroot	5 mL
1 tsp	toasted sesame oil	5 mL
	Sea salt	

1. In a large saucepan or deep skillet, combine carrots and rutabaga. Fill with just enough water to cover the vegetables. Bring to a boil over high heat. Cover, reduce heat to medium-low and simmer for 30 minutes or until the vegetables are tender when pierced with the tip of a knife. Drain and let cool slightly.

2. In blender, combine vegetables, orange zest (if using), orange juice, agave nectar, ginger, sesame oil and salt to taste. Blend or process until puréed or smooth. Serve immediately.

Nutrients per serving (1 of 6)

Calories	38
Fat	1 g
Carbohydrate	8 g
Fiber	1 g
Protein	1 g
Vitamin A	6015 IU
Iron	0.2 mg
Zinc	0.1 mg

Old English Celery Bake

Suitable for Phases 1, 2 & 3

This dish, adapted from a traditional English recipe, is a great accompaniment to just about anything, from roast poultry and meat to a rich, luscious vegetable stew. It's a great way to use up the less tender outer stalks of celery, which often linger in the crisper long after the tender heart has been used.

Tip

Large stalks of celery can be fibrous. For best results, use a vegetable peeler to remove the outer layer.

- Preheat oven to 325°F (160°C)
- Shallow 6-cup (1.5 L) baking dish, lightly greased

1 cup	Job's tears, soaked, rinsed and drained	250 mL
1	bay leaf	1
4	large stalks celery, diced (see tip, at left)	4
2½ cups	ready-to-use reduced-sodium vegetable or chicken broth (gluten-free, if needed) or water	625 mL

1. Spread Job's tears evenly over bottom of prepared baking dish. Place bay leaf in the center and arrange celery evenly over top. Add broth and bake in preheated oven until liquid is absorbed and the grain is tender, about 1½ hours.

Nutrients per serving

Calories	124
Fat	2 g
Carbohydrate	22 g
Fiber	1 g
Protein	5 g
Vitamin A	122 IU
Iron	6.6 mg
Zinc	0.0 mg

Braised Green Beans and Fennel

Suitable for Phases 1, 2 & 3

Mediterranean-style vegetables work beautifully as a warm-up starter salad or as a side to grilled meat or fish. Green beans provide the bulk, but it is the fresh fennel that gives the dish character.

Tip

The fennel bulb always comes attached to woody branches and thin leaves that look like dill. You'll need the leaves for the final garnish, so cut them off and set them aside. Cut off and discard the woody branches. Quarter the bulb vertically, then cut out and discard the hard triangular sections of core. What remains is the usable part of the fennel.

¼ cup	olive oil	60 mL
½ tsp	salt	2 mL
¼ tsp	freshly ground black pepper	1 mL
1 tsp	whole fennel seeds	5 mL
12 oz	green beans, trimmed	375 g
1	large or 2 small fennel bulbs, trimmed, cored and cut into ½-inch (1 cm) slices (see tip, at left)	1
1	small carrot, scraped and sliced into ¼-inch (0.5 cm) rounds	1
6	cloves garlic, thinly sliced	6
1 cup	water	250 mL
1 tbsp	balsamic vinegar	15 mL
	Few sprigs fennel greens, chopped	

1. In a large, deep frying pan, heat olive oil, salt and pepper over high heat for 1 minute. Add fennel seeds; stir-fry 1 minute or until just browning. Add green beans, fennel and carrots; stir-fry 3 minutes or until all the vegetables are shiny and beginning to sizzle. Add garlic; stir-fry for 1 more minute.

2. Immediately add water and vinegar; cook 2 minutes or until bubbling. Reduce heat to medium-low, cover pan tightly and cook 20 minutes.

3. Place a strainer over a bowl and strain contents of the pan. Transfer the strained vegetables onto a platter and keep warm. Transfer the liquid that has collected in the bowl back into the pan; bring to a boil and cook 6 to 7 minutes or until thick and syrupy.

4. Spoon the reduced sauce over the vegetables, garnish with the chopped fennel greens and serve immediately.

Adjustments for Phase 1

▶ Omit the pepper and garlic.

Advice for a Healthy Gut

▶ Choose extra virgin olive oil and natural balsamic vinegar (without color or sulfites).

Nutrients per serving (1 of 6)

Calories	121
Fat	9 g
Carbohydrate	9 g
Fiber	3 g
Protein	2 g
Vitamin A	1837 IU
Iron	1.1 mg
Zinc	0.3 mg

Simple Stir-Fried Kale

This recipe is a very easy way to prepare kale. Kale is an excellent source of potassium and anti-inflammatory carotenoids, including beta-carotene, which the body converts to vitamin A, a nutrient that helps heal and repair the gut.

Tips

Tahini is often used in Middle Eastern cooking and is an ingredient in hummus. It is made from ground sesame seeds and adds a nutty flavor to dishes.

Leave out the hot pepper sauce if your family does not like spice.

1 tbsp	vegetable oil	15 mL
1 tsp	sesame oil	5 mL
4 cups	julienned kale (tough center rib removed first)	1 L
2	leeks (white and light green parts only), julienned	2
1 tbsp	tahini	15 mL
2 tsp	hot pepper sauce	10 mL
2 tsp	soy sauce (gluten-free, if needed)	10 mL
	Freshly ground white or black pepper	

1. In a wok or large skillet, heat vegetable oil and sesame oil over high heat. Add kale and leeks; stir-fry for 3 to 5 minutes or until limp.

2. Combine tahini, hot pepper sauce and soy sauce; pour over vegetables. Season to taste with pepper. Serve warm.

This recipe courtesy of dietitian Gerry Kasten.

Adjustments for Phase 2

▸ Omit the hot pepper sauce and soy sauce, and increase the tahini to 2 tbsp (30 mL).

Advice for a Healthy Gut

▸ Use extra virgin olive oil, macadamia nut oil, grapeseed oil or avocado oil for the vegetable oil.

▸ Soy sauce is permitted in Phase 3, but make sure to use gluten-free soy sauce.

Nutrients per serving

Calories	126
Fat	7 g
Carbohydrate	14 g
Fiber	2 g
Protein	4 g
Vitamin A	11,050 IU
Iron	2.3 mg
Zinc	0.5 mg

Roasted Garlic Sweet Pepper Strips

Makes 4 servings

Suitable for Phases 2 & 3

This is a delicious and colorful way to serve sweet bell peppers. They can also be prepared ahead of time and served cold.

- **Preheat oven to 400°F (200°C)**

4	large bell peppers (combination of green, red and yellow)	4
2 tbsp	olive oil	30 mL
1½ tsp	crushed garlic	7 mL
1 tbsp	freshly grated Parmesan cheese	15 mL

1. On baking sheet, bake whole peppers for 15 to 20 minutes, turning occasionally, until blistered and blackened. Place in paper bag; seal and let stand for 10 minutes.

2. Peel off charred skin from peppers; cut off tops and bottoms. Remove seeds and ribs; cut into 1-inch (2.5 cm) wide strips and place on serving platter.

3. Mix oil with garlic; brush over peppers. Sprinkle with cheese.

Variation

Add a sprinkle of chopped fresh herbs, such as parsley or basil, to the oil mixture.

Adjustment for Phase 2

▶ Omit the Parmesan cheese.

Advice for a Healthy Gut

▶ Choose extra virgin olive oil or avocado oil.

Nutrients per serving

Calories	104
Fat	7 g
Carbohydrate	8 g
Fiber	2 g
Protein	2 g
Vitamin A	2077 IU
Iron	0.6 mg
Zinc	0.3 mg

Sautéed Spinach with Pine Nuts

Makes 4 servings

**Suitable for
Phases 2 & 3**

This is an easy way to add flavor to spinach. You can substitute Swiss chard, kale, rapini or mustard greens for the spinach. If you don't have pine nuts, try pecans or walnuts.

Tip

Stir-frying vegetables is a great way to preserve nutrients. When boiled, vegetables can lose up to 45% of vitamin C, compared with losing only 5% when stir-fried.

2 tsp	olive oil, divided	10 mL
¼ cup	pine nuts	60 mL
1	package (10 oz/300 g) fresh spinach, trimmed	1
1 tsp	minced garlic	5 mL
1 tsp	freshly squeezed lemon juice	5 mL
⅛ tsp	ground nutmeg	0.5 mL
	Freshly ground black pepper	

1. In a large nonstick skillet, heat 1 tsp (5 mL) oil over medium heat. Add pine nuts and cook, stirring constantly, for 2 to 3 minutes or until golden. Remove pine nuts from pan and set aside.

2. Add remaining oil to pan. Add spinach in several bunches (it will cook down quickly), stirring constantly. Add garlic and cook for 1 to 2 minutes. Stir in lemon juice and nutmeg. Season to taste with pepper. Add reserved pine nuts. Cook until heated through.

This recipe courtesy of dietitian Bev Callaghan.

Advice for a Healthy Gut

▶ Choose extra virgin olive oil or avocado oil.

Nutrients per serving	
Calories	97
Fat	8 g
Carbohydrate	5 g
Fiber	2 g
Protein	3 g
Vitamin A	6648 IU
Iron	2.4 mg
Zinc	0.9 mg

Italian Broiled Tomatoes

Makes 4 servings

Suitable for Phases 2 & 3

Serve this often during tomato season to accompany broiled or barbecued meat. Tomatoes are rich in vitamin C, which the body uses to produce collagen, an important protein in healing and repair.

Tip

Fresh tomatoes in season are a real treat. Store underripe tomatoes, unwashed, at room temperature away from sunlight until slightly soft. Room-temperature tomatoes will have more flavor than cold ones.

- Preheat broiler
- Shallow baking pan

2	large tomatoes	2
Pinch	garlic powder	Pinch
1 tbsp	chopped fresh parsley	15 mL
1 tsp	dried basil	5 mL
½ tsp	dried oregano	2 mL
	Freshly ground black pepper	
2 tbsp	bread crumbs	30 mL

1. Cut tomatoes in half crosswise. Place cut side up on rack in shallow baking pan. Sprinkle lightly with garlic powder. Combine parsley, seasonings and bread crumbs. Divide mixture over surface of tomato halves.

2. Place pan about 6 inches (15 cm) below broiler. Broil for 3 to 4 minutes until tomatoes are heated through, or cook on barbecue along with meat being grilled.

This recipe courtesy of dietitian Helen Haresign.

Advice for a Healthy Gut

▶ Make sure to choose gluten-free bread crumbs.

Nutrients per serving	
Calories	21
Fat	0 g
Carbohydrate	4 g
Fiber	1 g
Protein	1 g
Vitamin A	842 IU
Iron	0.6 mg
Zinc	0.2 mg

Summer Zucchini

Makes 4 servings

Suitable for Phases 1, 2 & 3

This is an ideal recipe for the vast quantities of lush, juicy zucchini we get every summer — mostly from our friends with vegetable patches.

4	young zucchini, preferably 2 each of green and yellow, less than 6 inches (15 cm) in length	4
3 tbsp	olive oil	45 mL
1/4 tsp	salt	1 mL
1/4 tsp	freshly ground black pepper	1 mL
1	red bell pepper, cut into thick strips	1
3	green onions, chopped	3
1 tbsp	freshly squeezed lemon juice	15 mL
	Few sprigs fresh basil and/or parsley, chopped	

1. Trim ends of zucchini and cut into ¾-inch (2 cm) chunks. Set aside.

2. In a large frying pan, heat olive oil over high heat for 30 seconds. Add salt and pepper and stir. Add zucchini chunks and red pepper strips. Stir-fry for 4 to 6 minutes until the zucchini have browned on both sides and the red pepper has softened. Add green onions and stir-fry for 30 seconds. Transfer to a serving dish and drizzle evenly with lemon juice. Garnish with basil and/or parsley and serve immediately.

Adjustments for Phase 1

▶ Omit the black pepper and green onions.

Adjustment for Phase 2

▶ Omit the green onions.

Advice for a Healthy Gut

▶ Choose extra virgin olive oil or avocado oil.

Nutrients per serving

Calories	121
Fat	11 g
Carbohydrate	6 g
Fiber	2 g
Protein	2 g
Vitamin A	1205 IU
Iron	0.7 mg
Zinc	0.5 mg

Sautéed Vegetables

Suitable for Phases 2 & 3

Chopped beets add an attractive rosy red color to this dish. The mix of vegetables provides an abundance of antioxidants and phytonutrients, plant compounds that support healing and overall health.

Tip

Fresh beets are delicious steamed or cold in salads. To maximize flavor and nutrition, cut the green tops from beets, leaving at least 1 inch (2.5 cm) attached. Don't remove the root end. This prevents the beet color and vitamins from being lost in the cooking water. Once the beets are cooked, rinse under cold water and slide off the skins, using rubber gloves if desired.

1/4 cup	sliced onion	60 mL
1 tbsp	olive oil	15 mL
1 cup	broccoli florets	250 mL
1 cup	cauliflower florets	250 mL
1 cup	cubed zucchini	250 mL
1/2 cup	chopped raw beets	125 mL
1 cup	ready-to-use chicken broth (gluten-free, if needed)	250 mL
1 cup	chopped Swiss chard or spinach (optional)	250 mL
1 cup	chopped tomatoes	250 mL
2 tbsp	water	30 mL
2 tsp	cornstarch	10 mL
	Salt and freshly ground black pepper	

1. In a large skillet over medium–high heat, cook onion in hot oil for about 5 minutes. Add broccoli, cauliflower, zucchini, beets and broth. Cook, covered, for about 3 minutes or until tender–crisp.

2. Stir in chard (if using) and tomatoes. Mix together water, cornstarch and seasonings; stir into vegetable mixture. Cook for about 2 minutes or until thickened.

This recipe courtesy of Jeanette Snowden.

Advice for a Healthy Gut

▶ Choose extra virgin olive oil or avocado oil.

Nutrients per serving	
Calories	53
Fat	3 g
Carbohydrate	6 g
Fiber	2 g
Protein	2 g
Vitamin A	646 IU
Iron	0.5 mg
Zinc	0.3 mg

Roasted Vegetables or Fruit

Suitable for Phases 1, 2 & 3

Thick, firm and juicy-fleshed antioxidant-rich fruit, such as plums, apricots and cherries, and all manner of vegetables, such as beets, onions, squash, turnips, carrots, parsnips, eggplant, sweet potatoes, corn on the cob and asparagus, benefit from roasting.

Tips

For the herbs, use rosemary, sage, thyme, oregano, chives, parsley, basil or savory.

Roasted fruit and vegetables blacken slightly around the edges and are shriveled in appearance, so use them in soups and puréed dishes.

- Preheat oven to 400°F (200°C)
- Baking sheet, lightly oiled

3 cups	roughly chopped or quartered vegetables or pitted fruit	750 mL
2 tbsp	olive oil	30 mL
¼ cup	chopped fresh herbs (see tip, at left)	60 mL

1. On prepared baking sheet, toss vegetables or fruit with oil and herbs. Roast in lower half of preheated oven for 25 to 45 minutes or until browned and tender. Root vegetables will take the full 45 minutes while tender vegetables like asparagus and zucchini will take less time.

Advice for a Healthy Gut

▶ Choose extra virgin olive oil or avocado oil.

Nutrients per serving (based on 1 cup/250 mL each onion, beet and turnip)

Calories	96
Fat	7 g
Carbohydrate	8 g
Fiber	2 g
Protein	1 g
Vitamin A	1925 IU
Iron	0.8 mg
Zinc	0.3 mg

Baked Parsnip Fries

Suitable for Phases 1, 2 & 3

Potatoes and sweet potatoes aren't the only vegetables that can be used to make fries. Parsnips are naturally sweet and offer a unique spin on a classic side.

- Preheat oven to 400°F (200°C)
- Large rimmed baking sheet, lined with foil and brushed with extra virgin olive oil

1 lb	parsnips, cut into 3-inch (7.5 cm) long by ¼-inch (0.5 cm) thick sticks	500 g
¼ tsp	fine sea salt	1 mL
⅛ tsp	freshly ground black pepper	0.5 mL
1 tbsp	extra virgin olive oil	15 mL
1 tbsp	chopped fresh flat-leaf (Italian) parsley	15 mL

1. In a large bowl, combine parsnips, salt, pepper and oil, tossing to coat. Spread in a single layer on prepared baking sheet.

2. Bake in preheated oven for 15 minutes. Gently turn parsnips over and bake for 12 to 17 minutes or until crisp. Serve immediately, sprinkled with parsley.

Adjustment for Phase 1

▶ Omit the pepper.

Nutrients per serving

Calories	115
Fat	4 g
Carbohydrate	21 g
Fiber	6 g
Protein	1 g
Vitamin A	80 IU
Iron	0.8 mg
Zinc	0.7 mg

Sweet Potato Fries

Makes 6 servings

Suitable for Phases 1, 2 & 3

Sweet potatoes become incredibly tasty when roasted at a high temperature. They are rich in carotenoids, especially beta-carotene, a potent antioxidant. The body converts beta-carotene to vitamin A, which is needed for healing and repair.

- Preheat oven to 450°F (230°C)
- Large rimmed baking sheet, lined with foil and brushed with extra virgin olive oil

4	sweet potatoes (each about 8 oz/250 g), peeled and cut into 3-inch (7.5 cm) long by 1/4-inch (0.5 cm) thick sticks	4
1/2 tsp	fine sea salt	2 mL
1/4 tsp	freshly ground black pepper	1 mL
4 tsp	vegetable oil	20 mL

1. In a large bowl, combine sweet potatoes, salt, pepper and oil, tossing to coat. Spread in a single layer on prepared baking sheet.
2. Bake in preheated oven for 20 minutes. Gently turn sweet potatoes over and bake for 12 to 17 minutes or until crisp. Serve immediately.

Adjustment for Phase 1

▶ Omit the pepper.

Advice for a Healthy Gut

▶ "Vegetable oil" is a catchall term for any edible oil from a plant source, whether it be a vegetable, fruit, nut or seed. While you are following the LGS Diet Plan, the best choices for this recipe are extra virgin olive oil, macadamia nut oil, grapeseed oil and avocado oil.

Nutrients per serving

Calories	102
Fat	3 g
Carbohydrate	18 g
Fiber	3 g
Protein	1 g
Vitamin A	12,296 IU
Iron	0.5 mg
Zinc	0.3 mg

Mashed Sweet Potatoes with Rosemary

Suitable for Phases 1, 2 & 3

For a twist on an old favorite, try this savory dish of mashed sweet potatoes, rich in potassium, vitamin C and beta-carotene.

2 lbs	sweet potatoes, peeled and diced	1 kg
2½ tsp	minced fresh rosemary	12 mL
¼ tsp	fine sea salt	1 mL
¼ tsp	freshly ground black pepper	1 mL
2 tsp	extra virgin olive oil	10 mL

1. Place sweet potatoes in a medium saucepan and cover with water. Bring to a boil over high heat. Boil for 8 minutes or until tender. Drain, reserving ⅓ cup (75 mL) of the cooking water.

2. In a large bowl, using an electric mixer on medium speed, beat sweet potatoes and reserved cooking liquid until smooth. Beat in rosemary, salt and pepper. Spoon into a bowl and drizzle with oil.

Adjustment for Phase 1

▶ Omit the pepper.

Nutrients per serving

Calories	120
Fat	2 g
Carbohydrate	25 g
Fiber	4 g
Protein	2 g
Vitamin A	22,674 IU
Iron	0.9 mg
Zinc	0.4 mg

Sweet Potato, Apple and Raisin Casserole

Makes 6 servings

Suitable for Phases 2 & 3

Sweet potatoes pair well with walnuts and apples for a dish that is as rich in flavor as it is in antioxidants.

Tips

The darker the skin of the sweet potato, the moister it is.

Chopped dates or apricots can replace the raisins.

You can prepare the casserole without apples the day before. Add apples, toss and bake just prior to serving.

- Preheat oven to 350°F (180°C)
- Baking dish, sprayed with nonstick vegetable spray

1 lb	sweet potatoes, peeled and cubed	500 g
¾ tsp	ground ginger	3 mL
¼ cup	liquid honey or pure maple syrup	60 mL
¾ tsp	ground cinnamon	3 mL
2 tbsp	margarine, melted	30 mL
¼ cup	raisins	60 mL
2 tbsp	chopped walnuts	30 mL
¾ cup	cubed peeled sweet apples	175 mL

1. Steam or microwave sweet potatoes just until slightly underdone. Place in baking dish.

2. In small bowl, combine ginger, honey, cinnamon, margarine, raisins, walnuts and apples; mix well. Pour over sweet potatoes and bake, uncovered, for 20 minutes or until tender.

Adjustment for Phase 2

▸ Replace the margarine with extra virgin olive oil, macadamia nut oil, grapeseed oil or avocado oil.

Advice for a Healthy Gut

▸ Extra virgin olive oil, macadamia nut oil, grapeseed oil and avocado oil continue to be the best fat choices, but in Phase 3, you may use organic butter instead, if desired.

▸ Choose unsweetened raisins.

Nutrients per serving	
Calories	187
Fat	6 g
Carbohydrate	34 g
Fiber	3 g
Protein	2 g
Vitamin A	10,736 IU
Iron	0.8 mg
Zinc	0.4 mg

Herbed Potatoes

Makes 4 servings

Suitable for Phases 1, 2 & 3

When the palate demands the wonderful taste of fried potatoes, try this zesty re-fry of parboiled potato. It uses a minimum of oil and delivers delightful flavors.

1 lb	new potatoes, unpeeled but well scrubbed (about 3)	500 g
¼ cup	olive oil	60 mL
¼ tsp	salt	1 mL
¼ tsp	freshly ground black pepper	1 mL
1 tbsp	grated lemon zest	15 mL
4	cloves garlic, finely chopped	4
	Few sprigs fresh parsley and/or rosemary, chopped	
2 tbsp	freshly squeezed lemon juice	30 mL

1. In a large saucepan, boil potatoes over high heat for 5 to 7 minutes, until they can just be pierced with a fork. Drain and refresh several times with cold water. Cut potatoes into ½-inch (1 cm) rounds.

2. In a large frying pan, heat oil over high heat for 30 seconds. Add salt and pepper and stir. Add potatoes in a single layer and fry for 2 to 3 minutes; reduce heat to medium–high, turn rounds over and fry other side for 2 to 3 minutes, then toss-fry for another 1 to 2 minutes until golden all over. (Some of the skins will have peeled off and fried to a crisp; don't worry, they'll add to the final appeal.)

3. Add lemon zest, garlic and most of the chopped herb(s), reserving some for the final garnish. Toss-fry for 1 to 2 minutes. Add lemon juice and toss-fry for 1 to 2 minutes, until the sizzle has stopped and the acidity of the lemon has mellowed. (Taste a piece.) Transfer potatoes to a serving bowl and garnish with the remainder of the herb(s). Serve immediately.

Adjustments for Phase 1

▶ Omit the pepper and garlic.

Advice for a Healthy Gut

▶ Choose extra virgin olive oil or avocado oil.

Nutrients per serving

Calories	214
Fat	14 g
Carbohydrate	22 g
Fiber	3 g
Protein	3 g
Vitamin A	5 IU
Iron	1.0 mg
Zinc	0.4 mg

Fragrant Coconut Rice

Makes 4 servings

Suitable for Phases 1, 2 & 3

This is deliciously rich rice — perhaps a bit too much for every day, but a wonderful treat now and again.

Tip

Coconut milk should be suitable for people who are allergic to gluten. However, some brands contain guar gum, which, although it does not contain gluten, is not recommended for people with celiac disease. Also it may be processed in a facility where gluten is present. Check the label.

1½ cups	coconut milk (see tip, at left)	375 mL
1 cup	water	250 mL
1	stick cinnamon, about 2 inches (5 cm) long	1
1 cup	brown basmati or brown long-grain rice, rinsed and drained	250 mL

1. In a saucepan over medium–high heat, bring coconut milk, water and cinnamon stick to a rapid boil. Stir in rice and return to a boil. Reduce heat to low. Cover and simmer until rice is tender and liquid is absorbed, about 50 minutes. Discard cinnamon stick.

Advice for a Healthy Gut

▶ Choose a carrageenan-free coconut milk.

Nutrients per serving

Calories	371
Fat	21 g
Carbohydrate	42 g
Fiber	4 g
Protein	5 g
Vitamin A	4 IU
Iron	2.0 mg
Zinc	0.6 mg

Italian-Style Green Rice

Suitable for Phases 1, 2 & 3

Here's a deliciously different rice that makes a perfect companion for grilled meats and fish. The short-grain rice is quite glutinous, and the results mimic risotto. You can fib and say you spent endless time stirring to produce such a stunning effect.

Tip

If your spinach has not been prewashed, be sure to rinse it thoroughly in a basin of lukewarm water. Swish it around to remove all traces of grit, then rinse it again in a colander under cold running water.

1 cup	short-grain brown rice	250 mL
1¼ cups	water, divided	300 mL
2 cups	ready-to-use reduced-sodium chicken or vegetable broth (gluten-free, if needed)	500 mL
1 lb	fresh spinach leaves, stems removed	500 g
	Salt and freshly ground black pepper	
2	green onions, white part only, finely chopped	2
2 tbsp	extra virgin olive oil	30 mL
¼ cup	freshly grated Parmesan cheese	60 mL

1. In a bowl, combine rice and 1 cup (250 mL) water. Stir well. Cover and set aside for at least 3 hours or overnight. Drain, reserving liquid.

2. In a heavy saucepan with a tight-fitting lid, combine broth and reserved soaking water. Bring to a boil. Stir in rice and return to a boil. Reduce heat to low. Cover and simmer for 35 minutes. Remove lid, stir well and simmer, uncovered, stirring occasionally, until liquid is absorbed and rice is tender, about 15 minutes.

3. When rice is almost cooked, in another saucepan over low heat, combine spinach and ¼ cup (60 mL) water. Cover and cook until wilted, about 5 minutes. Using a slotted spoon, transfer to a cutting board and chop finely. Transfer to a bowl. Season to taste with salt and pepper. Stir in green onions. Set aside.

4. *To serve:* Spread cooked rice evenly over a deep platter. Arrange spinach evenly over the center, leaving some rice exposed around the edge. Drizzle olive oil over the spinach and sprinkle with Parmesan. Serve immediately.

Adjustments for Phase 1

▶ Omit the pepper, green onions and Parmesan cheese.

Adjustment for Phase 2

▶ Omit the Parmesan cheese.

Advice for a Healthy Gut

▶ Choose extra virgin olive oil or avocado oil.

Nutrients per serving

Calories	205
Fat	7 g
Carbohydrate	29 g
Fiber	3 g
Protein	8 g
Vitamin A	7134 IU
Iron	2.8 mg
Zinc	0.6 mg

Cauliflower Rice

**Suitable for
Phases 2 & 3**

*This recipe is a light
and fluffy alternative to
starches such as potatoes
and rice. Cauliflower is
often underrated, but it's
rich in antioxidants and
has anti-inflammatory
properties.*

Tip

When pulsing the
cauliflower, be sure
not to overprocess.
Otherwise the cell
walls of the cauliflower
will break down
and the "rice" will
become soggy.

- **Food processor**

4 cups	chopped cauliflower florets	1 L
¼ cup	chopped fresh parsley	60 mL
2 tbsp	freshly squeezed lemon juice	30 mL
1 tsp	fine sea salt	5 mL

1. In food processor, pulse cauliflower until it breaks down to a rice-like consistency, 10 to 15 times (see tip, at left).
2. Transfer to a bowl. Add parsley, lemon juice and salt and stir well. Serve immediately or place in an airtight container and refrigerate for up to 4 days.

Variations

For a curry-style rice, add 1 tbsp (15 mL) curry powder, 1 tbsp (15 mL) chopped gingerroot, ½ tsp (2 mL) ground cumin and ¼ tsp (1 mL) ground turmeric with the parsley.

For Italian-style rice, add ¼ cup (60 mL) thinly sliced fresh basil leaves, 1 tbsp (15 mL) dried oregano and ½ tsp (2 mL) whole fennel seeds with the parsley.

Nutrients per serving	
Calories	30
Fat	0 g
Carbohydrate	6 g
Fiber	2 g
Protein	2 g
Vitamin A	321 IU
Iron	0.7 mg
Zinc	0.3 mg

Vegetable Rice

Suitable for Phases 1, 2 & 3

The spices in this nutrient-filled dish give it a unique flair.

Advice for a Healthy Gut

▸ Extra virgin olive oil continues to be the better fat choice, but in Phase 3, you may use organic butter in step 4, if desired.

¾ cup	trimmed green beans, cut into 1-inch (2.5 cm) pieces	175 mL
2 tsp	olive oil	10 mL
¾ cup	chopped peeled carrots	175 mL
1 cup	basmati rice	250 mL
1 tsp	butter	5 mL
4	whole allspice berries	4
1	cinnamon stick (about 3 inches/7.5 cm)	1
1 tsp	ground cumin	5 mL
1 tsp	ground cardamom	5 mL
2 cups	water	500 mL

1. Place beans in a small saucepan, add enough water to cover and bring to a boil over high heat. Reduce heat to medium and simmer for 10 to 15 minutes or until tender. Drain well and set aside.

2. In a medium skillet, heat oil over medium heat. Sauté beans and carrots for 5 to 10 minutes or until softened. Set aside.

3. Place rice in a medium bowl, add enough warm water to cover and let soak for 5 minutes. Drain well.

4. In a medium saucepan over medium heat, melt butter. Stir in allspice, cinnamon stick, cumin and cardamom and cook for 10 seconds. Stir in rice until coated with spice mixture.

5. Add water to rice mixture and bring to a boil. Boil for 3 to 4 minutes. Reduce heat to medium-low, cover and simmer for 15 to 20 minutes or until rice is tender. Remove from heat and let stand for 5 minutes.

6. Remove and discard cinnamon stick and allspice. Stir in bean mixture. Serve immediately.

Nutrients per serving

Calories	281
Fat	5 g
Carbohydrate	55 g
Fiber	4 g
Protein	5 g
Vitamin A	5573 IU
Iron	1.5 mg
Zinc	0.3 mg

Adjustment for Phase 1

▸ Omit the cumin.

Adjustments for Phases 1 & 2

▸ Choose extra virgin olive oil or avocado oil.

▸ Use an additional 1 tsp (5 mL) olive oil in place of the butter.

Wild Rice, Snow Pea and Almond Casserole

Makes 4 servings

Suitable for Phases 2 & 3

Wild rice adds color, texture and a uniquely chewy mouth-feel to this casserole.

Tips

This is delicious warm or cold. If serving cold, prepare early in the day and stir just prior to serving.

Toast almonds in a small skillet on the stovetop or in a 400°F (200°C) oven for 2 minutes.

For a special dinner menu, use 1 cup (250 mL) wild rice and omit the white rice.

2 tsp	margarine	10 mL
½ cup	chopped onion	125 mL
1 tsp	crushed garlic	5 mL
½ cup	wild rice	125 mL
½ cup	white rice	125 mL
3¼ cups	ready-to-use chicken broth (gluten-free, if needed)	800 mL
¾ cup	chopped snow peas	175 mL
¼ cup	finely chopped red bell pepper	60 mL
¼ cup	toasted sliced almonds (see tip, at left)	60 mL
1 tbsp	freshly grated Parmesan cheese	15 mL

1. In large nonstick saucepan, melt margarine; sauté onion and garlic until softened. Add wild and white rice; stir for 2 minutes.

2. Add broth; reduce heat, cover and simmer just until rice is tender and liquid is absorbed, 30 to 40 minutes.

3. Add snow peas, red pepper and almonds; cook for 2 minutes. Place in serving bowl and sprinkle with cheese.

Adjustments for Phase 2

▶ Substitute extra virgin olive oil for the margarine.

▶ Omit the Parmesan cheese.

Advice for a Healthy Gut

▶ Extra virgin olive oil continues to be the better fat choice, but in Phase 3, you may use organic butter instead, if desired.

Nutrients per serving

Calories	267
Fat	7 g
Carbohydrate	42 g
Fiber	3 g
Protein	11 g
Vitamin A	519 IU
Iron	2.4 mg
Zinc	2.0 mg

Quinoa Pilaf

Suitable for Phases 1, 2 & 3

Quinoa is a gluten-free, high-protein grain that is quickly gaining popularity.

2 tbsp	olive oil	30 mL
4	carrots, peeled and chopped	4
2	stalks celery, peeled and diced	2
1 cup	quinoa, rinsed	250 mL
2	bay leaves	2
2 cups	ready-to-use gluten-free vegetable broth	500 mL
2 cups	diced peeled butternut squash	500 mL
	Juice of 1 lemon	
	Salt and freshly ground black pepper	

1. In a large saucepan, heat oil over medium heat. Cook carrots and celery, stirring occasionally, for 10 minutes or until tender. Add quinoa and cook, stirring, for about 1 minute.

2. Add bay leaves, broth, squash and lemon juice and bring to a boil. Reduce heat to medium–low, cover and simmer for 15 to 20 minutes or until liquid has been absorbed and quinoa is tender. Remove and discard bay leaves. Season to taste with salt and pepper.

Adjustment for Phase 1

▶ Omit the pepper.

Advice for a Healthy Gut

▶ Choose extra virgin olive oil or avocado oil.

Nutrients per serving

Calories	188
Fat	6 g
Carbohydrate	29 g
Fiber	4 g
Protein	5 g
Vitamin A	11,989 IU
Iron	1.8 mg
Zinc	1.1 mg

Cilantro-Ginger Quinoa

Makes 4 servings

Suitable for Phases 1, 2 & 3

A stir-in of cilantro, sesame, ginger and lime transforms plain quinoa into a lively side that's an ideal accompaniment for Asian main dishes. Quinoa is rich in phytonutrients and magnesium.

● **Blender**

1 cup	black or white quinoa, rinsed	250 mL
2 cups	ready-to-use reduced-sodium chicken or vegetable broth (gluten-free, if needed)	500 mL
1	clove garlic, minced	1
1	1-inch (2.5 cm) piece gingerroot, roughly chopped	1
1 cup	packed fresh cilantro leaves	250 mL
2 tbsp	freshly squeezed lime juice	30 mL
1 tbsp	toasted sesame oil	15 mL
	Fine sea salt and freshly ground black pepper	

1. In a medium saucepan, combine quinoa and broth. Bring to a boil over medium–high heat. Reduce heat to low, cover and simmer for 12 to 15 minutes or until liquid is absorbed. Remove from heat and let stand, covered, for 5 minutes. Fluff with a fork. Transfer to a medium bowl.

2. Meanwhile, in blender, combine garlic, ginger, cilantro, lime juice and oil; pulse until smooth. Add to quinoa, tossing with a fork to combine. Season to taste with salt and pepper.

Adjustments for Phase 1

▶ Omit the garlic and pepper.

Nutrients per serving	
Calories	209
Fat	7 g
Carbohydrate	30 g
Fiber	3 g
Protein	9 g
Vitamin A	37 IU
Iron	2.2 mg
Zinc	1.5 mg

Roasted Cauliflower Quinoa

Suitable for Phases 2 & 3

Try this modern spin on roasted cauliflower. Green olives and golden raisins are the wild cards here, contributing unexpected depth of flavor. Both cauliflower and quinoa are rich in phytonutrients and antioxidants. Quinoa is also a good source of magnesium.

Tip

Chopped pitted brine-cured black olives (such as kalamata) may be used in place of the green olives.

- Preheat oven to 450°F (230°C)
- Large rimmed baking sheet, lined with foil and brushed with extra virgin olive oil

4 cups	roughly chopped cauliflower florets (about 1 medium head)	1 L
1 tbsp	olive oil	15 mL
	Fine sea salt and freshly cracked black pepper	
1 cup	quinoa, rinsed	250 mL
2 cups	ready-to-use reduced-sodium vegetable broth (gluten-free, if needed)	500 mL
½ cup	packed fresh flat-leaf (Italian) parsley leaves, chopped	125 mL
½ cup	chopped toasted walnuts	125 mL
¼ cup	chopped pitted green olives	60 mL
¼ cup	golden raisins	60 mL

1. In a large bowl, combine cauliflower and oil. Season to taste with salt and pepper. Spread in a single layer on prepared baking sheet. Roast in preheated oven for 20 to 25 minutes, stirring once or twice, until golden brown and tender.

2. Meanwhile, in a medium saucepan, combine quinoa and broth. Bring to a boil over medium–high heat. Reduce heat to low, cover and simmer for 12 to 15 minutes or until liquid is absorbed. Remove from heat and let stand, covered, for 5 minutes. Fluff with a fork.

3. To the quinoa, add roasted cauliflower, parsley, walnuts, olives and raisins, tossing to combine. Season to taste with salt and pepper.

Advice for a Healthy Gut

▸ Choose extra virgin olive oil.

▸ Choose unsweetened raisins.

Nutrients per serving

Calories	344
Fat	18 g
Carbohydrate	40 g
Fiber	5 g
Protein	11 g
Vitamin A	903 IU
Iron	3.1 mg
Zinc	2.0 mg

Sauces and Condiments

Melizzano Despina (Eggplant Dip)

Suitable for Phases 2 & 3

This smoky, oniony dip works wonderfully with raw vegetables and also as a spread on sandwiches.

Advice for a Healthy Gut

▸ "Vegetable oil" is a catchall term for any edible oil from a plant source, whether it be a vegetable, fruit, nut or seed. While you are following the LGS Diet Plan, the best choices for this recipe are extra virgin olive oil, macadamia nut oil, grapeseed oil and avocado oil.

▸ Choose extra virgin olive oil.

Nutrients per serving

Calories	175
Fat	15 g
Carbohydrate	11 g
Fiber	5 g
Protein	2 g
Vitamin A	38 IU
Iron	0.5 mg
Zinc	0.3 mg

• Preheat oven to 450°F (230°C)

1	eggplant (about 1 lb/500 g)	1
1 tsp	vegetable oil	5 mL
1	onion	1
2 tbsp	freshly squeezed lemon juice	30 mL
¼ cup	olive oil	60 mL
	Few sprigs fresh parsley, chopped	
	Salt and freshly ground black pepper	

1. Brush eggplant lightly with vegetable oil. Using a fork, pierce the skin lightly at 1-inch (2.5 cm) intervals. Place on a baking sheet and bake for 1 hour or until eggplant is very soft and the skin is dark brown and caved in.

2. Transfer eggplant to a working surface. Cut off 1 inch (2.5 cm) at the stem end and discard (this part never quite cooks through). Peel the eggplant by picking at an edge from the cut end, then pulling upward. The skin should come off easily in strips.

3. Cut the eggplant lengthwise and place each half with the interior facing you. With a spoon, scoop out the tongues of seed-pods, leaving as much of the flesh as possible. To remove the additional seed-pods hiding inside, cut each piece of eggplant in half and repeat the deseeding procedure. Once deseeded, let cleaned eggplant flesh sit to shed some of its excess water.

4. Transfer drained eggplant flesh to a bowl. Using a wooden spoon, mash and then whip the pulp until smooth and very soft. Coarsely grate onion directly into the eggplant (the onion juice that results is very important to this dip). Add lemon juice and whip with a wooden spoon until perfectly integrated. Keep beating and add olive oil in a very thin stream; the result should be a frothy, light colored emulsion. Season to taste with salt and pepper. Transfer to a serving bowl and garnish with chopped parsley.

Edamame Basil Spread

**Makes about
1²⁄₃ cups (400 mL)**

Suitable for
Phase 3

*This gorgeous green dip is
rich in folate, a B vitamin
that is needed for tissue
repair and healing.*

Tip

This spread can be
stored in an airtight
container in the
refrigerator for up to
3 days.

- Food processor

6	cloves garlic	6
12 oz	frozen shelled edamame	375 g
1 cup	packed fresh basil leaves	250 mL
½ tsp	fine sea salt	2 mL
3 tbsp	extra virgin olive oil	45 mL
3 tbsp	freshly squeezed lemon juice	45 mL

1. In a medium saucepan of boiling water, cook garlic
   and edamame for 7 to 10 minutes or until edamame
   are very tender. Drain, reserving ½ cup (125 mL)
   of the cooking liquid. Let cool.

2. In food processor, combine cooled garlic and
   edamame, basil, salt, half the reserved cooking liquid,
   oil and lemon juice; process until smooth. Add more
   reserved liquid, 1 tbsp (15 mL) at a time, until mixture
   is creamy. Transfer to a serving dish, cover and
   refrigerate for 30 minutes or until chilled.

Nutrients per 1 tbsp (15 mL)

Calories	30
Fat	2 g
Carbohydrate	2 g
Fiber	1 g
Protein	1 g
Vitamin A	86 IU
Iron	0.4 mg
Zinc	0.2 mg

Fresh Basil Pesto

Makes about ⅔ cup (150 mL)

Suitable for Phases 1, 2 & 3

Classic pesto sauce is rich in flavor and antioxidants. Fresh and dried herbs deserve the title of "superfood" just as much as kale, quinoa, broccoli and the like.

- Food processor

1	clove garlic	1
2 tbsp	pine nuts	30 mL
⅔ cup	firmly packed fresh basil leaves	150 mL
⅓ cup	extra virgin olive oil	75 mL
3 tbsp	freshly grated Parmesan cheese	45 mL
	Salt and freshly ground black pepper	

1. In food processor, process garlic and pine nuts until finely chopped. Add basil and process until finely chopped. With the motor running, slowly add oil through the feed tube.

2. Transfer to a bowl and stir in Parmesan, salt and pepper.

3. Store in an airtight container in the refrigerator for up to 1 week. Use in any recipe that calls for pesto.

Adjustments for Phase 1

▸ Omit the garlic, Parmesan cheese and pepper.

Adjustment for Phase 2

▸ Omit the Parmesan cheese.

Nutrients per 1 tbsp (15 mL)

Calories	83
Fat	9 g
Carbohydrate	1 g
Fiber	0 g
Protein	1 g
Vitamin A	163 IU
Iron	0.2 mg
Zinc	0.2 mg

Salsa Cynthia

Makes about 2 cups (500 mL)

Suitable for Phase 3

This spicy salsa is perfect as a dip for nachos and as an accompaniment to Mexican-style dishes like enchiladas, as well as avocado-based salsas and soups.

Tips

The flavor of this sauce improves if kept in the fridge for up to 3 or 4 days. Stir thoroughly before each use.

When working with hot peppers, be sure to wear gloves; otherwise, wash hands thoroughly.

• Food processor

4	ripe tomatoes	4
1	red or white onion, cut into eighths	1
2	cloves garlic, crushed	2
Pinch	salt	Pinch
5	jalapeño peppers	5
2 tbsp	vegetable oil	30 mL
1 tbsp	freshly squeezed lime juice	15 mL
	Few sprigs fresh coriander, chopped	

1. Blanch tomatoes in boiling water for 30 seconds. Over a bowl, peel, core and deseed them. Chop tomatoes roughly and put in food processor. Strain any accumulated tomato juices from bowl; add to food processor. Add onion pieces, garlic and salt.

2. Remove the stems of the jalapeños, and cut them into halves. Scoop out and discard the core and most of the seeds (the more seeds, the hotter your sauce; without any seeds, you'll have a mildly hot sauce). Chop the peppers roughly and add to the food processor, along with retained seeds. Pulse on and off until mixed and slightly chunky, but not puréed.

3. Transfer mixture to a saucepan, add vegetable oil, and cook over medium heat for 6 to 8 minutes, until mildly bubbling and foaming pinkly. Remove from heat and let salsa cool for at least 10 minutes.

4. Add lime juice and chopped coriander; stir well and serve.

Advice for a Healthy Gut

▸ Use extra virgin olive oil, macadamia nut oil, grapeseed oil or avocado oil for the vegetable oil.

▸ Start with $\frac{1}{2}$ to 1 jalapeño pepper and gauge your tolerance. Gradually increase the amount you use, monitoring your tolerance as your gut continues to heal.

Nutrients per $\frac{1}{4}$ cup (60 mL)

Calories	52
Fat	4 g
Carbohydrate	5 g
Fiber	1 g
Protein	1 g
Vitamin A	608 IU
Iron	0.2 mg
Zinc	0.2 mg

Pineapple Salsa

**Makes about
2¼ cups (550 mL)**

Suitable for
Phase 3

Pineapple is a vitamin C jackpot with a bonus: it has an enzyme that helps relieve indigestion, making it a snack your stomach will welcome.

Tips

For the best results, make this salsa at least 30 minutes ahead of time to allow the flavors to mingle.

This salsa can be stored in an airtight container in the refrigerator for up to 2 days.

1	small jalapeño pepper, seeded and minced	1
2 cups	diced fresh pineapple (see tip, page 231)	500 mL
¾ cup	packed fresh cilantro leaves, chopped	175 mL
¼ cup	finely chopped red onion	60 mL
1 tsp	finely grated lime zest	5 mL
1 tbsp	freshly squeezed lime juice	15 mL
⅛ tsp	fine sea salt	0.5 mL

1. In a medium bowl, combine jalapeño, pineapple, cilantro, red onion, lime zest, lime juice and salt.

Nutrients per ¼ cup (60 mL)

Calories	22
Fat	0 g
Carbohydrate	6 g
Fiber	1 g
Protein	0 g
Vitamin A	42 IU
Iron	0.1 mg
Zinc	0.1 mg

Plum Dipping Sauce

Makes 1 cup (250 mL)

Suitable for Phase 3

This quick, easy, rich, plum-colored sauce is wonderful with Cornish game hens (page 246), and kids will love it with baked chicken fingers.

Tips

This sauce can be stored, covered, in the refrigerator for up to 2 weeks.

To prevent cross-contamination, set out individual bowls of dipping sauces for each person.

Serve the sauce warm or cold — it's delicious either way!

- **Blender**

1	can (14 oz/398 mL) prune plums	1
⅓ cup	granulated sugar	75 mL
3 tbsp	white vinegar	45 mL

1. Drain plums, reserving 2 tbsp (30 mL) liquid. Remove pits from plums. In blender, purée plums and reserved liquid.

2. In a small saucepan, combine plum purée, sugar and vinegar. Heat over medium heat until mixture comes to a gentle boil. Remove from heat and let cool before serving.

Variation

In season, 8 fresh plums can be substituted for the canned plums. For an even quicker sauce, substitute one 7.5-oz (213 mL) jar of unsweetened gluten-free baby food strained plums.

Advice for a Healthy Gut

▶ While you are following the LGS Diet Plan, use liquid honey instead of granulated sugar as the sweetener in this recipe, and use rice vinegar instead of white vinegar.

Nutrients per 1 tbsp (15 mL)	
Calories	27
Fat	0 g
Carbohydrate	7 g
Fiber	0 g
Protein	0 g
Vitamin A	239 IU
Iron	0.0 mg
Zinc	0.0 mg

Garlic White Sauce

**Makes 2 cups
(500 mL)**

Suitable for
Phase 3

*Many casseroles, soups
and pasta dishes rely on
a white sauce to bind all
the ingredients. Here is
another basic, vegan white
sauce to have in your
recipe toolbox.*

- **Blender**

1 tbsp	olive oil	15 mL
½	onion, finely chopped	½
3 tbsp	finely chopped fresh parsley	45 mL
1	clove garlic, finely chopped	1
1½ cups	rice milk	375 mL
1	roasted eggplant, peeled (see Roasted Vegetables or Fruit, page 283)	1
1	head roasted garlic (see recipe, opposite)	1

1. In a saucepan, heat oil over medium heat. Add onion and cook, stirring occasionally, for 5 minutes or until slightly softened. Add parsley and garlic and cook, stirring frequently, for 3 to 4 minutes or until onion is soft.

2. In blender, combine onion mixture, rice milk, eggplant and garlic. Process until liquefied. Store sauce, tightly covered, in the refrigerator for up to 3 days.

> ### Advice for a Healthy Gut
> ▸ Choose extra virgin olive oil or avocado oil.
> ▸ Choose a carrageenan-free rice milk.

Nutrients per ¼ cup (60 mL)

Calories	90
Fat	5 g
Carbohydrate	12 g
Fiber	3 g
Protein	2 g
Vitamin A	230 IU
Iron	0.6 mg
Zinc	0.3 mg

Roasted Garlic

Suitable for Phase 3

Whole roasted garlic bulbs morph into a sweet and meltingly tender pulp with a deceptively mellow flavor.

Tip

Store whole roasted garlic head tightly covered in the refrigerator for up to 5 days. Or squeeze the cloves out of the skins, place in sealable freezer bags and freeze for up to 3 months.

- Preheat oven to 400°F (200°C)
- Small heatproof baking dish with lid or foil

1	whole head garlic	1
1 tsp	olive oil	5 mL

1. Remove loose, papery skin from garlic head. Slice off and discard ¼ inch (0.5 cm) from tops of the cloves in entire head. Place garlic head cut side up in baking dish and drizzle with oil. Cover with a lid or foil. Bake in preheated oven for about 40 minutes or until garlic is quite soft. Transfer to a wire rack and let cool. If using a clay garlic roaster with a lid, roast at 375°F (190°C) for 35 to 40 minutes or until garlic is quite soft.

2. When garlic is cool enough to handle, squeeze cloves from their skins. They are now ready to use in any recipe that calls for roasted garlic.

Advice for a Healthy Gut

▶ Choose extra virgin olive oil or avocado oil.

Nutrients per 1 tbsp (15 mL)

Calories	19
Fat	1 g
Carbohydrate	2 g
Fiber	0 g
Protein	0 g
Vitamin A	1 IU
Iron	0.1 mg
Zinc	0.1 mg

Roasted Vegetable Sauce

Makes about 1½ cups (375 mL)

Suitable for Phase 3

Vegetable sauce on vegetables is doubly healthy and doubly divine! The onion adds a subtle base and blends perfectly with the roasted broccoli. Scrumptious tossed with gluten-free pasta or on rice or baked potatoes.

- Preheat oven to 400°F (200°C)
- Baking sheet, lined with parchment paper
- Blender

4 cups	broccoli florets	1 L
½	onion, ends cut off, unpeeled, quartered	½
2	cloves garlic, unpeeled	2
2 tsp	olive oil	10 mL
½ cup	ready-to-use vegetable broth (gluten-free, if needed)	125 mL
¼ cup	plain hemp milk	60 mL
	Salt and freshly ground black pepper (optional)	

1. Place broccoli, onion and garlic on prepared baking sheet. Drizzle and toss with oil. Bake in preheated oven until tender, 20 to 25 minutes. Let cool.

2. When cool, peel onion and garlic and transfer with broccoli to blender. Add broth and milk and blend until smooth. Taste and add salt and pepper, if desired. Serve immediately or refrigerate in an airtight container for up to 2 days. Heat over low heat before using or serve chilled.

Variation

Substitute cauliflower, winter squash, carrots and ginger or your favorite vegetables.

Advice for a Healthy Gut

▶ Choose extra virgin olive oil or avocado oil.

▶ Choose a carrageenan-free hemp milk.

Nutrients per ¼ cup (60 mL)

Calories	37
Fat	2 g
Carbohydrate	4 g
Fiber	2 g
Protein	2 g
Vitamin A	1458 IU
Iron	0.6 mg
Zinc	0.3 mg

Pickled Pink Onion Relish

Makes about 1½ cups (375 mL)

Suitable for Phase 3

This bright pink relish is a perfect condiment for many sandwiches and salads. It is also a colorful way to top off hors d'oeuvres. It keeps in the refrigerator for a few weeks. One red onion goes a long way.

Tip

The color of this relish will deepen with time. Any juice left over once the onions have been used up can be used to make tasty salad dressings and marinades.

6 cups	water	1.5 L
1 tsp	salt	5 mL
1	red onion, cut in half from stem to root, then crosswise, and thinly sliced	1
½ cup	seasoned rice vinegar	125 mL

1. In a pot over high heat, bring water and salt to a boil. Add onion and return to a boil (about 45 seconds). Drain and immediately transfer to a nonreactive container. Add vinegar and toss to coat evenly.

2. Let cool to room temperature. Cover and refrigerate for 2 hours or until chilled and deep pink.

Variation

Add ½ tsp (2 mL) of your favorite dried herb, such as thyme, tarragon or basil, along with the vinegar.

Nutrients per 1 tbsp (15 mL)

Calories	7
Fat	0 g
Carbohydrate	2 g
Fiber	0 g
Protein	0 g
Vitamin A	0 IU
Iron	0.0 mg
Zinc	0.0 mg

Apple Butter

Makes about 4½ cups (1.125 L)

Suitable for Phases 1, 2 & 3

Apples are cooked with the skin to increase flavor and nutrients, so using scrubbed organic apples is best. The use of a food mill is required for this method. If you prefer to skip that step, see the variation, below.

Tips

About 12 medium apples will generally equal 4 lbs (2 kg).

To sterilize canning jars, immerse in a pot of simmering, not boiling, water for 10 minutes or wash using the sterilizing cycle in dishwasher. Keep hot until filling.

Nutrients per 1 tbsp (15 mL)

Calories	25
Fat	0 g
Carbohydrate	7 g
Fiber	1 g
Protein	0 g
Vitamin A	13 IU
Iron	0.0 mg
Zinc	0.0 mg

• **Food mill or small-holed colander**

4 lbs	sweet, tart apples, such as Granny Smith, Cortland or Pippin, cored and quartered	2 kg
1¾ cups	apple cider or juice	425 mL
¾ cup	agave nectar	175 mL
2 tbsp	freshly squeezed lemon juice	30 mL
1½ tsp	ground cinnamon	7 mL
1 tsp	ground cardamom	5 mL

1. In a large heavy-bottomed saucepan over medium-high heat, bring apples and apple cider to a boil. Reduce heat and simmer, stirring occasionally, until very soft, 25 to 30 minutes. Let cool.

2. Press softened apples through a food mill or small-holed colander to remove skins.

3. Transfer apple purée to a clean large heavy-bottomed saucepan over medium-high heat. Stir in agave, lemon juice, cinnamon and cardamom and bring to a boil, stirring frequently. Reduce heat and simmer, stirring frequently to prevent any sticking and adjusting heat as necessary as mixture thickens, until mixture is very thick and mounds on a spoon, about 1½ hours.

4. Remove from heat and let cool. Spoon into sterilized canning jars (see tip, at left) or airtight containers and refrigerate for up to 1 month or freeze for up to 3 months.

Variation

To avoid using a food mill to purée apples, peel, core and quarter apples and follow instructions through step 1. Skip step 2 and instead use a food processor to purée softened apples. Resume instructions at step 3.

Advice for a Healthy Gut

▶ Choose pure, unsweetened apple cider or juice.

Basic Almond Spread

Makes about 2 cups (500 mL)

Suitable for Phase 3

This recipe is so versatile and healthy. When savory herbs and garlic are used, it replaces commercial spreads and dips and sauces; if berries and soft fruits are added, it becomes a sweet topping or light pudding with all sorts of applications for healthy desserts.

- **Blender**

1 cup	whole almonds (unblanched)	250 mL
2 cups	water, divided	500 mL
2 tbsp	olive oil	30 mL
2 tbsp	freshly squeezed lemon juice (approx.)	30 mL
2	cloves garlic	2
½ tsp	salt (optional)	2 mL

1. In a small bowl, mix almonds with 1 cup (250 mL) water. Cover and let stand in the refrigerator for at least 6 hours or overnight.

2. Drain and rinse almonds well. Place the remaining water in blender. Add almonds, olive oil, lemon juice, garlic and salt (if using), and process for 30 seconds or until mixture is smooth and creamy. Taste and add more salt or lemon juice, if required. Use right away or store, tightly covered, in the refrigerator for up to 5 days.

Variation

In step 2 after processing, fold in ¼ cup (60 mL) chopped toasted almonds.

Advice for a Healthy Gut

▸ Choose extra virgin olive oil or avocado oil.

Nutrients per 1 tbsp (15 mL)

Calories	33
Fat	3 g
Carbohydrate	1 g
Fiber	1 g
Protein	1 g
Vitamin A	0 IU
Iron	0.2 mg
Zinc	0.1 mg

Cashew Cream

**Makes 1⅓ cups
(325 mL)**

Suitable for Phase 3

Use this gut-friendly dairy-free substitute wherever half-and-half (10%) cream is called for. You can make the sauce thicker by using another ½ cup (125 mL) cashews. It can then substitute for heavy (whipping) cream in recipes. Only one other nut may be substituted for the cashews in this versatile cook's tool, and that is macadamia.

• **Blender**

⅓ cup	cashews	75 mL
1 cup	rice milk or soy milk	250 mL

1. In blender, combine cashews and milk. Blend until nuts are completely puréed and cream is smooth.

2. Store cream tightly covered in the refrigerator for up to 4 days. Shake well before using.

Advice for a Healthy Gut

▶ Choose a carrageenan-free rice milk.

Nutrients per 1 tbsp (15 mL)

Calories	17
Fat	1 g
Carbohydrate	2 g
Fiber	0 g
Protein	0 g
Vitamin A	23 IU
Iron	0.2 mg
Zinc	0.1 mg

Desserts

Citrus Mint Toss

Makes 2 servings

Suitable for Phase 3

This salad is reminiscent of Mediterranean dishes, bursting with fresh green herbs and sweet citrus, and is packed with vitamin C, which is both an antioxidant and a cofactor in healing.

Tip

To prepare the citrus segments for this recipe, place fruit on a cutting board and remove a bit of skin from each end to create a flat surface — this will reveal the thickness of the pith. Using a sharp knife in a downward motion, remove the skin and the pith. Shave off any remaining bits of pith, then cut between the membranes to produce wedges of pure citrus flesh.

½ cup	orange segments (see tip, at left)	125 mL
½ cup	grapefruit segments	125 mL
¼ cup	lemon segments	60 mL
1 cup	finely sliced fresh mint leaves	250 mL
2 tbsp	cold-pressed (extra virgin) olive oil	30 mL
¼ tsp	fine sea salt	1 mL

1. In a bowl, combine orange, grapefruit and lemon segments and mint. Add oil and salt. Toss well. Serve immediately or transfer to an airtight container and refrigerate for up to 2 days.

Variation

Substitute an equal quantity of lime segments for the lemon.

Nutrients per serving

Calories	176
Fat	14 g
Carbohydrate	14 g
Fiber	3 g
Protein	2 g
Vitamin A	1184 IU
Iron	1.0 mg
Zinc	0.2 mg

Watermelon and Cashew Salad

Suitable for Phase 3

Watermelon pairs beautifully with nuts, seeds and spices and is wonderfully refreshing on a warm summer's day.

Tips

Cashews provide protein, copper, zinc, phosphorus, potassium and magnesium and are a source of healthy monounsaturated fat.

You may substitute 2 tbsp (30 mL) thinly sliced fresh oregano leaves for the dried oregano.

- **Food processor**

1/2 cup	whole raw cashews	125 mL
1 tbsp	cold-pressed (extra virgin) olive oil	15 mL
1 tsp	dried oregano	5 mL
1/4 tsp	fine sea salt	1 mL
2 cups	cubed seeded watermelon	500 mL
2 tbsp	finely sliced green onion (green part only)	30 mL

1. In food processor, process cashews until roughly chopped. Add oil, oregano and salt. Process until just combined, about 5 seconds, or until cashews just begin to stick together.

2. In a bowl, combine watermelon and green onion. Toss well. Using a fine-mesh sieve, drain off any excess liquid and discard. Add cashew mixture to watermelon and mix well. Serve immediately or cover and refrigerate for up to 2 days.

Nutrients per serving	
Calories	305
Fat	23 g
Carbohydrate	24 g
Fiber	2 g
Protein	6 g
Vitamin A	936 IU
Iron	2.7 mg
Zinc	2.1 mg

Creamy Cashew Maple Dip with Apples

Apples are a great source of fiber, which helps with regularity. They also provide an abundance of phytonutrients called polyphenols, which help to reduce inflammation.

Tip

This dip can be stored in an airtight container in the refrigerator for up to 1 week. The apples are best prepared just before serving.

- **Blender or food processor**

3	tart-sweet apples (such as Gala, Braeburn or Honeycrisp), cored and each cut into 8 slices	3
	Ice water	
½ cup	cashews	125 mL
Pinch	fine sea salt	Pinch
½ cup	water	125 mL
1 tbsp	pure maple syrup	15 mL
½ tsp	vanilla extract (gluten-free, if needed)	2 mL

1. Place apple slices in a large bowl and add enough ice water to cover. Refrigerate for at least 30 minutes or until apples are very crisp. Drain and pat dry with paper towels.

2. In blender, combine cashews, salt, water, maple syrup and vanilla; blend until very smooth and creamy.

3. Transfer dip to a serving dish. Serve with apple slices for dipping.

Nutrients per serving	
Calories	92
Fat	4 g
Carbohydrate	14 g
Fiber	2 g
Protein	2 g
Vitamin A	37 IU
Iron	0.6 mg
Zinc	0.6 mg

Banana Soup with Raspberry and Mint Relish

Suitable for Phase 3

When you grow tired of banana bread, here's another creative way to use over-ripe bananas. If the ingredients are already chilled, this soup takes very little time to prepare.

Tip

The soup can be prepared up to 2 hours ahead; cover and refrigerate until ready to serve.

• **Food processor or blender**

4	chilled very ripe bananas, halved	4
2 cups	chilled unsweetened apple juice	500 mL
1/2 cup	chilled freshly squeezed orange juice	125 mL
2 tbsp	freshly squeezed lemon juice (approx.)	30 mL
Pinch	salt	Pinch
2 tbsp	liquid honey (optional)	30 mL
1	very ripe banana, diced	1
1 cup	raspberries	250 mL
2 tbsp	chopped fresh mint	30 mL

1. In food processor, purée halved bananas and apple juice until smooth. Transfer to a large bowl and stir in orange juice, lemon juice and salt. Taste and add honey or more lemon juice if necessary.

2. In a small bowl, combine diced banana, raspberries and mint.

3. Ladle soup into chilled bowls and top with raspberry and mint relish.

Variation

For a smoothie-like rendition of this summer cooler, add 1 cup (250 mL) yogurt or non-dairy yogurt alternative and reduce the apple juice by half.

Nutrients per serving	
Calories	147
Fat	1 g
Carbohydrate	37 g
Fiber	4 g
Protein	2 g
Vitamin A	135 IU
Iron	0.6 mg
Zinc	0.3 mg

The Ultimate Baked Apples

Makes 8 servings

Suitable for Phase 3

These luscious apples are the definitive autumn dessert, a tasty way to benefit from their anti-inflammatory phytonutrients. For added decadence, serve with a dollop of Coconut Whipped Cream (page 322).

Tips

You can halve this recipe, but be sure to use a smaller oval slow cooker (approx. 3 quarts) that will comfortably accommodate 4 apples.

When buying nuts, be sure to source them from a purveyor with high turnover. Because nuts are high in fat (but healthy fat), they tend to become rancid very quickly.

Nutrients per serving	
Calories	182
Fat	5 g
Carbohydrate	36 g
Fiber	5 g
Protein	3 g
Vitamin A	117 IU
Iron	0.6 mg
Zinc	0.4 mg

- **Large (minimum 5-quart) oval slow cooker**

½ cup	chopped toasted walnuts	125 mL
½ cup	dried cranberries	125 mL
2 tbsp	coconut sugar	30 mL
1 tsp	grated orange zest	5 mL
8	apples, cored	8
1 cup	pure pomegranate juice	250 mL

1. In a bowl, combine walnuts, cranberries, sugar and orange zest. To stuff the apples, hold your hand over the bottom of the apple and, using your fingers, tightly pack core space with filling. One at a time, place filled apples in slow cooker stoneware. Drizzle pomegranate juice evenly over tops.

2. Cover and cook on Low for 6 hours or on High for 3 hours, until apples are tender.

3. Transfer apples to a serving dish and spoon cooking juices over them. Serve hot.

> ## Advice for a Healthy Gut
> ▶ Choose unsweetened dried cranberries.

Gingery Pears Poached in Green Tea

Makes 8 servings

Suitable for Phase 3

Ginger and pears combine in this light but delicious dessert. Sprinkle with toasted almonds and top with a dollop of Coconut Whipped Cream for a perfect finish to a substantial meal.

Tips

You can halve this recipe, but be sure to use a small (1½- to 2-quart) slow cooker.

These pears have a strong ginger taste, but you can vary the amount of ginger to suit your preference.

This dessert should be made early in the day or the night before so it can be well chilled before serving.

Nutrients per serving	
Calories	175
Fat	0 g
Carbohydrate	46 g
Fiber	6 g
Protein	1 g
Vitamin A	41 IU
Iron	0.8 mg
Zinc	0.2 mg

- **Small (maximum 3½-quart) slow cooker**

4 cups	boiling water	1 L
2 tbsp	green tea leaves	30 mL
1 to 2 tbsp	grated gingerroot	15 to 30 mL
½ cup	liquid honey	125 mL
1 tsp	pure almond extract	5 mL
1 tsp	grated lemon zest	5 mL
8	firm pears, such as Bosc, peeled, cored and cut into quarters lengthwise	8

Topping (optional)

Toasted sliced almonds

Coconut Whipped Cream (page 322)

1. In a pot, combine boiling water and green tea leaves. Cover and let steep for 5 minutes. Strain through a fine sieve into slow cooker stoneware.

2. Add ginger, honey, almond extract and lemon zest and stir well. Add pears. Cover and cook on Low for 6 hours or on High for 3 hours, until pears are tender. Transfer to a serving bowl, cover and chill thoroughly.

3. If desired, serve garnished with toasted almonds and a dollop of Coconut Whipped Cream.

Poached Quinces

Makes 4 to 6 servings

Suitable for Phase 3

Quinces are fabulous winter fruit that are made for the slow cooker, because they demand cooking. Raw, the quince is a tough, fibrous ball. Softened by slow cooking, it turns a beautiful shade of pink and melts in your mouth, releasing a panoply of complex flavors.

Tip

You can halve this recipe, but be sure to use a small (1½- to 2-quart) slow cooker.

- **Small to medium (2- to 4-quart) slow cooker**

½ cup	water	125 mL
½ cup	liquid honey	125 mL
	Zest of 1 orange	
4	quinces (about 2 lbs/1 kg), peeled, cored and sliced	4
	Coconut Whipped Cream (page 322)	
	Toasted chopped walnuts or toasted coconut (optional)	

1. In slow cooker stoneware, combine water, honey and orange zest. Add quinces and stir well. Cover and cook on Low for about 8 hours, until quinces are tender and turn pink. Serve warm or chilled. To serve, top with Coconut Whipped Cream. Sprinkle with walnuts, if desired.

Nutrients per serving (1 of 6)

Calories	120
Fat	0 g
Carbohydrate	32 g
Fiber	1 g
Protein	0 g
Vitamin A	25 IU
Iron	0.6 mg
Zinc	0.1 mg

Apple-Cranberry Compote

A medley of flavorful fruits makes this dessert a tasty way to get an abundance of anti-inflammatory polyphenols, which help to heal the gut.

Tips

Fresh, frozen or even dried cranberries may be used in this autumn dish. If using dried cranberries, reduce the amount to ⅔ cup (150 mL).

Store compote, tightly covered, in the refrigerator for up to 5 days.

1 cup	cranberries (see tips, at left)	250 mL
2	apples, peeled and sliced	2
¼ cup	dried cherries or chopped dried apricots	60 mL
¼ cup	apple juice or white wine	60 mL
2 tbsp	butter	30 mL
¼ cup	organic cane sugar	60 mL
1 tbsp	chopped fresh lemon balm or sweet cicely	15 mL

1. In a saucepan, combine cranberries, apples, cherries and apple juice. Bring to a boil over medium-high heat. Reduce heat and simmer for 7 minutes or until fruit is soft.

2. Add butter, sugar and lemon balm and simmer for 2 minutes.

Variations

Use black currants, elderberries, gooseberries or chopped rhubarb in place of the cranberries.

Use 1½ cups (375 mL) chopped fresh pineapple instead of the apples.

Adjustments for Phases 1 & 2

▶ Use apple juice (not white wine).

▶ Substitute virgin coconut oil or grapeseed oil for the butter.

▶ Replace the cane sugar with an equal amount of liquid honey.

Advice for a Healthy Gut

▶ Choose unsweetened dried fruit.

▶ Virgin coconut oil and grapeseed oil continue to be the best fat choices, but in Phase 3, you may use organic butter instead, if desired.

▶ Continue to use honey as the sweetener in this recipe while you are following the LGS Diet Plan.

Nutrients per ¼ cup (60 mL)

Calories	128
Fat	4 g
Carbohydrate	24 g
Fiber	4 g
Protein	0 g
Vitamin A	400 IU
Iron	0.8 mg
Zinc	0.1 mg

Pineapple Coconut Crumble

Suitable for Phase 3

This sweet, crumbly treat is a blend of juicy pineapple and rich coconut oil topped with a crisp almond and coconut crust.

Tips

When shopping for dates, always look for the Medjool variety. They are larger, softer and more flavorful.

Coconut oil is solid at room temperature but has a melting temperature of 76°F (24°C), so it is easy to liquefy. To melt it, place in a shallow glass bowl over a pot of simmering water.

Use unsweetened medium-shred unsulfured coconut.

- Blender
- Food processor
- 4-inch (10 cm) square glass baking dish

2 cups	pineapple cut into 1-inch (2.5 cm) pieces, divided	500 mL
1/4 cup	filtered water	60 mL
9	chopped pitted dates, divided	9
3 tbsp	melted coconut oil (see tip, at left)	45 mL
1 1/2 cups	whole raw almonds	375 mL
1/2 cup	dried shredded coconut (see tip, at left)	125 mL
Pinch	fine sea salt	Pinch

1. In blender, combine 1 cup (250 mL) pineapple, water, a third of the dates and the coconut oil. Blend on high speed until smooth. Fold in remaining pineapple. Transfer to baking dish and spread over bottom of dish.

2. In food processor, process almonds, shredded coconut and salt until just combined (you want to retain some texture). Add remaining dates and pulse until combined.

3. Spread almond mixture on top of pineapple mixture. Refrigerate for 10 minutes or until set. Serve immediately or cover and refrigerate for up to 3 days.

Nutrients per serving

Calories	411
Fat	35 g
Carbohydrate	22 g
Fiber	8 g
Protein	10 g
Vitamin A	40 IU
Iron	2.2 mg
Zinc	1.6 mg

Carrot Cake

Suitable for Phase 3

This cake, a blend of sweet carrots, rich coconut and fragrant cinnamon, is sure to be a crowd-pleaser no matter where you go.

Tips

To soak the raisins, place in a bowl with ½ cup (125 mL) hot water. Cover and set aside for 10 minutes. Drain, discarding soaking liquid.

To remove excess water from shredded carrots, place them in a piece of cheesecloth and, using your hands, squeeze out the moisture. You can also use a nut-milk bag if you have one, or you can place the carrots in a fine-mesh sieve and use the back of a ladle to press out the excess water.

Nutrients per serving	
Calories	422
Fat	22 g
Carbohydrate	57 g
Fiber	9 g
Protein	8 g
Vitamin A	18,386 IU
Iron	2.0 mg
Zinc	1.4 mg

- Food processor
- 4-inch (10 cm) square glass baking dish

1 cup	raw walnut halves	250 mL
¾ cup	chopped pitted dates	175 mL
¼ cup	raisins, soaked (see tip, at left)	60 mL
1 tsp	ground cinnamon	5 mL
3 cups	grated carrots, excess water removed (see tip, at left)	750 mL

1. In food processor, process walnuts, dates, soaked raisins and cinnamon until coarsely chopped (you want to retain some texture). Add shredded carrots and pulse to combine, about 8 to 10 times.

2. Transfer to baking dish and press down firmly, especially at the edges. Refrigerate for about 10 minutes or until firm throughout. Serve immediately or cover and refrigerate for up to 3 days.

Variation

Add a pinch of ground nutmeg and 3 tbsp (45 mL) dried shredded coconut in step 1.

Coconut Whipped Cream

Suitable for Phase 3

Coconut whipped cream is a great dairy-free finish for many desserts. The secret to a successful result is ensuring that your coconut milk and the bowl and beaters used for whipping are all thoroughly chilled.

Tip

You can vary the flavor of the cream to complement the dish you are serving it with. Substitute pure maple syrup and maple extract for the coconut sugar and vanilla or, for a more intense coconut flavor, substitute coconut extract for the vanilla.

1	can (14 oz/400 mL) coconut milk, refrigerated for at least 4 hours	1
2 tsp	coconut sugar	10 mL
½ tsp	vanilla extract (gluten-free, if needed)	2 mL

1. Skim off the thick layer of cream on top of the milk and transfer to a chilled mixing bowl. (Save the remaining liquid for another use.) Add sugar and vanilla and, using an electric mixer, beat on low speed to incorporate ingredients. Increase speed to high and beat until peaks form, about 2 minutes. Serve immediately.

Advice for a Healthy Gut

▶ Choose a carrageenan-free coconut milk.

Nutrients per 1 tbsp (15 mL)

Calories	66
Fat	7 g
Carbohydrate	2 g
Fiber	0 g
Protein	1 g
Vitamin A	0 IU
Iron	1.1 mg
Zinc	0.2 mg

Beverages

Almond Milk

**Suitable for
Phases 1, 2 & 3**

*This recipe is very simple
to make and, after soaking
the almonds, takes no
time at all. Use this in
smoothies and soups or as
a refreshing pick-me-up
any time of the day. If you
are feeling a bit peckish or
having a slight slump, a
glass of cold almond milk
will provide instant energy.*

Tip

A nut milk bag, which
is used to squeeze the
liquid from the pulp
when making nut or
seed milks, is typically
made from nylon mesh.
They are available from
specialty raw food
dealers and most health
food stores.

Nutrients per 1 cup (250 mL)

Calories	206
Fat	18 g
Carbohydrate	8 g
Fiber	0 g
Protein	8 g
Vitamin A	0 IU
Iron	1.3 mg
Zinc	1.1 mg

- Blender
- Nut milk bag or cheesecloth (see tip, at left)

1 cup	whole raw almonds	250 mL
6 cups	filtered water, divided	1.5 L

1. Place almonds in a bowl and add 2 cups (500 mL)
   filtered water. Cover and set aside for at least
   30 minutes or up to 12 hours. If you are soaking
   the nuts at room temperature, change the water
   every 3 hours (if they are refrigerated, this step isn't
   necessary). Drain, discard the soaking water and rinse
   under cold running water until the water runs clear.

2. In blender, combine almonds and the remaining water.
   Blend on high speed for 30 to 60 seconds or until the
   liquid becomes milky white and no visible pieces of
   almond remain.

3. If using a nut milk bag, place the bag over a pitcher
   large enough to accommodate the liquid, pour in the
   almond mixture and strain. Starting at the top of the
   bag and using your hands, squeeze in a downward
   direction to extract the remaining milk. (If you do
   not have a nut milk bag, line a sieve with two layers of
   cheesecloth and place it over a bowl or pitcher. Pour in
   the almond mixture and strain. Use a wooden spoon to
   press out the liquid, extracting as much of it as possible.
   Collect the corners of the cheesecloth and twist them
   to form a tight ball. Using your hands, squeeze out the
   remaining liquid.)

4. Cover and refrigerate the milk for up to 3 days.
   Discard the pulp or save it for another use (see tip,
   at left.)

Variation

Sweetened Almond Milk: After straining, return milk
to the blender and add a chopped pitted date, a dash
of raw vanilla extract and a pinch of sea salt. Blend
until smooth.

Pecan Milk

Suitable for Phases 2 & 3

Pecans are a great option for making a dairy-free milk, suitable if you have a milk allergy or simply want to avoid milk. Pecan milk is lower in protein than dairy milk, but it contains the phytonutrients found in pecans.

- **Blender**

2 cups	boiling water, divided	500 mL
¾ cup	finely chopped pecans	175 mL
1 tbsp	chopped raisins	15 mL
1 tbsp	chopped vanilla bean	15 mL

1. In blender, combine 1 cup (250 mL) boiling water, pecans, raisins and vanilla bean. Secure lid and blend (from low to high if using a variable-speed blender) until smooth.

2. With blender still running, add remaining boiling water through opening in center of lid. Blend until smooth. Let cool. Cover and refrigerate for up to 3 days.

Advice for a Healthy Gut

▶ Choose unsweetened raisins.

Nutrients per 1 cup (250 mL)

Calories	296
Fat	29 g
Carbohydrate	12 g
Fiber	4 g
Protein	4 g
Vitamin A	23 IU
Iron	1.1 mg
Zinc	1.9 mg

Coconut Milk

**Makes about
4 cups (1 L)**

Suitable for
Phases 2 & 3

*Coconut milk is higher in
fat than other raw milks,
which makes it perfect for
adding to tea and other
warm beverages.*

Tip

After refrigeration, a
small layer of fat will
form at the top of
the container. Simply
stir this fat back into
the liquid, using a
small whisk or fork,
before drinking.

- Blender
- Nut milk bag or cheesecloth (see tip, page 324)

1 cup	unsweetened dried shredded coconut	250 mL
6 cups	filtered water, divided	1.5 L
Pinch	fine sea salt	Pinch

1. Place coconut in a bowl and add 2 cups (500 mL) water. Cover and set aside for 30 minutes. Drain and rinse under cold running water until the water runs clear.

2. In blender, combine coconut, salt and the remaining water. Blend on high speed for 1 minute or until the liquid becomes milky white and no visible pieces of coconut remain.

3. Pour into a nut milk bag placed over a pitcher large enough to accommodate the liquid, and strain. Starting at the top of the bag and using your hands, squeeze in a downward direction to extract the remaining milk (for cheesecloth instructions, see step 3, page 324). Cover and refrigerate the milk for up to 3 days.

Variation

Strawberry Chocolate Coconut Milk: After straining the coconut milk, return it to the blender. Add ½ cup (125 mL) chopped hulled strawberries, 3 tbsp (45 mL) liquid honey and 2 tbsp (30 mL) cacao powder and blend again until smooth.

Nutrients per 1 cup (250 mL)

Calories	71
Fat	7 g
Carbohydrate	3 g
Fiber	2 g
Protein	1 g
Vitamin A	0 IU
Iron	0.5 mg
Zinc	0.3 mg

Hemp Milk

Makes about 4 cups (1 L)

Suitable for Phases 1, 2 & 3

Hemp has a very distinctive flavor, and raw milk made from hemp seeds has a nuttier flavor than most. Hemp milk, like the seeds it is made from, is rich in omega-3 fats. Use hemp milk on cereal, in smoothies or simply as a drink.

Tip

Shelled hemp seeds are soft and small enough to make straining unnecessary. However, if you prefer, strain the milk through a nut milk bag. Starting at the top of the bag, use your hands to squeeze in a downward direction to extract the milk. Discard the solids.

Nutrients per 1 cup (250 mL)

Calories	43
Fat	3 g
Carbohydrate	1 g
Fiber	0 g
Protein	3 g
Vitamin A	0 IU
Iron	0.9 mg
Zinc	0.0 mg

- **Blender**

4 cups	filtered water	1 L
3 tbsp	raw shelled hemp seeds	45 mL

1. In blender, combine water and hemp seeds. Blend on high speed for 30 to 45 seconds or until the liquid becomes milky white and no visible pieces of hemp seeds remain. Transfer to a pitcher, cover and refrigerate for up to 3 days.

Variation

Cinnamon-Strawberry Hemp Milk: After processing the hemp milk, add ½ cup (125 mL) chopped hulled strawberries and 2 tsp (10 mL) ground cinnamon. Blend on high speed until smooth.

Basic Nut Milk Smoothie

Suitable for Phases 2 & 3

This basic smoothie, made with nut milk, mango and banana, is a good source of potassium and vitamin C. Orange fruits such as mangos are an excellent source of beta-carotene, a powerful antioxidant. Bananas are a good source of a type of fiber that helps to maintain healthy bacteria in your gut.

- **Blender**

1½ cups	Almond Milk (page 324)	375 mL
1	mango, peeled, seeded and chopped	1
1	banana	1
4	strawberries	4

1. In blender, combine almond milk, mango, banana and strawberries. Blend on high speed until smooth.

Variations

Substitute an equal quantity of Coconut Milk (page 326) or Hemp Milk (page 327) in this smoothie.

Substitute other fleshy orange fruits for the mango. In season, use 2 peaches or nectarines or 4 apricots, with stones removed. An orange tropical fruit such as papaya will also work well.

You can substitute other berries for the strawberries. Try blueberries, raspberries, blackberries or even a "bumbleberry" combination of berries. If the fruit is not as sweet as you would like or if you prefer a sweeter drink, add a pitted soft date.

To boost the protein content, add 1 to 2 tbsp (15 to 30 mL) of your favorite nut butter.

Nutrients per serving	
Calories	316
Fat	14 g
Carbohydrate	47 g
Fiber	8 g
Protein	8 g
Vitamin A	1867 IU
Iron	1.5 mg
Zinc	1.1 mg

Chocolate Pecan Smoothie

Suitable for Phases 2 & 3

This smoothie is rich in antioxidants and phytonutrients from the pecan milk, peaches and pineapple. If you use cocoa powder, it adds even more antioxidants and phytonutrients and is a great source of magnesium.

- **Blender**

¾ cup	Pecan Milk (page 325)	175 mL
½ cup	frozen peach slices	125 mL
½ cup	chopped pineapple	125 mL
1 tbsp	carob powder or unsweetened cocoa powder	15 mL
4	frozen juice cubes or ice cubes	4

1. In blender, combine pecan milk, peaches, pineapple, carob powder and juice cubes. Secure lid and blend (from low to high if using a variable-speed blender) until smooth.

Nutrients per serving	
Calories	346
Fat	22 g
Carbohydrate	41 g
Fiber	6 g
Protein	4 g
Vitamin A	430 IU
Iron	1.4 mg
Zinc	1.6 mg

Basic Berry Smoothie

**Suitable for
Phases 2 & 3**

*This smoothie is high in
potassium, vitamin C and
healthy carbohydrates.*

Nutrients per serving	
Calories	132
Fat	1 g
Carbohydrate	32 g
Fiber	4 g
Protein	2 g
Vitamin A	330 IU
Iron	0.7 mg
Zinc	0.3 mg

- **Blender**

1 cup	freshly squeezed orange juice	250 mL
12	strawberries	12
8	blackberries	8
1	banana	1
1	pitted soft date, chopped	1

1. In blender, combine orange juice, strawberries, blackberries, banana and date. Blend on high speed until smooth.

Variations

Substitute pineapple juice for the orange juice.

Try different mixes of berries.

Autumn Refresher

**Suitable for
Phases 2 & 3**

*Here's a source of fiber,
to promote healthy
gut bacteria.*

Nutrients per serving	
Calories	133
Fat	0 g
Carbohydrate	35 g
Fiber	6 g
Protein	1 g
Vitamin A	209 IU
Iron	0.5 mg
Zinc	0.2 mg

- **Blender**

¼ cup	freshly squeezed orange juice	60 mL
3 tbsp	freshly squeezed lime juice	45 mL
2	pears, quartered	2
1	peach, chopped	1
1	apple, quartered	1

1. In blender, combine orange juice, lime juice, pears, peach and apple. Secure lid and blend (from low to high if using a variable-speed blender) until smooth.

Apple Beet Pear Smoothie

Makes 3 to 4 servings

Suitable for Phases 2 & 3

Nutrients per serving (1 of 4)

Calories	79
Fat	0 g
Carbohydrate	20 g
Fiber	4 g
Protein	1 g
Vitamin A	69 IU
Iron	1.5 mg
Zinc	0.2 mg

- **Blender**

1	can (14 or 15 oz/398 or 425 mL) diced beets in water	1
1 tbsp	freshly squeezed lemon juice	15 mL
¼ cup	apple juice	60 mL
1	pear, quartered	1
1	apple, quartered	1
1 tsp	chopped fresh savory	5 mL

1. In blender, combine beets with liquid, lemon juice, apple juice, pear, apple and savory. Secure lid and blend (from low to high if using a variable-speed blender) until smooth.

Orange Zinger

Makes 1 serving

Suitable for Phases 2 & 3

Carrots are rich in anti-inflammatory beta-carotene.

Nutrients per serving

Calories	164
Fat	1 g
Carbohydrate	40 g
Fiber	6 g
Protein	3 g
Vitamin A	26,869 IU
Iron	1.1 mg
Zinc	0.4 mg

- **Blender**

½ cup	freshly squeezed orange juice	125 mL
1 cup	cooked chopped carrots	250 mL
½ cup	seedless red grapes	125 mL
1	½-inch (1 cm) piece gingerroot, peeled	1

1. In blender, combine orange juice, carrots, grapes and gingerroot. Secure lid and blend (from low to high if using a variable-speed blender) until smooth.

Avocado Orange Smoothie

Makes 2 to 3 servings

Suitable for Phases 2 & 3

Nutrients per serving (1 of 3)

Calories	193
Fat	5 g
Carbohydrate	38 g
Fiber	7 g
Protein	3 g
Vitamin A	282 IU
Iron	0.8 mg
Zinc	0.5 mg

- **Blender**

½ cup	freshly squeezed orange juice	125 mL
2 tbsp	freshly squeezed lemon juice	30 mL
1	orange, sectioned and seeded	1
4	fresh or dried figs, quartered	4
½	avocado	½
2	frozen banana chunks	2

1. In blender, combine orange juice, lemon juice, orange, figs, avocado and banana. Secure lid and blend (from low to high if using a variable-speed blender) until smooth.

Creamy Fennel Smoothie

Makes 1 to 2 servings

Suitable for Phases 2 & 3

Nutrients per serving (1 of 2)

Calories	202
Fat	15 g
Carbohydrate	20 g
Fiber	5 g
Protein	2 g
Vitamin A	109 IU
Iron	1.6 mg
Zinc	0.6 mg

- **Blender**

½ cup	coconut milk	125 mL
1 cup	chopped fennel bulb	250 mL
1	apple, quartered	1
1 tsp	fennel seeds	5 mL

1. In blender, combine coconut milk, chopped fennel, apple and fennel seeds. Secure lid and blend (from low to high if using a variable-speed blender) until smooth.

Advice for a Healthy Gut

▶ Use carrageenan-free canned coconut milk or homemade Coconut Milk (page 326) in this smoothie.

Beet Juice

Makes 1 to 2 servings

Suitable for Phases 2 & 3

Nutrients per serving (1 of 2)	
Calories	155
Fat	1 g
Carbohydrate	39 g
Fiber	8 g
Protein	2 g
Vitamin A	10,316 IU
Iron	1.1 mg
Zinc	0.5 mg

- Juicer

2	beets, tops intact	2
2	carrots	2
2	apples	2

1. Using a juicer, process beets, beet tops, carrots and apples. Whisk and pour into glasses.

Celery Juice

Makes 1 serving

Suitable for Phases 2 & 3

This juice is full of anti-inflammatory nutrients.

Nutrients per serving	
Calories	98
Fat	1 g
Carbohydrate	21 g
Fiber	8 g
Protein	3 g
Vitamin A	21,183 IU
Iron	1.5 mg
Zinc	0.6 mg

- Juicer

4	stalks celery	4
2	carrots	2
$\frac{1}{4}$	fresh fennel bulb	$\frac{1}{4}$
$\frac{1}{2}$ tsp	ground cumin	2 mL

1. Using a juicer, process celery, carrots and fennel. Whisk and pour into a glass. Whisk in cumin.

Cucumber Fuzz

**Suitable for
Phases 2 & 3**

*Cucumber makes for
a uniquely refreshing
beverage.*

Nutrients per serving

Calories	113
Fat	1 g
Carbohydrate	25 g
Fiber	5 g
Protein	4 g
Vitamin A	1143 IU
Iron	1.1 mg
Zinc	0.8 mg

- **Juicer**

2	peaches, pitted	2
2	stalks celery	2
1	cucumber	1

1. Using a juicer, process peaches, celery and cucumber. Whisk and pour into a glass.

Spin Doctor

Makes 1 serving

**Suitable for
Phases 2 & 3**

*Here's a truly antioxidant-
rich beverage.*

Nutrients per serving

Calories	178
Fat	1 g
Carbohydrate	43 g
Fiber	10 g
Protein	4 g
Vitamin A	24,317 IU
Iron	2.2 mg
Zinc	0.8 mg

- **Juicer**

1 cup	fresh spinach	250 mL
2	carrots	2
1	apple	1
1	tomato	1
½ tsp	ground turmeric	2 mL

1. Using a juicer, process spinach, carrots, apple and tomato. Whisk together with turmeric and pour into a glass.

Nip of Goodness

Suitable for Phases 2 & 3

Turnip and parsnips offer a uniquely refreshing flavor.

Nutrients per serving

Calories	222
Fat	1 g
Carbohydrate	55 g
Fiber	13 g
Protein	4 g
Vitamin A	177 IU
Iron	1.6 mg
Zinc	1.1 mg

- **Juicer**

1	turnip	1
3	parsnips	3
1	apple	1
1/4	fresh fennel bulb	1/4

1. Using a juicer, process turnip, parsnips, apple and fennel. Whisk and pour into a glass.

Fennel Fantasy

Suitable for Phases 2 & 3

Digestive issues meet their match in this fennel-rich juice.

Nutrients per serving

Calories	279
Fat	1 g
Carbohydrate	73 g
Fiber	13 g
Protein	3 g
Vitamin A	405 IU
Iron	1.6 mg
Zinc	0.4 mg

- **Juicer**

1/2	fresh fennel bulb, cut in half	1/2
2	apples	2
1/2 cup	red grapes	125 mL
1/4 tsp	ground cinnamon	1 mL
Pinch	ground fennel (optional)	Pinch

1. Using a juicer, process fennel, apples and grapes. Whisk together with cinnamon and ground fennel (if using), and pour into a glass.

Orange Sunrise

**Makes 1 to
2 servings**

**Suitable for
Phases 2 & 3**

Nutrients per serving (1 of 2)

Calories	284
Fat	2 g
Carbohydrate	71 g
Fiber	13 g
Protein	4 g
Vitamin A	9160 IU
Iron	1.4 mg
Zinc	0.6 mg

- **Juicer**

2	oranges	2
2	kiwifruits	2
1	papaya, seeded	1
1	carrot	1

1. Using a juicer, process oranges, kiwifruits, papaya and carrot. Whisk and pour into glasses.

Deep Orange Heart

**Makes 1 to
2 servings**

**Suitable for
Phases 2 & 3**

Nutrients per serving (1 of 2)

Calories	166
Fat	1 g
Carbohydrate	41 g
Fiber	5 g
Protein	3 g
Vitamin A	4364 IU
Iron	0.6 mg
Zinc	0.4 mg

- **Juicer**

1	mango, pitted	1
1	wedge cantaloupe	1
2	fresh apricots, pitted	2
1	orange	1

1. Using a juicer, process mango, cantaloupe, apricots and orange. Whisk and pour into glasses.

Berry Fine

Makes 1 serving

**Suitable for
Phases 2 & 3**

*This refreshing juice
delivers vitamin C,
potassium and antioxidants.*

Nutrients per serving

Calories	190
Fat	1 g
Carbohydrate	49 g
Fiber	8 g
Protein	3 g
Vitamin A	303 IU
Iron	1.5 mg
Zinc	0.6 mg

- **Juicer**

1 cup	red grapes	250 mL
1/2 cup	blueberries	125 mL
1/2 cup	blackberries	125 mL
1/2	lemon	1/2

1. Using a juicer, process grapes, blueberries, blackberries and lemon. Whisk and pour into a glass.

Green Tea and Blueberries

Makes 2 servings

**Suitable for
Phases 2 & 3**

*This anti-inflammatory
juice offers a large dose
of antioxidants.*

Nutrients per serving

Calories	104
Fat	1 g
Carbohydrate	25 g
Fiber	6 g
Protein	2 g
Vitamin A	422 IU
Iron	0.8 mg
Zinc	0.6 mg

- **Juicer**

1 cup	blueberries	250 mL
1 cup	blackberries	250 mL
2	black plums, pitted	2
1/2 cup	green tea, steeped and chilled	125 mL

1. Using a juicer, process blueberries, blackberries and plums. Whisk together with green tea and pour into glasses.

Contributing Authors

Alexandra Anca and Theresa Santandrea-Cull
Complete Gluten-Free Diet & Nutrition Guide
A recipe from this book is found on page 170.

Byron Ayanoglu
The New Vegetarian Gourmet
A recipe from this book is found on page 298.

Byron Ayanoglu with contributions from Algis Kemezys
125 Best Vegetarian Recipes
Recipes from this book are found on pages 192, 194, 196, 201, 276, 281, 288 and 301.

Pat Crocker
The Juicing Bible, Second Edition
Recipes from this book are found on pages 333–37.

Pat Crocker
The Smoothies Bible, Second Edition
Recipes from this book are found on pages 325, 329, 330 (bottom) and 331–32.

Pat Crocker
The Vegan Cook's Bible
Recipes from this book are found on pages 187, 209, 212, 274, 283, 304–5 and 310.

Pat Crocker
The Vegetarian Cook's Bible
Recipes from this book are found on pages 178, 180, 184, 186, 207, 309 and 319.

Dietitians of Canada
Cook Great Food
Recipes from this book are found on pages 227, 229, 232, 235, 248, 254, 273, 279–80 and 282.

Dietitians of Canada
Simply Great Food
Recipes from this book are found on pages 158, 191, 204, 211, 220, 230, 236, 241, 250–51 and 277.

Maxine Effenson-Chuck and Beth Gurney
125 Best Vegan Recipes
Recipes from this book are found on pages 202–3, 208, 217 and 307.

Judith Finlayson
150 Best Slow Cooker Recipes
A recipe from this book is found on page 271.

Judith Finlayson
The 163 Best Paleo Slow Cooker Recipes
Recipes from this book are found on pages 256, 268, 316–18 and 322.

Judith Finlayson
The Complete Gluten-Free Whole Grains Cookbook
Recipes from this book are found on pages 161, 275, 289 and 290.

Judith Finlayson
The Complete Whole Grains Cookbook
Recipes from this book are found on pages 164–65.

Judith Finlayson
The Healthy Slow Cooker,
Second Edition
Recipes from this book are found on pages 243 and 252.

Douglas McNish
Eat Raw, Eat Well
Recipes from this book are found on pages 166, 291, 324, 326–28 and 330 (top).

Douglas McNish
Raw, Quick & Delicious!
Recipes from this book are found on pages 190, 193, 197, 198–200, 312, 313 and 320–21.

Dr. Maitreyi Raman, Angela Sirounis & Jennifer Shrubsole
The Complete IBS Health & Diet Guide
Recipes from this book are found on pages 185, 221–22, 234, 244, 258, 260–61, 292 and 294.

Deb Roussou
350 Best Vegan Recipes
Recipes from this book are found on pages 181–82, 206, 210, 214, 216, 218, 270, 306 and 308.

Camilla V. Saulsbury
5 Easy Steps to Healthy Cooking
Recipes from this book are found on pages 226, 262, 264, 266, 284–86, 299, 302 and 314.

Camilla V. Saulsbury
500 Best Quinoa Recipes
Recipes from this book are found on pages 159–60, 162, 167–69, 213, 231 and 295–96.

Camilla V. Saulsbury
Recipes written by this author for *The Total Food Allergy Health and Diet Guide* by Alexandra Anca with Dr. Gordon L. Sussman are found on pages 172–76

Andrew Schloss with Ken Bookman
2500 Recipes
Recipes from this book are found on pages 224–25, 228, 238, 239–40, 263, 265, 267 and 300.

Carla Snyder and Meredith Deeds
300 Sensational Soups
A recipe from this book is found on page 315.

Donna Washburn and Heather Butt
The Best Gluten-Free Family Cookbook
Recipes from this book are found on pages 242, 246 and 303.

Katherine E. Younker, Editor
America's Complete Diabetes Cookbook
Recipes from this book are found on pages 179, 188, 245, 272, 278, 287 and 293.

References

Ak T, Gülçin I. Antioxidant and radical scavenging properties of curcumin. *Chem Biol Interact*, 2008 Jul 10; 174 (1): 27–37. doi: 10.1016/j.cbi.2008.05.003. Epub 2008 May 7.

Assimakopoulos SF, Tsamandas AC, Tsiaoussis GI, et al. Altered intestinal tight junctions' expression in patients with liver cirrhosis: A pathogenetic mechanism of intestinal hyperpermeability. *Eur J Clin Invest*, 2012 Apr; 42 (4): 439–46. doi: 10.1111/j.1365-2362.2011.02609.x. Epub 2011 Oct 24.

Balakrishnan M, Floch MH. Prebiotics, probiotics and digestive health. *Curr Opin Clin Nutr Metab Care*, 2012 Nov; 15 (6): 580–85. doi: 10.1097/MCO.0b013e328359684f.

Banerjee M, Siddique S, Mukherjee S, et al. Hematological, immunological, and cardiovascular changes in individuals residing in a polluted city of India: A study in Delhi. *Int J Hyg Environ Health*, 2012 Apr; 215 (3): 306–11. doi: 10.1016/j.ijheh.2011.08.003. Epub 2011 Sep 16.

Barreau F, Hugot JP. Intestinal barrier dysfunction triggered by invasive bacteria. *Curr Opin Microbiol*, 2014 Feb; 17: 91–98. doi: 10.1016/j.mib.2013.12.003. Epub 2014 Jan 14.

Beguin P, Errachid A, Larondelle Y, et al. Effect of polyunsaturated fatty acids on tight junctions in a model of the human intestinal epithelium under normal and inflammatory conditions. *Food Funct*, 2013 Jun; 4 (6): 923–31. doi: 10.1039/c3fo60036j. Epub 2013 May 9.

Berant M, Khourie M, Menzies IS. Effect of iron deficiency on small intestinal permeability in infants and young children. *J Pediatr Gastroenterol Nutr*, 1992 Jan; 14 (1): 17–20.

Bornstein, JC. Serotonin in the gut: What does it do? *Front Neurosci*, 2012 Feb 6; 6: 16. doi: 10.3389/fnins.2012.00016. eCollection 2012.

Brusca SB, Abramson SB, Scher JU. Microbiome and mucosal inflammation as extra-articular triggers for rheumatoid arthritis and autoimmunity. *Curr Opin Rheumatol*, 2014 Jan; 26 (1): 101–7. doi: 10.1097/BOR.0000000000000008.

Campos-Rodríguez R, Godínez-Victoria M, Abarca-Rojano E, et al. Stress modulates intestinal secretory immunoglobulin A. *Front Integr Neurosci*, 2013 Dec 2; 7: 86. doi: 10.3389/fnint.2013.00086.

Carroll IM, Maharshak N. Enteric bacterial proteases in inflammatory bowel disease: Pathophysiology and clinical implications. *World J Gastroenterol*, 2013 Nov 21; 19 (43): 7531–43.

Costedio MM, Hyman N, Mawe GM. Serotonin and its role in colonic function and in gastrointestinal disorders. *Dis Colon Rectum*, 2007 Mar; 50 (3): 376–88.

Davis DL, Kesari S, Soskolne CL, et al. Swedish review strengthens grounds for concluding that radiation from cellular and cordless phones is a probable human carcinogen. *Pathophysiology*, 2013 Apr; 20 (2): 123–29. doi: 10.1016/j.pathophys.2013.03.001. Epub 2013 May 7.

De-Souza DA, Greene LJ. Intestinal permeability and systemic infections in critically ill patients: Effect of glutamine. *Crit Care Med*, 2005 May; 33 (5): 1125–35.

Dhaliwal SK, Hunt RH. Doctor-patient interaction for irritable bowel syndrome in primary care: A systematic perspective. *Eur J Gastroenterol Hepatol*, 2004 Nov; 16 (11): 1161–66.

Di Raimondo D, Tuttolomondo A, Buttà C, et al. Metabolic and anti-inflammatory effects of a home-based programme of aerobic physical exercise. *Int J Clin Pract*, 2013 Dec; 67 (12): 1247–53. doi: 10.1111/ijcp.12269.

Dobreva ZG, Kostadinova GS, Popov BN, et al. Proinflammatory and anti-inflammatory cytokines in adolescents from Southeast Bulgarian cities with different levels of air pollution. *Toxicol Ind Health*, 2013 Jun 14. [Epub ahead of print]

El-Tawil AM. Zinc supplementation tightens leaky gut in Crohn's disease. *Inflamm Bowel Dis*, 2012 Feb; 18 (2): E399. doi: 10.1002/ibd.21926. Epub 2011 Oct 12.

Epstein MD, Tchervenkov JI, Alexander JW, et al. Increased gut permeability following burn trauma. *Arch Surg*, 1991 Feb; 126 (2): 198–200.

Farhadi A, Fields JZ, Keshavarzian A. Mucosal mast cells are pivotal elements in inflammatory bowel disease that connect the dots: Stress, intestinal hyperpermeability and inflammation. *World J Gastroenterol*, 2007 Jun 14; 13 (22): 3027–30.

Finamore A, Massimi M, Conti Devirgiliis L, et al. Zinc deficiency induces membrane barrier damage and increases neutrophil transmigration in Caco-2 cells. *J Nutr*, 2008 Sep; 138 (9): 1664–70.

Fink MP. Intestinal epithelial hyperpermeability: Update on the pathogenesis of gut mucosal barrier dysfunction in critical illness. *Curr Opin Crit Care*, 2003 Apr; 9 (2): 143–51.

Forsyth CB, Shannon KM, Kordower JH, et al. Increased intestinal permeability correlates with sigmoid mucosa alpha-synuclein staining and endotoxin exposure markers in early Parkinson's disease. *PLoS One*, 2011; 6 (12): e28032. doi: 10.1371/journal.pone.0028032. Epub 2011 Dec 1.

Gareau MG, Silva MA, Perdue MH. Pathophysiological mechanisms of stress-induced intestinal damage. *Curr Mol Med*, 2008 Jun; 8 (4): 274–81.

Gecse K, Róka R, Séra T, et al. Leaky gut in patients with diarrhea-predominant irritable bowel syndrome and inactive ulcerative colitis. *Digestion*, 2012; 85 (1): 40–46. doi: 10.1159/000333083. Epub 2011 Dec 14.

Guo H, Jiang T, Wang J, et al. The value of eliminating foods according to food-specific immunoglobulin G antibodies in irritable bowel syndrome with diarrhoea. *J Int Med Res*, 2012; 40 (1): 204–10.

Gupta SC, Patchva S, Aggarwal BB. Therapeutic roles of curcumin: Lessons learned from clinical trials. *AAPS J*, 2013 Jan; 15 (1): 195–218. doi: 10.1208/s12248-012-9432-8. Epub 2012 Nov 10.

Hadhazy A. Think twice: How the gut's "second brain" influences mood and well-being. *Scientific American*, 2010 Feb 12, accessed Nov 2014, www.scientificamerican.com/article/gut-second-brain.

Halpert A, Godena E. Irritable bowel syndrome patients' perspectives on their relationships with healthcare providers. *Scand J Gastroenterol*, 2011 Jul; 46 (7–8): 823–30. doi: 10.3109/00365521.2011.574729. Epub 2011 May 11.

Hanai H, Sugimoto K. Curcumin has bright prospects for the treatment of inflammatory bowel disease. *Curr Pharm Des*, 2009; 15 (18): 2087–94.

Hardell L, Carlberg M, Hansson Mild K. Use of mobile phones and cordless phones is associated with increased risk for glioma and acoustic neuroma. *Pathophysiology*, 2013 Apr; 20 (2): 85–110. doi: 10.1016/j.pathophys.2012.11.001. Epub 2012 Dec 21.

Hollander D. Intestinal permeability, leaky gut, and intestinal disorders. *Curr Gastroenterol Rep*, 1999 Oct; 1 (5): 410–16.

Holton KF, Taren DL, Thomson CA, et al. The effect of dietary glutamate on fibromyalgia and irritable bowel symptoms. *Clin Exp Rheumatol*, 2012 Nov–Dec; 30 (6 Suppl 74): 10–17. Epub 2012 Dec 14.

Hoskin-Parr L, Teyhan A, Blocker A, et al. Antibiotic exposure in the first two years of life and development of asthma and other allergic diseases by 7.5 yr: A dose-dependent relationship. *Pediatr Allergy Immunol*, 2013 Dec; 24 (8): 762–71. doi: 10.1111/pai.12153. Epub 2013 Dec 2.

Iebba V, Nicoletti M, Schippa S. Gut microbiota and the immune system: An intimate partnership in health and disease. *Int J Immunopathol Pharmacol*, 2012 Oct–Dec; 25 (4): 823–33.

Ito Y, Sasaki M, Funaki Y, et al. Nonsteroidal anti-inflammatory drug-induced visible and invisible small intestinal injury. *J Clin Biochem Nutr*, 2013 Jul; 53 (1): 55–59. doi: 10.3164/jcbn.12-116. Epub 2013 Apr 9.

Johnston JD, Harvey CJ, Menzies IS, et al. Gastrointestinal permeability and absorptive capacity in sepsis. *Crit Care Med*, 1996 Jul; 24 (7): 1144–49.

Konturek PC, Brzozowski T, Konturek SJ. Stress and the gut: Pathophysiology, clinical consequences, diagnostic approach and treatment options. *J Physiol Pharmacol*, 2011 Dec; 62 (6): 591–99.

Kronman MP, Zaoutis TE, Haynes K, et al. Antibiotic exposure and IBD development among children: A population-based cohort study. *Pediatrics*, 2012 Oct; 130 (4): e794–803. doi: 10.1542/peds.2011-3886. Epub 2012 Sep 24.

Kumar A, Purwar B, Shrivastava A, et al. Effects of curcumin on the intestinal motility of albino rats. *Indian J Physiol Pharmacol*, 2010 Jul–Sep; 54 (3): 284–88.

Levinson W, Roter D. Physicians' psychosocial beliefs correlate with their patient communication skills. *J Gen Intern Med*, 1995 Jul; 10 (7): 375–79.

Lim SG, Menzies IS, Lee CA, et al. Intestinal permeability and function in patients infected with human immunodeficiency virus: A comparison with coeliac disease. *Scand J Gastroenterol*, 1993 Jul; 28 (7): 573–80.

Lima AA, Anstead GM, Zhang Q, et al. Effects of glutamine alone or in combination with zinc and vitamin A on growth, intestinal barrier function, stress and satiety-related hormones in Brazilian shantytown children. *Clinics (Sao Paulo)*, 2014 Apr; 69 (4): 225–33.

Liu XJ, Zhu TT, Zeng R, et al. [An epidemiological study of food intolerance in 2434 children]. [Article in Chinese]. *Zhongguo Dang Dai Er Ke Za Zhi*, 2013 Jul; 15 (7): 550–54.

Liu Y, Chen F, Odle J, et al. Fish oil enhances intestinal integrity and inhibits TLR4 and NOD2 signaling pathways in weaned pigs after LPS challenge. *J Nutr*, 2012 Nov; 142 (11): 2017–24. doi: 10.3945/jn.112.164947. Epub 2012 Sep 26.

Liu Z, Li N, Neu J. Tight junctions, leaky intestines, and pediatric diseases. *Acta Paediatr*, 2005 Apr; 94 (4): 386–93.

Luckey D, Gomez A, Murray J, et al. Bugs & us: The role of the gut in autoimmunity. *Indian J Med Res*, 2013 Nov; 138 (5): 732–43.

Luo B, Xiang D, Nieman DC, et al. The effects of moderate exercise on chronic stress-induced intestinal barrier dysfunction and antimicrobial defense. *Brain Behav Immun*, 2014 Jul; 39: 99–106. doi: 10.1016/j.bbi.2013.11.013. Epub 2013 Nov 27.

Majamaa H, Isolauri E. Evaluation of the gut mucosal barrier: Evidence for increased antigen transfer in children with atopic eczema. *J Allergy Clin Immunol*, 1996 Apr; 97 (4): 985–90.

Marcinowicz L, Chlabicz S, Grebowski R. Patient satisfaction with healthcare provided by family doctors: Primary dimensions and an attempt at typology. *BMC Health Serv Res*, 2009 Apr 16; 9: 63. doi: 10.1186/1472-6963-9-63.

Mayer EA, Savidge T, Shulman RJ. Brain-gut microbiome interactions and functional bowel disorders. *Gastroenterology*, 2014 May; 146 (6): 1500–1512. doi: 10.1053/j.gastro.2014.02.037. Epub 2014 Feb 28.

Molenda M, Bober J, Stańkowska-Walczak D, et al. [Cigarette smoking as a promoting factor for nonspecific inflammatory bowel disease]. [Article in Polish]. *Ann Acad Med Stetin*, 2010; 56 (3): 50–54.

Navarro F, Bacurau AV, Pereira GB, et al. Moderate exercise increases the metabolism and immune function of lymphocytes in rats. *Eur J Appl Physiol*, 2013 May; 113 (5): 1343–52. doi: 10.1007/s00421-012-2554-y. Epub 2012 Dec 2.

Neal KR, Barker L, Spiller RC. Prognosis in post-infective irritable bowel syndrome: A six year follow up study. *Gut*, 2002 Sep; 51 (3): 410–13.

Odenwald MA, Turner JR. Intestinal permeability defects: Is it time to treat? *Clin Gastroenterol Hepatol*, 2013 Sep; 11 (9): 1075–83. doi: 10.1016/j.cgh.2013.07.001. Epub 2013 Jul 12.

Pácha J, Sumová A. Circadian regulation of epithelial functions in the intestine. *Acta Physiol (Oxf)*, 2013 May; 208 (1): 11–24. doi: 10.1111/apha.12090. Epub 2013 Mar 22.

Persborn M, Gerritsen J, Wallon C, et al. The effects of probiotics on barrier function and mucosal pouch microbiota during maintenance treatment for severe pouchitis in patients with ulcerative colitis. *Aliment Pharmacol Ther*, 2013 Oct; 38 (7): 772–83. doi: 10.1111/apt.12451. Epub 2013 Aug 19.

Pusztai A, Grant G. Assessment of lectin inactivation by heat and digestion. *Methods Mol Med*, 1998; 9: 505–14. doi: 10.1385/0-89603-396-1:505.

Quan ZF, Yang C, Li N, et al. Effect of glutamine on change in early postoperative intestinal permeability and its relation to systemic inflammatory response. *World J Gastroenterol*, 2004 Jul 1; 10 (13): 1992–94.

Rapin JR, Wiernsperger N. Possible links between intestinal permeablity and food processing: A potential therapeutic niche for glutamine. *Clinics (Sao Paulo)*, 2010 June; 65 (6): 635–43.

Rhodes JM, Campbell BJ, Yu LG. Lectin-epithelial interactions in the human colon. *Biochem Soc Trans*, 2008 Dec; 36 (Pt 6): 1482–86. doi: 10.1042/BST0361482.

Roos N, Sørensen JC, Sørensen H, et al. Screening for anti-nutritional compounds in complementary foods and food aid products for infants and young children. *Matern Child Nutr*, 2013 Jan; 9 Suppl 1: 47–71. doi: 10.1111/j.1740-8709.2012.00449.x.

Roy SK, Behrens RH, Haider R, et al. Impact of zinc supplementation on intestinal permeability in Bangladeshi children with acute diarrhoea and persistent diarrhoea syndrome. *J Pediatr Gastroenterol Nutr*, 1992 Oct; 15 (3): 289–96.

Rutten EP, Lenaerts K, Buurman WA, et al. Disturbed intestinal integrity in patients with COPD: Effects of activities of daily living. *Chest*, 2014 Feb 1; 145 (2): 245–52. doi: 10.1378/chest.13-0584.

Rycerz K, Jaworska-Adamu JE. Effects of aspartame metabolites on astrocytes and neurons. *Folia Neuropathol*, 2013; 51 (1): 10–17.

Salim SY, Söderholm JD. Importance of disrupted intestinal barrier in inflammatory bowel diseases. *Inflamm Bowel Dis*, 2011 Jan; 17 (1): 362–81. doi: 10.1002/ibd.21403. Epub 2010 Aug 19.

Savelkoul FH, Van Der Poel AF, Tamminga S. The presence and inactivation of trypsin inhibitors, tannins, lectins and amylase inhibitors in legume seeds during germination: A review. *Plant Foods Hum Nutr*, 1992 Jan; 42 (1): 71–85.

Schab DW, Trinh NH. Do artificial food colors promote hyperactivity in children with hyperactive syndromes? A meta-analysis of double-blind placebo-controlled trials. *J Dev Behav Pediatr*, 2004 Dec; 25 (6): 423–34.

Serghini M, Karoui S, Boubaker J, et al. [Post-infectious irritable bowel syndrome].[Article in French]. *Tunis Med*, 2012 Mar; 90 (3): 205–13.

Sevastiadou S, Malamitsi-Puchner A, Costalos C, et al. The impact of oral glutamine supplementation on the intestinal permeability and incidence of necrotizing enterocolitis/septicemia in premature neonates. *J Matern Fetal Neonatal Med*, 2011 Oct; 24 (10): 1294–300. doi: 10.3109/14767058.2011.564240. Epub 2011 Apr 4.

Shimizu K, Kimura F, Akimoto T, et al. Effect of moderate exercise training on T-helper cell subpopulations in elderly people. *Exerc Immunol Rev*, 2008; 14: 24–37.

Shulman RJ, Jarrett ME, Cain KC, et al. Associations among gut permeability, inflammatory markers, and symptoms in patients with irritable bowel syndrome. *J Gastroenterol*, 2014 Nov; 49 (11): 1467–76. doi: 10.1007/s00535-013-0919-6. Epub 2014 Jan 17.

Sindhu KN, Sowmyanarayanan TV, Paul A, et al. Immune response and intestinal permeability in children with acute gastroenteritis treated with lactobacillus rhamnosus GG: A randomized, double-blind, placebo-controlled trial. *Clin Infect Dis*, 2014 Apr; 58 (8): 1107–15. doi: 10.1093/cid/ciu065. Epub 2014 Feb 5.

Soffritti M, Padovani M, Tibaldi E, et al. The carcinogenic effects of aspartame: The urgent need for regulatory re-evaluation. *Am J Ind Med*, 2014 Apr; 57 (4): 383–97. doi: 10.1002/ajim.22296. Epub 2014 Jan 16.

Steptoe A, Wardle J. Locus of control and health behaviour revisited: A multivariate analysis of young adults from 18 countries. *Br J Psychol*, 2001 Nov; 92 (Pt 4): 659–72.

Summa KC, Voigt RM, Forsyth CB, et al. Disruption of the circadian clock in mice increases intestinal permeability and promotes alcohol-induced hepatic pathology and inflammation. *PLoS One*, 2013 Jun 18; 8 (6): e67102. Print 2013.

Teixeira TF, Collado MC, Ferreira CL, et al. Potential mechanisms for the emerging link between obesity and increased intestinal permeability. *Nutr Res*, 2012 Sep; 32 (9): 637–47. doi: 10.1016/j.nutres.2012.07.003. Epub 2012 Sep 7.

Vaarala O. Is the origin of type 1 diabetes in the gut? *Immunol Cell Biol*, 2012 Mar; 90 (3): 271–76. doi: 10.1038/icb.2011.115. Epub 2012 Jan 31.

Van Wijck K, Lenaerts K, Van Bijnen AA, et al. Aggravation of exercise-induced intestinal injury by ibuprofen in athletes. *Med Sci Sports Exerc*, 2012 Dec; 44 (12): 2257–62. doi: 10.1249/MSS.0b013e318265dd3d.

Vanuytsel T, van Wanrooy S, Vanheel H, et al. Psychological stress and corticotropin-releasing hormone increase intestinal permeability in humans by a mast cell–dependent mechanism. *Gut*, 2014 Aug; 63 (8): 1293–99. doi: 10.1136/gutjnl-2013-305690. Epub 2013 Oct 23.

Wekerle H, Berer K, Krishnamoorthy G. Remote control–triggering of brain autoimmune disease in the gut. *Curr Opin Immunol*, 2013 Dec; 25 (6): 683–89. doi: 10.1016/j.coi.2013.09.009. Epub 2013 Oct 23.

Whiteley P, Shattock P, Knivsberg AM, et al. Gluten- and casein-free dietary intervention for autism spectrum conditions. *Front Hum Neurosci*, 2013 Jan 4; 6: 344. doi: 10.3389/fnhum.2012.00344. eCollection 2012.

Wu HJ, Wu E. The role of gut microbiota in immune homeostasis and autoimmunity. *Gut Microbes*, 2012 Jan–Feb; 3 (1): 4–14. doi: 10.4161/gmic.19320. Epub 2012 Jan 1.

Xiao G, Tang L, Yuan F, et al. Eicosapentaenoic acid enhances heat stress–impaired intestinal epithelial barrier function in Caco-2 cells. *PLoS One*, 2013 Sep 16; 8 (9): e73571. doi: 10.1371/journal.pone.0073571. eCollection 2013.

Yamaguchi N, Sugita R, Miki A, et al. Gastrointestinal Candida colonisation promotes sensitisation against food antigens by affecting the mucosal barrier in mice. *Gut*, 2006 Jul; 55 (7): 954–60. Epub 2006 Jan 19.

Yang CM, Li YQ. [The therapeutic effects of eliminating allergic foods according to food-specific IgG antibodies in irritable bowel syndrome]. [Article in Chinese]. *Zhonghua Nei Ke Za Zhi*, 2007 Aug; 46 (8): 641–43.

Other Resources

Lab Testing

Doctor's Data:
www.doctorsdata.com
Genova Diagnostics: www.gdx.net
Rocky Mountain Analytical:
www.rmalab.com
US Biotek Laboratories:
www.usbiotek.com

Metaphysical Guides

Dolores Cannon:
www.dolorescannon.com
Dr. Wayne W. Dyer:
www.drwaynedyer.com
Louise Hay: www.louisehay.com
Caroline Myss: www.myss.com

Index

A

abscesses, 34
acesulfame potassium (acesulfame-K), 108
acupuncture, 93–94, 96
Agave Flax Muffins, 174
air pollution, 53
alcohol, 110, 111, 130
allergens, 14
allergies, 55, 57. *See also* food sensitivities
allicin, 105–6
almonds and almond butter
  Almond Milk, 324
  Basic Almond Spread, 309
  Big-Batch Seed and Nut Granola, 158
  Chewy Coconut Quinoa Bars, 169
  Mushroom-Almond Bisque, 184
  Nutty Tofu and Green Vegetable Stir-Fry, 220
  Pineapple Coconut Crumble, 320
  Wild Rice, Snow Pea and Almond Casserole, 293
aloe vera gel, 88
amaranth. *See* grains
anemia, 19
anger, 83–84
ankylosing spondylitis, 19
antibiotics, 53–54
antigens, 14
anxiety, 82
apples and applesauce. *See also* fruit juices
  Apple Beet Pear Smoothie, 331
  Apple Butter, 308
  Apple-Cranberry Compote, 319
  Applesauce Raisin Muffins, 172
  Autumn Refresher, 330
  Baked Apples, The Ultimate, 316
  Beet Juice, 333
  Borscht, 180
  Braised Red Cabbage, 273
  Creamy Cashew Maple Dip with Apples, 314
  Creamy Fennel Smoothie, 332
  Fennel Fantasy, 335
  Health Salad, 203
  Mixed Fruit, Chia and Flaxseed Porridge, 166
  Multigrain Quinoa Muffins, 175
  Nip of Goodness, 335
  Spin Doctor, 334
  Sweet Potato, Apple and Raisin Casserole, 287
apricots
  Apple-Cranberry Compote, 319
  Basic Nut Milk Smoothie (variation), 328
  Deep Orange Heart, 336
  Moroccan-Style Lamb with Raisins and Apricots, 252
  Roast Lamb with Marrakech Rub, 250
  Spiced Fruit and Grain Cereal, 160
  Sweet Potato, Apple and Raisin Casserole (tip), 287
  Toasted Sesame Quinoa Bars, 168
arame. *See* sea vegetables
arthritis, 19
artichoke hearts
  Hearts of Palm and Artichoke, 191
  Vegetable Paella, 216
asparagus
  Asparagus and Leek Soup, 179
  Balsamic Asparagus with Walnuts, 270
  Cedar-Baked Salmon, 229
  Foil-Roasted Halibut and Asparagus, 226
  Vegetable Paella, 216
aspartame, 108
asthma, 54
attitude adjustment, 77–86
autism spectrum disorder, 35
autoimmune diseases, 14, 19, 79. *See also specific conditions*
Autumn Refresher, 330
avocado
  Avocado Orange Smoothie, 332
  Avocado Salad, 192
  Creamy Cherry Tomato Salad, 198
  Hearts of Palm and Artichoke, 191
  Quinoa Salad with Grapefruit and Avocado, 202

B

bacon. *See* pork
bacteria
  antibiotic-resistant, 92
  beneficial, 29, 46, 54, 90
  dysbiotic, 46
  overgrowth of, 16, 37, 46
Balsamic Asparagus with Walnuts, 270
bananas
  Avocado Orange Smoothie, 332
  Banana Soup with Raspberry and Mint Relish, 315
  Basic Berry Smoothie, 330
  Basic Nut Milk Smoothie, 328
  Mixed Fruit, Chia and Flaxseed Porridge, 166
  Pumpkin Spice Muffins, 176
  Sugar-Free Quinoa Granola Bars, 167
Basic Berry Smoothie, 330
Basic Nut Milk Smoothie, 328
basil. *See also* herbs
  Big-Batch Oven-Roasted Ratatouille, 211
  Cauliflower Rice (variation), 291
  Cedar-Baked Salmon, 229
  Edamame Basil Spread, 299
  Fresh Basil Pesto, 300
  Salmon, Potato and Green Bean Salad, 235
beans
  Braised Green Beans and Fennel, 276
  Edamame Basil Spread, 299
  Nutty Tofu and Green Vegetable Stir-Fry, 220
  Salmon, Potato and Green Bean Salad, 235
  Vegetable Paella, 216
  Vegetable Rice, 292
beef, 130
  Beef and Quinoa Power Burgers, 262
  Beef with Baby Bok Choy, 258
  Beef with Cumin and Lime, 260
  Blackened Cajun Burgers, 263
  Ginger Beef, 261
beets
  Apple Beet Pear Smoothie, 331
  Beet Juice, 333

Library and Archives Canada Cataloguing in Publication

Trotter, Makoto, 1977–, author
    The complete leaky gut health & diet guide : improve everything from autoimmune conditions to eczema by healing your gut / Dr. Makoto Trotter, BSc (Hons), ND ; with Doug Cook, RD.

Includes index.
Includes 150 recipes.
ISBN 978-0-7788-0501-4 (pbk.)

1. Gastrointestinal system — Diseases. 2. Gastrointestinal system — Diseases — Diet therapy — Recipes.
3. Gastrointestinal system — Diseases — Alternative treatment. 4. Autoimmune diseases — Diet therapy — Recipes.
5. Autoimmune diseases — Alternative treatment. 6. Cookbooks.
I. Cook, Doug, 1964–, author II. Title.

RC806.T76 2015   616.3'30654   C2015-900146-3